A Life Course Approach to Healthy Ageing

Edited by

Diana Kuh[1]

Rachel Cooper[1]

Rebecca Hardy[1]

Marcus Richards[1]

Yoav Ben-Shlomo[2]

[1]Medical Research Council Unit for Lifelong Health and Ageing at UCL

[2]Department of Social Medicine, School of Social and Community Medicine, University of Bristol

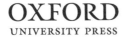

OXFORD
UNIVERSITY PRESS

OXFORD
UNIVERSITY PRESS

Great Clarendon Street, Oxford, OX2 6DP,
United Kingdom

Oxford University Press is a department of the University of Oxford.
It furthers the University's objective of excellence in research, scholarship,
and education by publishing worldwide. Oxford is a registered trade mark of
Oxford University Press in the UK and in certain other countries

© Oxford University Press 2014

The moral rights of the authors have been asserted

First Edition published in 2014

Impression: 1

Published in the United States of America by Oxford University Press
198 Madison Avenue, New York, NY 10016, United States of America

British Library Cataloguing in Publication Data
Data available

Library of Congress Control Number: 2013942969

ISBN 978–0–19–965651–6

Printed in Great Britain by
Clays Ltd, St Ives plc

Foreword

A healthy old age is a widespread ambition, one that accumulating knowledge from a wide array of disciplines has made increasingly feasible. Developments ranging from molecular biology and appreciation of epigenetic forces at the one extreme to policy decisions bearing on health at the other have induced a major shift in perspective. At the individual level, stochastic processes and good luck are undeniably important and will always remain so. At the population level, healthy ageing is increasingly understood as the culminations of a wide variety of risks, protections, and environmental exposures operating over long periods, often from early in the life course.

Extraordinary gains in life expectancy over the past century, amounting to some 30 years in economically developed countries, have resulted in an expanding population living to advanced ages. While there are wide variations in health and functionality among older populations, high degrees of physical, cognitive, and social functioning are enjoyed by some. Understanding the causes of this heterogeneity is a central theme of the research agenda on ageing and energizes the search for interventions that will lead to lengthening trajectories of healthy ageing for more people, i.e. the compression of morbidity into progressively later years of the life course. This, of necessity, will involve multiple actors in interlocking health-relevant sectors extending from the at-risk individual, who must be engaged to a greater degree than ever before in the management of his or her health, to the clinical sector, the public health enterprise, the environmental health sciences and others, extending to the policy community. In addition, research priorities must reflect and include this array of disciplines. We must learn how to move to a more syncytial view of health and of the problems and opportunities before us. A greater degree of interdisciplinarity is clearly required, a need that will increase steadily in the years ahead. In the process, new and more effective interventions will emerge.

It has become clear that the determinants of the erosion of health prospects in later life emerge irregularly across the life course, starting with the intrauterine environment and even earlier, as intergenerational factors operate. The life course approach to the epidemiology of ageing adds coherence and richness to understanding the importance of long latency in the impact of early risks and determinants on health in later life, as for example in the association of low birth weight and risk of the elements of the metabolic syndrome in adult life, or the correlation of childhood socioeconomic deprivation with functional ageing, or the connection between cerebral vascular disease in mid-life and later cognitive deficits.

Chronic diseases are of particular concern with regard to the quality of life in the later years. These diseases are for the most part characterized by early onset, prolonged pre-symptomatic courses, multiple risk factors which often act synergistically, and important social forces. These features parallel to a considerable degree the determinants of health in ageing, and in similar fashion help to frame opportunities for interventions as well as research pathways.

This volume presents a wide-ranging and authoritative overview of the current terrain relating to the preservation of health across the life course, and includes a consideration of research methods for life course studies. It offers, therefore, a basis for extension of understanding of important phenomena of ageing as well as for the formulation of new questions and interventions.

Jeremiah A Barondess, M.D.
Professor of Clinical Public Health
Weill-Cornell Medical College

Professor of Clinical Epidemiology
Mailman School of Public Health
Columbia University

President Emeritus
New York Academy of Medicine

Acknowledgements

We wish to acknowledge the New Dynamics of Ageing cross council programme (http://www.newdynamics.group.shef.ac.uk/) which funded the Healthy Ageing across the Life Course (HALCyon) research programme (http://www.halcyon.ac.uk) and the Medical Research Council Population Health Sciences Research Network which funded the Measurement and Modelling across the Life Course (FALCon) research programme.

The editors would like to thank Dr Stephanie Pilling for her invaluable support in co-ordinating many aspects of the manuscript preparation.

Contents

Part IV **The way we live**

Abbreviations

ADL	Activities of daily living
ALSPAC	The Avon Longitudinal Study of Parents and Children
BCS70	1970 British Cohort Study
BIC	Bayesian information criterion
BMC	Bone mineral content
aBMD	Areal bone mineral density
vBMD	Volumetric bone mineral density
BMI	Body mass index
BP	Blood pressure
CaPS	Caerphilly Prospective Study
CAR	Cortisol awakening response
CBG	Cortisol binding globulin
C. elegans	Caenorhabditis elegans
CFAS	Cognitive Function and Ageing Study
CHD	Coronary heart disease
CI	Confidence interval
CIMT	Carotid Intima Media Thickness
COHORTS	Consortium of health-orientated research in transitioning societies
CRF	Cardio-respiratory fitness
CSMA	Cross-sectional muscle area
DAGs	Directed acyclic graphs
DBP	Diastolic blood pressure
DHEA-S	Dehydroepiandrosterone-sulphate
DNA	Deoxyribonucleic acid
DXA	Dual energy X-ray absorptiometry
EPIC	European Prospective Investigation into Nutrition and Cancer Study
ELSA	English Longitudinal Study of Ageing
FEM	Finite element modelling
FEV	Forced expiratory volume
FEV1	Forced expiratory volume in the first second
GEE	Generalized estimating equations
GH	Growth hormone
GMM	Growth mixture models
GWAS	Genome-Wide Association Study
HALCyon	Healthy Ageing across the Life Course Research Collaboration
HCS	Hertfordshire Cohort Study
HDLc	High density lipoprotein cholesterol
Health ABC study	Health, Aging, and Body Composition study
HEPESE	Hispanic Established Populations for Epidemiologic Studies of the Elderly
HPA-axis	Hypothalamic-pituitary-adrenal axis
HR	Hazard ratio
HR-pQCT	High resolution peripheral quantitative computed tomography
IADL	Instrumental activities of daily living
IALSA	Integrative Analysis of Longitudinal Studies of Aging
IGF-I	Insulin-like growth factor-I
InCHIANTI study	Invecchiare in Chianti study
LASA	Longitudinal Aging Study Amsterdam
LCGA	Latent class growth analysis
LDLc	Low density lipoprotein cholesterol
LGM	Latent growth models
LIFE study	Lifestyle Interventions and Independence for Elders study
LIFE-P study	Lifestyle Interventions and Independence for Elders pilot study

LMIC	Low and middle income country	PHV	Peak height velocity
MAR	Missing at random	pQCT	Peripheral quantitative computed tomography
MCAR	Missing completely at random	P_T	Propensity score
MET	Metabolic equivalent tasks	QCT	Quantitative computed tomography
MIDUS	Midlife in the US study	RCT	Randomized controlled trial
MLM	Multilevel models	RE	Random effects
MMSE	Mini-Mental State Examination	REE	Resting energy expenditure
MNAR	Missing not at random	SALSA	Sacramento Area Latino Study on Aging
MPA	Moderate intensity physical activity	SD	Standard deviation
MR	Mendelian randomization	SEM	Structural equation models
MRC	Medical Research Council	SEP	Socioeconomic position
MRI	Magnetic resonance imaging	SF-36	Short-Form 36
MRS	Magnetic resonance spectroscopy	SITAR	SuperImposition by Translation and Rotation
MSEM	Multilevel structural equation models	SNP	Single nucleotide polymorphism
MSM	Multistate models	SPPB	Short physical performance battery
MSS	Model sum of squares	SRH	Self-rated health
MVPA	Moderate to vigorous physical activity	SUTVA	Stable unit treatment value assumption
n-3 LCPs	Omega-3 long-chain polyunsaturated fatty acids	T4	Thyroxine
NCDS	National Child Development Study	TC	Total cholesterol
		TICS	Telephone Interview for Cognitive Status
NGS	Next generation sequencing	TSH	Thyroid-stimulating hormone
NIH	National Institutes of Health		
NSDE	National Study of Daily Experiences	TVC	Time varying covariate
		VFA	Vertebral fracture assessment
NSHD	National Survey of Health and Development	VPA	Vigorous intensity physical activity
NT-proBNP	N-terminal prohormone of brain natriuretic peptide	WAIS-S	Weschler Adult Intelligence Scale—Similarities index
		WEMWBS	Warwick-Edinburgh Mental Wellbeing Scale
PAEE	Physical activity energy expenditure	WHII	Whitehall II study

Contributors

Judith E Adams
Consultant and Honorary Professor
of Diagnostic Radiology, Clinical Radiology,
and Manchester Academic Health Science
Centre, Central Manchester University
Hospitals NHS Foundation Trust and
University of Manchester, Manchester, UK.

Avan Aihie Sayer
MRC Clinical Scientist and Professor
of Geriatric Medicine, MRC Lifecourse
Epidemiology Unit, University of
Southampton, Southampton, UK.

Tamuno Alfred
ESRC-funded PhD student, School of Social
and Community Medicine, University of
Bristol, Bristol, UK.

Yoav Ben-Shlomo
Professor of Clinical Epidemiology, School
of Social & Community Medicine, University
of Bristol, Bristol, UK.

JD Carpentieri
Senior Policy and Research Officer, Institute
of Education, London, UK.

Sean AP Clouston
Assistant Professor, Public Health Program
and the Department of Preventative Medicine,
Stony Brook University, New York, USA.

Cyrus Cooper
Director and Professor of Rheumatology,
MRC Lifecourse Epidemiology Unit, and
Vice Dean, Faculty of Medicine, University
of Southampton, Southampton, UK, and
Professor of Musculoskeletal Science,
University of Oxford, Oxford, UK.

Rachel Cooper
MRC Programme Leader Track and Senior
Lecturer, MRC Unit for Lifelong Health and
Ageing at UCL, London, UK.

Teri-Louise Davies
MRC-funded PhD student in the Bristol
Centre for Systems Biomedicine (BCSBmed)
doctoral training centre, Bristol Genetic
Epidemiology Laboratories, School of Social
and Community Medicine, University
of Bristol, Bristol, UK.

Ian NM Day
Professor of Genetics and Molecular
Epidemiology, Bristol Genetic Epidemiology
Laboratories, School of Social and
Community Medicine, University of Bristol,
Bristol, UK.

Ian J Deary
Professor of Differential Psychology,
and Director of the Centre for Cognitive
Ageing and Cognitive Epidemiology,
Department of Psychology, University
of Edinburgh, Edinburgh, UK.

Ulf Ekelund
Professor, Department of Sport Medicine,
Norwegian School of Sport Sciences, Oslo,
Norway, and MRC Epidemiology Unit,
University of Cambridge, Cambridge, UK.

Jane Elliott
Director of the Centre for Longitudinal
Studies, and the Director of the
Collaborative CLOSER (Cohorts and
Longitudinal Studies Enhancement
Resources) Programme, Institute of
Education, London, UK.

Anne C Ferguson-Smith
Professor of Genetics and Head of
Department, Department of Genetics
University of Cambridge, Cambridge, UK.

Catharine R Gale
Reader, Centre for Cognitive Ageing and
Cognitive Epidemiology, Department

of Psychology, University of Edinburgh, Edinburgh, UK, and MRC Lifecourse Epidemiology Unit, University of Southampton, Southampton, UK.

Michael Gardner
Research Associate in Epidemiology, School of Social & Community Medicine, University of Bristol, Bristol, UK.

James Goodwin
Visiting Professor in Physiology of Ageing, Loughborough University, and Head of Research, Age UK.

Paul Haggarty
Professor and Head of Lifelong Health, Rowett Institute of Nutrition and Health, University of Aberdeen, Aberdeen, UK.

Rebecca Hardy
MRC Programme Leader and Professor of Epidemiology and Medical Statistics, MRC Unit for Lifelong Health and Ageing at UCL London, UK.

Scott Hofer
Professor, Harald Mohr, MD and Wilhelma Mohr, MD Research Chair in Adult, Development and Aging, Department of Psychology and Center on Aging, Department of Psychology, University of Victoria, British Columbia, Canada. Principal Investigator, IALSA network.

Diana Kuh
MRC Unit Director and Professor of Life Course Epidemiology, MRC Unit for Lifelong Health and Ageing at UCL, London, UK. Principal Investigator, HALCyon network.

Debbie A Lawlor
Professor of Epidemiology, MRC University of Bristol Unit for Integrated Epidemiology, School of Social and Community Medicine, University of Bristol, Bristol, UK.

Stafford Lightman
Professor of Medicine, Director of the Henry Wellcome Laboratories for Integrative Neuroscience and Endocrinology, University of Bristol, Bristol, UK.

Carmen Martin-Ruiz
Senior Research Associate, Institute for Ageing and Health, Newcastle University, Newcastle, UK.

Seema Mihrshahi
Lecturer, School of Population Health, University of Queensland, Australia.

Gita Mishra
Professor of Life Course Epidemiology, Co-Director of Centre for Longitudinal and Life Course Research, School of Population Health, University of Queensland, Australia.

Graciela Muniz-Terrera
MRC Programme Leader Track and Lecturer, MRC Unit for Lifelong Health and Ageing at UCL, London, UK.

Emily T Murray
Research Fellow, Division of Population Health Sciences and Education, Population Health Research Centre, St George's University of London, London, UK.

Ann Prentice
MRC Unit Director, MRC Human Nutrition Research, Cambridge, UK.

Marcus Richards
MRC Programme Leader and Professor of Psychology in Epidemiology, MRC Unit for Lifelong Health and Ageing at UCL, London, UK.

Mai Stafford
Programme Leader Track and Reader, MRC Unit for Lifelong Health and Ageing at UCL, London, UK.

Alison Stephen
Principal Investigator Scientist, MRC Human Nutrition Research, Cambridge, UK.

Kate Tilling
Professor of Medical Statistics, School
of Social and Community Medicine,
University of Bristol, Bristol, UK.

Thomas von Zglinicki
Professor of Cell Gerontology, Institute for
Ageing and Health, Newcastle University,
Newcastle, UK.

Kate A Ward
MRC Senior Investigator Scientist,
MRC Human Nutrition Research,
Cambridge, UK.

Andrew Wills
Lecturer in Applied Statistics, School
of Clinical Sciences, University of Bristol,
Bristol, UK.

Part I

The life course perspective on healthy ageing

Chapter 1

Life course epidemiology, ageing research, and maturing cohort studies: a dynamic combination for understanding healthy ageing

Diana Kuh, Marcus Richards, Rachel Cooper, Rebecca Hardy, and Yoav Ben-Shlomo

'Old age is like everything else. To make a success of it, you've got to start young.'

(Theodore Roosevelt 1858–1919)

1.1 Setting the scene

Population ageing is a feature of all developed countries and many developing countries. Its simplest manifestation is in the changing demographic dependency ratio, which typically shows the proportion of people aged 65 and older in a population as a ratio of those of working age (usually taken as 15–64 years). In 27 countries of the European Union (EU-27), for example, between 2010 and 2050 this ratio is set to double from 26% to 50% [1]. Population ageing is occurring because of the remarkable improvements in life expectancy since the nineteenth century, driven first by increased child survival, and then increased survival at older ages; the lower fertility rates in younger generations have also contributed [2]. While these upward trends show striking parallelism across Western Europe and North America, there is clearly variation (and periods of stagnation) among countries, and there are some notable exceptions elsewhere of periods of declining life expectancy, for example in Eastern Europe and sub-Saharan Africa [3].

Increased life expectancy can be viewed as a success of human endeavour in improving the environment, whether through better childhood nutrition, education, medical science, public health, or lifestyle change. To make a success of this demographic shift requires major changes in our attitudes to ageing [4]. However population ageing is usually viewed at best as a grand challenge, and at worst as a social problem. The debate focuses on the expected increase in health and welfare expenditure required to care for the post-war baby boom generations now reaching retirement, and how resourcing this additional expenditure may impact negatively on economic growth and disadvantage later-born generations.

The implications of population ageing could be viewed more positively if there was evidence that healthy life expectancy (the expected years of remaining life in good health) or disability-free life expectancy (expected years of remaining life free from limiting longstanding illness or disability) was increasing faster than life expectancy, leading to a compression of morbidity or disability [5]. In regard to disease trends, the evidence from the US and Europe suggests a rise in chronic diseases among older people [2]. This is likely to reflect increased duration of time living with disease because of earlier diagnosis, improved medical care resulting in reduced case fatality, and the ever widening boundaries of definitions of diseases or disorders that are seen to require medical intervention. In terms of disability, US data show a decline in late life disability since the 1980s, although recent trends in younger adults are not so encouraging [6]. These trends were based on reports of limitations in personal care activities such as bathing, eating, toileting, and dressing (commonly called the activities of daily living) and in activities related to independent living such as shopping, preparing meals, doing housework, and managing money (commonly called the instrumental activities of daily living). However, a study of 12 OECD countries found clear evidence of a decline in late life severe disability in only five [7]. Robine and colleagues [8] concluded that as of 2009 there was no strong evidence of compression of morbidity or disability in developed countries with the lowest mortality; the three countries where there was evidence of a compression of disability in recent decades, Denmark, the Netherlands, and the US, had all lagged behind the low mortality countries in terms of life expectancy at age 65. The recently updated Global Burden of Disease study provides the opportunity to compare health performance across countries based on the health loss due to diseases, injuries, and risk factors from which measures of healthy life expectancy, years lived with disability and disability-adjusted life are derived sytematically [9]; however the definitions of disability and methods used are not comparable with those used in national studies with time trend data.

Within country trends reveal striking social inequalities, with more educated and socially advantaged groups being more likely to experience a compression of morbidity or disability than less educated or socially disadvantaged groups [10]. Social inequalities appear to be particularly strong for disability and mortality and weaker for doctor diagnosed chronic disease because of earlier diagnosis and better access to health care for more advantaged social groups. For example, the average difference in disability-free life expectancy is 17 years between people living in poor and rich areas of England [11].

1.2 The need for an interdisciplinary and life course approach to healthy ageing

Increasing the proportion of healthy and active older people who remain independent for longer is seen as the main way to relieve the costs of an ageing population, and enhance individual wellbeing; research into ageing has become a political and a scientific priority. There is a growing consensus from international health organizations [12], national policymakers [13], research funders [14], and scientists that ageing itself needs to be studied from an interdisciplinary and life course perspective, to inform intervention strategies. There are a number of key elements of this approach.

First, given that the biggest risk factor for the non-communicable chronic diseases of later life is age itself, a research priority is to understand better the underlying biological processes of ageing at the body system, cellular and molecular levels; and then to undertake interdisciplinary research that investigates how these processes integrate the rather separate research on specific age-related diseases, and how they relate to ageing measured at the individual and population levels. In short, mechanistic and population science need to work more closely together.

Second, there is now broad recognition that understanding health and ageing requires inter-disciplinary research in the broadest sense, encompassing social, psychological and biological approaches. The development of interdisciplinary theories and studies of ageing has been a key trend over the last decade [15]. Explanations for the striking social inequalities in mortality and disability within countries require an understanding of how social structure and social interaction affect individual behaviour and 'get under the skin' to leave biological imprints with lasting effects on social inequalities in health [16].

Third, there is an increased interest in studying the whole spectrum of health and ageing, from those with the best health or ageing well to those with the worst health or experiencing accelerated ageing, and seeing what can be learnt from the highest functioning individuals. Healthy ageing has been a neglected area of ageing research, particularly in the UK, where the traditional focus has been on specific chronic diseases of later life. Measures of healthy ageing are required to increase the chance of identifying new intervention targets beyond those already employed in chronic dis-ease epidemiology [17]. These should include objective measures of function. In this respect we note the development of the NIH toolbox, set to provide brief but comprehensive instruments to measure, motor, cognitive, sensory, and emotional function (http://www.nihtoolbox.org); and the UK Medical Research Council is developing guidance on healthy ageing indicators.

Fourth, there is growing interest in a life course approach to ageing because of accumulating evidence that factors from early life, even *in utero* [18], and intergenerational factors [19] influ-ence an individual's chance of developing a number of chronic diseases in later life. There is much excitement about elucidating the biological mechanisms [20,21]; equal attention needs to be paid to the social and psychological pathways. We also need to know whether early experiences and exposures influence the chance of healthy ageing or explain social inequalities in healthy ageing, and how they modify later life risk.

Fifth, scientists are harnessing the power of cohort studies that follow a sample of people through their lives as this is a powerful way to identify factors earlier in life that impact on healthy biological ageing or active ageing. Increasingly information from several cohorts is examined together to increase the power to detect associations between risk or protective factors and ageing outcomes, and to test whether these associations are robust and generalizable across cohorts, or differ in response to changing societal conditions.

1.3 Aims of this book

This book aims to review the evidence for biological, psychological, and social factors operating from early life that influence the chance of healthy ageing and healthy living in later life. We focus on functional measures of healthy ageing and on the evidence revealed by human cohort studies, especially those that have followed individuals for all or most of their lives, while referencing other study designs as appropriate. We pay particular attention to evidence from cross cohort studies to assess to what extent these associations are consistent and generalizable. We start by introducing the life course approach and defining the key terms used in this book as our aim is to reach a wide readership, and to promote interdisciplinarity.

1.4 Life course concepts and definitions of healthy ageing

Social, behavioural and biomedical scientists have long promoted a life course or a lifespan con-ceptual framework for organizing research on human development, maturation and ageing. In the past, the emphasis was on the distinctive features of this approach in each discipline; for example stressing the differences between life course sociology and lifespan developmental psychology [22]. However, recent debate emphasizes what these different approaches have in common [23], and how the life course perspective can be used as a common conceptual framework to integrate and guide the development of interdisciplinary theories and studies of ageing.

Reflecting this interdisciplinary trend, contributors to the following chapters draw on relevant elements of the life course perspective from a range of disciplines; but life course epidemiology is central for them all. A life course approach in epidemiology investigates the biological, behavioural, and social pathways that link physical and social exposures and experiences during gestation, childhood, adolescence, and adult life, and across generations, to changes in health and disease risk later in life [24,25]. Epidemiologists were late converts to the life course perspective and have drawn on relevant theories and concepts from other disciplines [26], but are increasingly recognized by these other disciplines for their contributions (see, for example, Alwin [23]). Initially, the focus was on chronic disease epidemiology where the life course perspective was used to integrate and extend three broad and apparently conflicting theories of disease aetiology. The fetal origins of adult disease hypothesis, proposed by David Barker [18], which evolved into the wider developmental origins of health and disease framework [27] acted as a catalyst for life course epidemiology which then drew attention to potential sensitive periods in childhood and adolescence as well as *in utero,* and developed life course models and ways of testing these. In respect of the adult lifestyle and social causation theories of chronic disease [28], life course epidemiology drew attention to the early acquisition of lifestyle and its cumulative effects, and to the impact of the socioeconomic environment in childhood as well as in adult life.

Increasingly life course epidemiology has widened its gaze from chronic disease to health and ageing, supporting a concept of *health* that is multidimensional, including how we feel or how we function (at the individual down to the molecular level), as well as what diseases or disorders we have, and how long we live. Health is captured too often at only one point in time ('health status'), or conceptualized as an ideal state of complete physical, mental, and social wellbeing [29]. Rather, health reflects the ability of the organism to respond adaptively to ever changing environmental challenges [30,31]. This chimes with the early nineteenth century view that health represents a 'delicate equilibrium' between the disturbing influences of the environment and the individual's constitution, a view which has its origins in the work of Galen, Aristotle and Hippocrates [32]. In the twenty-first century, we need to develop a dynamic concept of lifelong health, one that includes some assessment of health capital or reserve built up, and of future health potential: for those at the beginning of life it is the chance of full physical and mental development; post-maturity, it is the chance of healthy and active ageing. *Development* and *ageing* are thus dynamic concepts referring to the *changes* in health as we grow older. More specifically, *biological ageing* captures the progressive generalized impairment of function ('senescence') that occurs post-maturity, whether studied at the individual, body system, cellular or molecular level. According to the generally accepted evolutionary senescence theory, this is due to a decline in the force of natural selection in the post-reproductive phase of life [33]. There are many hypotheses of how (as opposed to why) we age at the body system, cellular, or molecular level which are not necessarily mutually exclusive [34]; some of these are discussed in the following chapters.

Life course epidemiologists make use conceptually and empirically of functional trajectories across life as a dynamic way of studying lifetime influences on health and disease risk (Figure 1.1). Life course trajectories of body functions (e.g. muscle, lung) or structures (e.g. bone mass) capture the natural history of biological systems which display rapid growth and development during the prenatal, pre-pubertal, and pubertal periods, reaching a peak or plateau at maturity ('structural

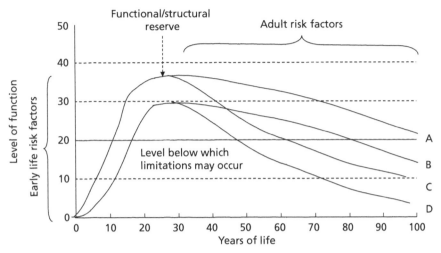

Figure 1.1 Life course functional trajectories.

Adapted from Yoav Ben-Shlomo and Diana Kuh, A life course approach to chronic disease epidemiology: conceptual models, empirical challenges and interdisciplinary perspectives, *International Journal of Epidemiology*, Volume **31**, Issue 2, pp. 285–293, Copyright © International Epidemiological Association 2002, by permission of Oxford University Press.

or functional reserve') and a gradual decline with age (line A). Exposures in early life, particularly during a critical developmental window, may leave imprints on the structure or function of body systems; and epigenetic mechanisms may contribute to these processes. This developmental plasticity may affect reserve without appreciable effects on the rate of decline (line B), or may interact with biological ageing processes to accelerate functional decline (line C). Exposures after the developmental period can only affect the timing and rate of decline. Adverse exposures across life may affect the reserve and accelerate functional decline (line D)

Thus *healthy biological ageing* includes three main hierarchical and dynamic components: first, survival to old age; second, delay in the onset of chronic disease or disability; and third, optimal functioning for the maximal period of time. Our preferred terms to describe functioning at the individual level are *physical and cognitive capability*, the capacity to undertake the physical and mental tasks of daily living; these terms emphasize the positive end of the spectrum and are distinguished from the functioning of body systems. In contrast we use the term *active ageing* to refer to the continued participation of the individual in valued social roles, engaging with others, whether in paid work, volunteering, or leisure pursuits, leading physically active and meaningful lives, and maintaining autonomy and independence.

In taking a life course approach to healthy biological ageing, the following chapters concentrate on functioning because of the relative paucity of research on this component of healthy biological ageing, and because improvements in functioning would be expected to delay onset of disease and disability and improve survival. However, we should note that even in high income countries more than one in ten people do not have much chance of healthy ageing because they die before 65 years, notwithstanding the tremendous improvements in survival rates up to age 65 (from 42.0% at the beginning of the twentieth century to 87.8% in 2005–9 [35]). In terms of chronic disease or disability, recent cohort studies suggest that already by early old age, only a minority of participants have no chronic disease or disability. Even for the relatively privileged Whitehall II study, only 30% were free of any chronic disease or disability at 60 years or older [17]. In the oldest and nationally representative British cohort study, the MRC National Survey of Health and Development, participants aged 60–64 years had two out of 15 common disorders on average, and only 15% were disorder-free [36]. A cluster of one in five of these participants had a high probability of cardio-metabolic disorders and were twice as likely than others to have been in the poorest health when assessed 30 years earlier; this finding is of considerable interest from a life course and early intervention perspective. Thus most older people are either 'survivors' (those living with age-related chronic disease diagnosed before old age), or 'delayers' (age-related disease diagnosed after the average life expectancy of their birth cohort). Few are likely to be 'escapers' (those who attain very old age without any major disease: evidence from the Newcastle 85 + study shows this clearly [37]). If most people age with some form of disorder or disability, there are two main policy implications: first to find ways to reduce symptom severity; second to find ways to support active ageing, despite the challenges of morbidity or disability.

1.4.1 Studies of healthy or successful ageing

There has been a strong focus on the concept of 'successful ageing', particularly in the US, a term used by Havinghurst in the first issue of *The Gerontologist* in 1961 [38]. The most referenced classification of successful ageing is that offered by Rowe and Kahn [39] and featured in the MacArthur Foundation research programme on successful ageing in the 1990s. The components included are: (1) low probability of disease and disease-related disability; (2) high cognitive and physical functional capacity; and (3) active engagement with life. Some researchers include all three areas in their definition of successful or healthy ageing; others prefer to keep active engagement as separate from healthy ageing.

While there may be some agreement of the broad constructs that make up successful or healthy ageing, most studies that have tried to operationalize these constructs use different measures and cutpoints. In a comprehensive review of such studies between 1978 and 2005, 28 studies covering 29 different definitions of healthy or successful ageing [40] were identified. In defining a group who are ageing well, these studies often relied on negative criteria, i.e. excluding those with disease, disability or self-reported functional limitations, usually at one point in time, rather than positive criteria that identified high functioning individuals at the top end of the spectrum, and those who have maintained good function over time. Thus, the research on successful or healthy ageing has been limited by the lack of standard definitions; the reliance on self-reported measures that do not discriminate the full spectrum of function or activity and just exclude the most adverse groups; and the cross-sectional nature of most operational definitions that take no account of an individual's trajectory over time, and do not incorporate those who have died as part of the denominator. The need for longitudinal objective measures is now better recognized [41], and these are increasingly being incorporated into some of the more recent studies of healthy ageing.

More generally, 'successful ageing' carries moral overtones with often unattainable ideals of success and inappropriate concepts of failure, and underlying questionable assumptions that 'success' is primarily the responsibility of the individual, and make assumptions that healthy ageing is mainly about older people acting like younger people for as long as possible.

Clearly then, the study of how healthy biological ageing and active ageing are maintained, improved, and restored requires longitudinal data on individual change, preferably in life course studies that have followed individuals from birth, or at least across a number of life stages (infancy, childhood, adolescence, early adulthood, midlife, and later adulthood). These longitudinal studies have an important contribution to make to the growing evidence that the ability to respond adaptively, either biologically, mentally or socially, is governed not only by current environmental challenges and genetic factors, but also by the response to earlier life challenges, especially at times of developmental plasticity when environmental exposures have greater and potentially lifelong impact than exposures during other periods of life.

1.5 Further development of an integrated life course model of ageing

We have previously defined four broad life course models to test the importance of timing and duration of exposures on later health and disease risk: (1) a 'critical or sensitive period model' when an exposure in earlier life has lifelong effects on structure or function that are not modified by later experience (also known as biological programming); (2) a 'critical or sensitive period with later effect modifiers model' when exposures in later life interact with earlier life exposures to exacerbate or diminish these effects (an extension of the first model); (3) an 'accumulation of risk model' where there is cumulative damage to biological systems over the life course; and (4) a 'chain of risk model' which is a version of the accumulation model where there is a sequence of linked exposures that lead to impaired function [26]. Critical periods of development are times of rapid change when there are rapid and usually irreversible intrinsic changes towards greater complexity taking place. Sensitive periods may also be times of rapid change but in this case there is more scope to modify or even reverse the changes outside the developmental time window. These life course models and illustrative examples are discussed extensively elsewhere [42]; and a novel structured modelling approach has been developed to distinguish between these different models [43], which has been applied in a number of research studies [44–46] and is discussed in Chapter 7.

These original life course models focused on lifetime exposures but they need to be developed to take more account of intrinsic ageing processes. One important process is 'compensatory reserve', that is the ability of body systems to compensate physiologically with varying degrees of success when faced with acute or chronic low level challenges in order to maintain function or limit decline. Functional trajectories post-maturity capture this dynamic interplay. There may or may not be an association between structural reserve (Figure 1.1) and compensatory reserve. For example, individuals with better synaptic connectivity may also be more able to reconnect adjacent circuits after a cerebrovascular event; hence they start with better structural reserve and have a better compensatory response. However, it is also possible that any cellular repair response is independent of the pre-existing structural reserve. We envisage compensatory reserve as an intrinsic biological phenomenon which preserves functional capacity but deteriorates with age, probably in a non-linear fashion and possibly in parallel across multiple domains (e.g. vascular, neurological, immune, homeostatic systems) in those who will become frail. In addition, the individual may show extrinsic responses when faced with age-related declines ('adaptations'), by altering behaviour or the environment to modify the effect of functional decline on activities of daily living and social participation. These adaptations could also slow the rate of decline by changing the level of exposures.

Our extended integrated life course model of ageing is illustrated in Figure 1.2. An important element of this model is that it captures the whole spectrum of health, and changes in health, during development, maturity, and ageing, in order to focus on the promotion of good health and not just the decline in health with age [17,47]. The figure illustrates the possibility of physiological compensation or psychological and social adaptation through feedback loops at all stages (labelled F1–5 in the diagram). We separate out lifetime physical and social environments

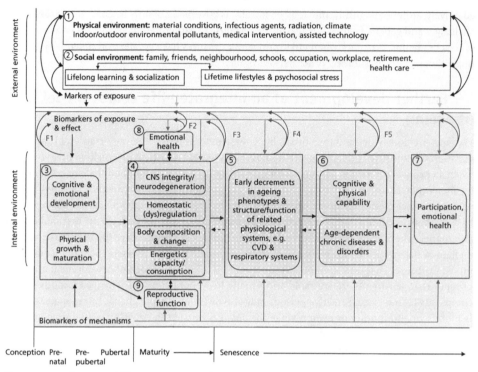

Figure 1.2 An integrated life course approach to ageing.

(boxes 1 and 2) but show strong links between the two given the impact of socioeconomic position on material conditions and other physical exposures that can affect the ageing trajectory, and the impact of these conditions on the social environment. The social environment also affects the ageing trajectory through influencing lifelong learning and socialization, lifetime lifestyles, and exposure to psychosocial stress.

To understand better the links between growth and development (box 3), and physical and cognitive capability, and age-dependent disease in later life (box 6) we have interposed four phenotypes (box 4) that capture the four key interlocking domains affected by molecular and cellular ageing [48]: (1) central nervous system (CNS) integrity and neurodegeneration (discussed in Chapter 3); (2) homeostatic regulation and age-related dysregulation in signalling pathways that maintain homeostasis (encompassing both the endocrine and immunological systems) (discussed in Chapter 10); (3) body composition and age-related change in muscle, fat, and bone (see Chapter 12); and (4) energetics and age-related changes in energy production and consumption (discussed briefly in Chapter 2) [49].

An important element of this general model is the lag time between decrements in these ageing phenotypes (box 4), and in related physiological systems such as the cardiovascular and respiratory systems (box 5), and the phenotypic emergence of their consequences for physical and cognitive capability or age-dependent disease (box 6). The model shows the close connections between the decline in (or maintenance of) physical and cognitive capability and the development (or absence) of age-dependent diseases. The more we understand the pathology of age-dependent disease, the more the distinction between ageing and these diseases becomes blurred.

One of the cornerstones of the life course perspective on ageing is being able to detect early markers of an accelerated trajectory of decline, because this offers an opportunity to delay the onset of decline or its rate of change through preventive strategies. Another is the ability to capture environmental characteristics before impairments emerge, facilitating a better understanding of the unfolding interaction between individuals and their environments. The differential effects of socioeconomic factors in childhood and adult life on ageing outcomes provide clues to the timing of modifiable risk factors at the individual and societal levels.

Our model of ageing also encompasses the emotional health of older people and their continued participation in society, both as a consequence of capability and chronic disease (box 7), and as a determinant or modifier (box 8) (discussed further in Chapters 3 and 4). It is important to study life course emotional health because early emotional development predicts adult emotional health and life chances, and lifetime emotional health influences physiological ageing and determines individual capacity for psychological and social adaptation.

The model assumes an intimate connection between brain and body ageing, and between physical and cognitive capability. Cohorts with repeated data across life can make an important contribution to questions about the nature and degree of interdependency across these domains and to the search for common causal mechanisms A common causal account of ageing may operate at various levels, from brain circuitry and brain pathology to the loss of molecular fidelity [50,51]. We return to this in the concluding chapter of this book and in the supplementary web material (at www.halcyon.ac.uk).

Reproductive function (box 9) needs to be considered if we are integrating our life course model of ageing with the broader evolutionary framework. The adaptations made during developmental plasticity are to promote the subsequent reproductive capacity of the organism; the deleterious effects of these adaptations on ageing post-maturity that are observed are of less evolutionary concern [31]. A woman's physiological response to the challenge of pregnancy and childbirth provides clues to adaptive capacity that may then impact on general ageing; thus reproductive characteristics (such as hypertension in pregnancy, offspring low birth weight, and early menopause) may act as sentinels for later disease and accelerated ageing [52,53]. Cohort studies with data on reproductive histories and timing of menopause and other menopausal characteristics may provide potential insights into the ageing of the cardiovascular and other physiological systems, and perhaps even into the decline in capability (Chapter 11).

The model promotes a life course perspective for both the internal and external environment, reflecting the growing interest in the 'exposome' to complement the genome [54]. There is active development of sophisticated tools to characterize better: (1) the external environment using, for example, sensor technologies to measure environmental pollutants or physical activity, or portable computerized devices for capturing behaviour and experiences (markers of exposure); and (2) the internal environment using, for example, biomarkers of effect to measure environmental effects on intermediate phenotypes and biomarkers of mechanisms to capture causal processes involved. New data on metabolomics and epigenomics to complement the genomic data in a number of cohorts will provide powerful tools for studies of ageing mechanisms (Chapters 14 and 15).

Finally, the influence of stochastic events and processes must be recognized in any general life course model of ageing [55,56]. The effects of such processes mean that, while any model is unlikely to predict individual outcomes, it can still provide insight into the lifetime characteristics of individuals and their environments that drive ageing, and that could be targeted to extend healthy active lives, and into the reasons for systematic variation in ageing between men and women, by social and cultural groups, and across birth cohorts. Systematic gender and socioeconomic differences in ageing outcomes are highlighted in this book; ethnicity, while equally important, is not comprehensively included, because the cohort studies from which much of the evidence will be drawn do not have sizeable ethnic groups.

1.6 **Content of this book**

In this book we mean healthy ageing to encompass healthy biological ageing and high levels of psychological and social wellbeing. In the remaining chapters in Part I, we examine healthy ageing at the individual level, first in relation to physical and cognitive capability (Chapters 2 and 3); and then in relation to psychological and social wellbeing, covering positive emotions and personal fulfilment, and how one feels or functions in relation to other people (Chapter 4). The reasons for including wellbeing as an aspect of healthy ageing are the prominence given to wellbeing by individuals themselves when asked to define healthy or successful ageing, and the need to understand whether the lifetime determinants of wellbeing are (or are not) a mirror image of the lifetime determinants of mental disorders [57]. However, unlike physical and cognitive capability, there is little evidence for a decline in psychological and social wellbeing until very old age. Like others, we prefer to study capability and wellbeing separately because of these different relationships with age, and to facilitate the study of any bidirectional links and shared lifetime influences.

The five chapters in Part II are methodological, and outline the study designs, quantitative longitudinal methods, and the qualitative narrative approach for the life course study of healthy ageing within and across cohorts. The six chapters in Part III investigate the underlying biology of ageing in terms of the role of key body systems (neuroendocrine, metabolic, and vascular, musculoskeletal) and of biomarkers, genetics, and epigenetics. The three chapters in Part IV examine how the way we live (in terms of diet, physical activity and area characteristics) affects the chance of healthy ageing, and the life course influences that determine the way we live. The concluding chapter highlights the key findings and emerging themes and places these within a knowledge transfer framework, given that the overriding reason for seeking to identify factors that influence health at older ages is to guide the design and implementation of preventive and therapeutic interventions.

The contributors to this book include investigators of maturing birth cohort and ageing studies, cross-cutting methodologists, and specialists in specific ageing outcomes, risk factors, and policy research. They share a common interest in characterizing ageing trajectories, and understanding reasons for variation within and between individuals, and across gender and social groups. Many of the contributors have been working together over the last few years on three interconnected research programmes that bring cohort studies together for the scientific discovery of lifetime influences on ageing: the Healthy Ageing across the Life Course (HALCyon) collaborative programme led by Diana Kuh and funded by the UK research councils under the New Dynamics of Ageing programme; the Measurement and Modelling of Functional Trajectories across the Life Course (FALCon) research project, led by Rebecca Hardy and funded the UK Medical Research Council; and the Integrative Analysis of Longitudinal Studies of Ageing (IALSA), an international network led by Scott Hofer, and funded primarily by the US National Institutes of Health. The authors present the results of these collaborations in the following chapters, and enhance them by drawing on the wider evidence, particularly from systematic and narrative reviews.

The HALCyon and FALCon research programmes draw mainly on the wealth of UK prospective cohort studies. These include the two oldest national birth cohort studies: the MRC National Survey of Health and Development (NSHD) and the National Child Development Study (NCDS), with samples recruited from those born in a week in March 1946 and 1958, respectively, and prospectively followed since. It also includes Avon Longitudinal Study of Parents and Children

(ALSPAC), which is a large regional based cohort of births in the 1990s, and followed prospectively since. There are regionally based historical cohort studies where those with health records at birth or in infancy (the Hertfordshire Cohort and Ageing studies), or records of cognitive tests in childhood (Lothian and Aberdeen cohort studies) or childhood diets (Boyd Orr cohort study) were traced and followed up later in life. Finally there are the adult cohort studies with long-term follow-up and repeated relevant measures, usually based on general adult populations with varying age ranges (the Caerphilly Prospective study, English Longitudinal Study of Ageing and Twenty-07 studies). A short description of these cohorts can be found on the HALCyon website (www.halcyon.ac.uk).

References

1 Wöss J, Türk E. Dependency ratios and demographic change. The labour market as a key element. European Trade Union Institute Policy Brief. European Economic and Employment Policy. Brussels: European Trade Union Institute; 2011. ISSN 2031-8782. <http://www.etui.org/Publications2/Policy-Briefs/European-Economic-and-Employment-Policy/Dependency-ratios-and-demographic-change.-The-labour-market-as-a-key-element>

2 Christensen K, et al. Ageing populations: the challenges ahead. *Lancet* 2009;**374**:1196–208.

3 Leon DA. Trends in European life expectancy: a salutary view. *Int J Epidemiol* 2011;**40**:271–7.

4 House of Lords Select Committee on Public Service and Demographic Change. Ready for Ageing? Report of session 2012–2013. <http://www.publications.parliament.uk/pa/ld201213/ldselect/ldpublic/140/140.pdf>

5 Fries JF, et al. Compression of morbidity 1980–2011: a focused review of paradigms and progress. *J Aging Res* 2011;**2011**:261702.

6 Martin LG, et al. Trends in health of older adults in the United States: past, present, future. *Demography* 2010;**47**:S17–40.

7 Lafortune G, et al. Trends in severe disability among elderly people: assessing the evidence in 12 OECD countries and the future implications. OECD Health Working Papers. 26th ed; 2007.

8 Robine J, et al. The relationship between longevity and healthy life expectancy. *Qual Ageing* 2012;**10**:5–14.

9 Murray CJL, et al. UK health performance: findings of the Global Burden of Disease study. *Lancet* 2013;**381**:997–1020 .

10 Deeg D. Compression of disability—privilege of the well-educated. In: McDaniel S, Zimmer Z, editors. Global Ageing in the Twenty-First Century: Challenges, Opportunities and Implications. Farnham, Surrey: Ashgate Publishing; 2012.

11 Marmot M. Fair Society, Healthy Lives: The Marmot Review. London: UCL Institute of Health Equity; 1–2–2010.

12 World Health Organization. Good Health Adds Life to Years: Global Brief for World Health Day. WHO; 2012.

13 House of Lords Science and Technology Committee. Ageing: Scientific Aspects. 21–7–2005. <http://www.publications.parliament.uk/pa/ld200506/ldselect/ldsctech/20/20i.pdf>

14 Medical Research Council. Research changes lives. MRC Strategic Plan 2009–2014. MRC; 10–6–2009.

15 Bengtson V, et al. Theories about age and aging. In: Bengtson V, Silverstein M, Putney N, Gans D, editors. Handbook of Theories of Aging. 2nd ed. New York: Springer; 2008:3–25.

16 Hertzman C, Boyce T. How experience gets under the skin to create gradients in developmental health. *Annu Rev Public Health* 2010;**31**:329–47.

17 Kivimaki M, Ferrie JE. Epidemiology of healthy ageing and the idea of more refined outcome measures. *Int J Epidemiol* 2011;**40**:845–7.

18 Barker D. Mothers, Babies and Health in Later Life. 2nd ed. Edinburgh: Churchill Livingstone; 1998.

19 **Lawlor D, Mishra G.** Family Matters: Designing, Analysing and Understanding Family Based Studies in Life Course Epidemiology. 1st ed. Oxford: Oxford University Press; 2009.

20 **Waterland RA, Michels KB.** Epigenetic epidemiology of the developmental origins hypothesis. *Annu Rev Nutr* 2007;**27**:363–88.

21 **Ng JW, et al.** The role of longitudinal cohort studies in epigenetic epidemiology: challenges and opportunities. *Genome Biol* 2012;**13**:246.

22 **Mayer K.** The sociology of the life course and life span psychology: diverging or converging pathways? In: Staudinger U, Lindenberger U, editors. Understanding Human Development: Dialogues with Lifespan Psychology. New York: Kluwer Academic; 2003:463–81.

23 **Alwin DF.** Integrating varieties of life course concepts. *J Gerontol B Psychol Sci Soc Sci* 2012;**67**:206–20.

24 **Kuh D, Ben-Shlomo Y.** A Life Course Approach to Chronic Disease Epidemiology: Tracing the Origins of Ill-health from Early to Adult Life. 2nd ed. Oxford: Oxford University Press; 2004.

25 **Kuh D, et al.** Life course epidemiology and analysis. In: The Oxford Textbook of Public Health. Oxford: Oxford University Press. In press.

26 **Kuh D, et al.** Life course epidemiology. *J Epidemiol Community Health* 2003;**57**:778–83.

27 **Gluckman PD, Hanson MA.** Developmental Origins of Health and Disease. Cambridge University Press; 2006.

28 **Krieger N.** Epidemiology and the People's Health: Theory and Context. New York: Oxford University Press; 2013.

29 **Official Records of the World Health Organization.** No. 2. Proceeding and Final Acts of the International Health Conference Held in New York from 19 June to 22 July 1946. United Nations: WHO Interim Commission; 1946.

30 **Dubos R.** Man Adapting. New Haven and London: Yale University Press; 1965.

31 **Gluckman PD, et al.** Towards a new developmental synthesis: adaptive developmental plasticity and human disease. *Lancet* 2009;**373**:1654–7.

32 **Hamlin C.** Predisposing causes and public health in early nineteenth-century medical thought. *Soc Hist Med* 1992;**5**:43–70.

33 **Austad SN.** Making sense of biological theories of aging. In: Bengtson V, Silverstein M, Putney N, Gans D, editors. Handbook of Theories of Aging. 2nd ed. New York: Springer; 2008:147–162.

34 **Weinert B, Timiras P.** Invited review: theories of aging. *J Appl Physiol* 2003;**95**:1706–16.

35 **Eggleston K, Fuchs V.** The new demographic transition: most gains in life expectancy now realized late in life. Asia Health Policy Program Working Paper #29; 11–6–2012.

36 **Pierce MB, et al.** Clinical disorders in a post war British cohort reaching retirement: evidence from the First National Birth Cohort Study. *PLoS One* 2012;**7**:e44857.

37 **Collerton J, et al.** Health and disease in 85 year olds: baseline findings from the Newcastle 85 + cohort study. *BMJ* 2009;**339**:b4904.

38 **Havinghurst R.** Successful ageing. *Gerontologist* 1961;**1**:4–7.

39 **Rowe JW, Kahn RL.** Successful aging. *Gerontologist* 1997;**37**:433–40.

40 **Depp CA, Jeste DV.** Definitions and predictors of successful aging: a comprehensive review of larger quantitative studies. *Am J Geriatr Psychiatry* 2006;**14**:6–20.

41 **Fiocco AJ, Yaffe K.** Defining successful aging: the importance of including cognitive function over time. *Arch Neurol* 2010;**67**:876–80.

42 **Ben-Shlomo Y, et al.** Life course epidemiology. In: Ahrens W, Pigeot I, editors. Handbook of Epidemiology. 2nd ed. New York: Springer Publishing Company; 2013.

43 **Mishra G, et al.** A structured approach to modelling the effects of binary exposure variables over the life course. *Int J Epidemiol* 2009;**38**:528–37.

44 **Murray ET, et al.** Life course models of socioeconomic position and cardiovascular risk factors: 1946 birth cohort. *Ann Epidemiol* 2011;**21**:589–97.

45 **Cooper R, et al.** Physical activity across adulthood and physical performance in midlife: findings from a British birth cohort. *Am J Prev Med* 2011;**41**:376–84.

46 **Birnie K, et al.** Socio-economic disadvantage from childhood to adulthood and locomotor function in old age: a lifecourse analysis of the Boyd Orr and Caerphilly prospective studies. *J Epidemiol Community Health* 2011;**65**:1014–23.

47 **Lowry KA, et al.** Successful aging as a continuum of functional independence: lessons from physical disability models of aging. *Aging Dis* 2012;**3**:5–15.

48 **Ferrucci L, Studenski S.** Clinical problems in aging. In: Harrison's Principles of Internal Medicine. 18th ed. New York: McGraw-Hill; 2012:570–85.

49 **Schrack JA, et al.** The energetic pathway to mobility loss: an emerging new framework for longitudinal studies on aging. *J Am Geriatr Soc* 2010;**58**:S329–36.

50 **Hayflick L.** Debates: the not-so-close relationship between biological aging and age-associated pathologies in humans. *J Gerontol A Biol Sci Med Sci* 2004;**59**:B547–50.

51 **Farooqui T, Farooqui AA.** Aging: an important factor for the pathogenesis of neurodegenerative diseases. *Mech Ageing Dev* 2009;**130**:203–15.

52 **Fraser A, et al.** Associations of gestational weight gain with maternal body mass index, waist circumference, and blood pressure measured 16 y after pregnancy: the Avon Longitudinal Study of Parents and Children (ALSPAC). *Am J Clin Nutr* 2011;**93**:1285–92.

53 **Rich-Edwards JW, et al.** Breathing life into the lifecourse approach: pregnancy history and cardiovascular disease in women. *Hypertension* 2010;**56**:331–4.

54 **Wild CP.** The exposome: from concept to utility. *Int J Epidemiol* 2012;**41**:24–32.

55 **Davey Smith G.** Epidemiology, epigenetics and the Gloomy Prospect: embracing randomness in population health research and practice. *Int J Epidemiol* 2011;**40**:537–62.

56 **Kirkwood TB.** Commentary: ageing—what's all the noise about? Developments after Gartner. *Int J Epidemiol* 2012;**41**:351–2.

57 **Karestan K, et al.** A Life Course Approach to Mental Disorders. Oxford: Oxford University Press. In press.

Chapter 2

A life course approach to physical capability

Rachel Cooper, Rebecca Hardy, Avan Aihie Sayer, and Diana Kuh

2.1 Introduction

Maintaining physical capability, the capacity to undertake the physical tasks of daily living, for the maximal period of time is one of the key components of healthy biological ageing (Chapter 1). Higher levels of physical capability have also been linked to higher survival rates [1] and to delays in the onset of chronic disease, and disability [2,3], other components of healthy biological ageing. The inclusion of physical capability and/or physical disability in the majority of existing studies that have attempted to operationalize healthy ageing exemplifies their perceived importance within the research community [4]. Qualitative work also demonstrates the value that older people themselves place on maintaining physical capability; in interviews undertaken with subsamples of the MRC National Survey of Health and Development (NSHD) and the Hertfordshire Cohort Study, physical decline and changes in capability were frequently cited self-perceived disadvantages of ageing [5]. Short quotes from two of these interviews exemplify this:

> '. . . old age doesn't come alone, . . . it brings with it all sorts of physical reductions'
> '. . . it's a bit frightening the prospect of losing my mobility'.

We use the generic term physical capability rather than physical functioning to emphasize healthy biological ageing at the individual level and to delineate it from the physiological functions of each body system [6]. To sustain performance for most physical tasks (such as rising from a chair or walking at normal speed) requires several body functions to operate. We include muscle strength as well as physical performance under the generic term physical capability because of the widespread use of strength as a measure of overall physical capability. In this chapter we focus on objective measures of physical capability with the reasons for this outlined in Section 2.2.

2.2 Assessment of physical capability

2.2.1 History of assessment

Earlier assessments of physical capability were usually based on self-reports of functional limitations or ability to perform activities of daily living (ADL). However, since the late 1980s objective assessments have come to be widely used, first in large population-based studies in North America and more recently in other countries. Objective tests of physical capability with standardized assessment criteria were introduced, to complement self-reports and to improve validity and reproducibility, more accurately capture change over time, and reduce the influence of cognitive function, culture, language, and education that may affect self-reported, subjective assessments, and limit comparability across studies [7]. While caution is required in using performance on objective tests to make direct inferences about individuals' abilities to undertake the tasks of daily living [7], poor performance on objective tests of physical capability, including slow walking speed and weak grip strength, are commonly used as components of operational definitions of disability and frailty [8,9]. These tests also allow performance to be measured along a continuum; Healthy Ageing across the Life Course research collaboration (HALCyon) systematic reviews have shown that lower levels of performance on these tests are linked with higher subsequent risk of a range of other health outcomes and lower survival rates in older community-dwelling populations [1,2] and may also be linked to lower levels of wellbeing (Chapter 4). From the perspective of healthy ageing, these objective tests enable the study of variation in functioning across the full spectrum of ability and the identification of people performing most well; this is not possible with self-reported measures, that primarily aim to capture loss of function. From a life course perspective, the use of objective physical capability measures facilitates the study of social, behavioural, and biological processes from early life onwards, prior to the manifestation of disability or frailty.

2.2.2 **Objective tests of physical capability**

One of the most commonly used tests of lower body function is walking speed, which involves recording the time taken to walk at a specified pace over a fixed short distance or to get up from a chair, walk a set distance (usually 3 metres), turn around and sit back in the chair (a variant called the 'timed get up and go test'). Other commonly used measures of lower body function are: chair stands which involve recording the time taken to stand from a chair and sit back down again a set number of times (usually one, five, or ten) or the number of stands completed in a set time period; and standing balance which is assessed in a number of different ways, including recording the length of time up to a maximum (often 30 seconds) that a one legged stand can be maintained with eyes open or closed. Upper body function is commonly measured by grip strength (i.e. muscle force) using a handheld dynamometer [10], but can also be assessed using tests of dexterity and functional reach including measurement of the speed pegs are moved on a pegboard, and the time taken to put on and take off a cardigan or shirt [11]. While there is considerable variability in the protocols of assessment [10,12] attempts are being made to standardize these, through initiatives such as the National Institutes of Health (NIH) toolbox <http://www.nihtoolbox.org>, which address many previous methodological concerns.

A set of different objective physical capability tests are often administered together [13], such as the short physical performance battery (SPPB) which includes tests of balance, walking, and chair rising [8,11,14]. An overall performance score may be most useful for the purposes of clinical assessment and prediction, but from an aetiological perspective there is often benefit in studying the measures separately, as each test measures somewhat different underlying constructs and so their lifetime determinants could be disguised by combining measures.

Within a healthy population, variation between individuals in physical capability is related, to varying degrees, to the normal functioning of each body system, especially the musculoskeletal, cardiovascular, respiratory, and nervous systems. Grip strength is a measure of isometric muscle strength (muscle force), often used as an indicator of overall body strength and viewed as a direct measure of musculoskeletal system function [15]. It is under direct command from the motor cortex through motor-neurones, fine-tuned at the spinal level; good performance is thus dependent not only on characteristics of the musculoskeletal system but also the nervous system [16]. Successful performance in tests of standing balance also depends primarily on the musculoskeletal and nervous systems including functions such as mental concentration, subtle motor control, good vestibular function, and lower limb strength. Chair rising and walking require energy, good balance and strength, power and speed in the extensor muscles of the lower body and, due to the aerobic challenge that these tests provide, they are also directly dependent on the function of the cardiovascular and respiratory systems. These differences between the measures provide a useful tool for helping to elucidate the underlying pathways of association with factors across life; similarities and differences in findings may provide clues as to the likely body systems and pathways involved.

Performance also depends on participant motivation, as maximal performance is usually required, and this may be affected by mental health and personality characteristics. It also relies on participants having sufficiently high levels of cognitive function to be able to understand the instructions provided and having no medical conditions that prevent participation.

2.3 Patterns of change in physical capability over the life course

It has been proposed that objectively assessed physical capability and many of the physiological systems on which it depends increase with age during growth and development until a peak or plateau at maturity is achieved, followed by decline in later life (Figure 1.1) [6]. The path an individual follows during each of these different stages of the trajectory and the timing of the transitions (e.g. from plateau to decline) will therefore influence the level of physical capability observed at any one point in time.

As grip strength is assessed in a wider range of study populations of different ages, there is currently most evidence on the average patterns of population level change in this measure. Empirical data from studies of children and adolescents confirm that there are steady age-related increases in grip strength during these early phases of life [17–19]. In studies combining longitudinal and cross-sectional data covering most of adulthood there is consistent evidence that after adolescence average population levels of grip strength continue to increase with a peak level reached in both sexes in the late thirties [20–22]. Data from the Baltimore Longitudinal Study of Aging [20,21] suggest that having achieved a peak, average levels of grip strength begin to decline in the forties, whereas data from the Fels Longitudinal Study suggest that grip strength plateaus for longer and the decline begins later, at an average age of 50 years in women and 56 years in men (Figure 2.1) [22]. Despite this slight inconsistency in estimates of the average timing of the onset of decline, in both these studies [20–22] and a number of others [12,23–25], there is evidence that from the fifties and sixties onwards average levels of grip strength are declining in both sexes. At all ages, average grip strength is found to be higher in males than females and there is also evidence of gender differences in the average age at onset and/or rate of decline with women often reported to have an earlier onset but men experiencing greater rates of decline [21–23,26,27]. When the gender difference in grip strength by age was examined in cross-sectional analyses of the HALCyon cohorts it was found that with increasing age the gender difference in grip strength diminished, which could be explained by the greater rates of decline among men [12].

There are much less empirical data on the average patterns of change in other objective measures of physical capability across life, because these measures have primarily been used in studies of older people. However, in analyses of the HALCyon cohorts and other studies, based mainly on cross-sectional data, older age is associated with slower walking and chair rise speeds and poorer standing balance performance and, at all ages women are usually reported to have lower levels than men [12,28–33].

Differences in physical capability by age observed using cross-sectional data may not be solely the result of longitudinal age-related changes. Secular increases in peak grip strength, not fully explained by the secular increases in body size, have recently been reported [22] and demonstrate

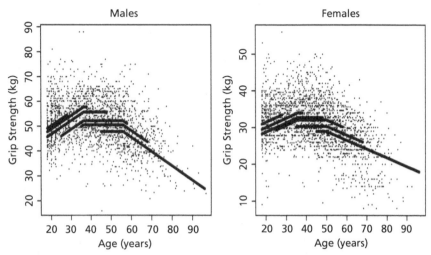

Figure 2.1 Grip strength age trajectories by sex in the Fels Longitudinal Study [22]. These plots assume BMI at age 45 is 25 kg/m², all continuous covariates at their sex-specific means, and all categorical covariates at their reference levels. The black lines represent estimated trajectories by birth cohort plotted over the range of ages observed for each cohort. From left to right, the lines are therefore in the birth cohort order 1980–1989 to 1905–1939.

the importance of considering sources of variation in physical capability by birth cohort and period.

A number of factors are likely to contribute to the age-related declines in physical capability observed across studies including: 'normal' ageing processes such as reductions in muscle mass and quality and other detrimental changes to the musculoskeletal system [34], and to neurological [16], hormonal, and cardiovascular function; detrimental changes in weight and health behaviours; and the increasing risk of developing chronic conditions.

As more longitudinal studies covering a wider range of different ages and drawn from a wider range of countries begin to include and repeat objective measures of physical capability it will be possible to characterize better, at the population level, life course trajectories of physical capability and also birth cohort, period, and country effects. It will also be possible to study different patterns of within-individual change. Even if mean levels of a measure are declining with age within a population, not all individuals will necessarily be experiencing a decline. The characteristics of those people who are maintaining or even improving their physical capability with increasing age need investigating.

2.4 **Factors across life associated with physical capability in adulthood**

Heritability studies of physical capability, which have usually been conducted in populations of older twins, suggest that genetic factors account for only an estimated 30 to 65% of the variation in grip strength [35,36], with similar or slightly lower estimates reported for other physical capability measures (Chapter 14) [37,38]. Therefore, as for most other complex traits, genetic factors alone cannot explain all of the population level variation in physical capability observed, confirming the important role of environmental factors across life at the social, individual, and cellular level.

We cannot comprehensively assess the evidence on all factors across life that may be associated with physical capability. We have chosen to focus on a set of potentially modifiable factors to which a life course perspective has most often been applied. These are lifetime socioeconomic position (SEP), lifestyle factors, and body size. Gender and age differences in associations have been considered but are only reported where they have been observed and formally tested.

2.4.1 Lifetime socioeconomic position

Studies have consistently found striking social inequalities in disability and functional limitations. However, less work has been done in relation to objective measures of physical capability. Most existing studies that have tested associations between socioeconomic position and physical capability have used education, occupational level, income, and wealth as markers of adult SEP [39–48]. Many of these report socioeconomic gradients in physical capability in later life, with people of lower SEP generally found to have lower levels of capability than people of higher SEP. However, results are not always consistent, for example, not all indicators of SEP tested are always associated with the outcomes studied [47,48] and some studies have found associations between SEP and physical capability at baseline but no evidence of associations with subsequent change in capability [42,45], whereas other studies have found an influence of SEP on decline [39], although this is not always in the expected direction [41]. In addition, studies of associations between SEP and grip strength are less consistent [40,42,44,47,49,50] suggesting that the influence of SEP on grip strength may be more specific to certain contexts, and more likely to vary by age than associations of SEP with other physical capability measures.

In a systematic review and meta-analyses of the associations between childhood SEP and objectively assessed physical capability in adulthood [51] only six papers (based on findings from four studies) which had previously been published (up to May 2010) were identified. However, through inclusion of data from two additional sources: (1) all the HALCyon cohorts with relevant data and; (2) contact with investigators from all other potential eligible studies worldwide, it was possible to include 19 studies in meta-analyses (grip strength, 12 studies, N = 1,061,855; walking speed, 13 studies, N = 20,770; chair rise time, 7 studies, N = 17,215; and standing balance, 11 studies, N = 22,156). Lower childhood SEP was found, in age and sex-adjusted models, to be associated with poorer physical capability in adulthood (Figure 2.2). After adjustment for indicators of adult SEP and body size, modest associations of childhood SEP with walking speed and chair rise time were maintained. While 11 of the 19 included studies were British, studies from other countries (USA, South Korea, Switzerland, Denmark, Sweden, Puerto Rico, Barbados, Cuba, Mexico, Chile, and Brazil) were also included. There were also differences in the methods of ascertaining information on childhood circumstances (i.e. in the indicator used and whether they were collected prospectively or retrospectively), and in the protocols used to assess physical capability. It is therefore not surprising that considerable heterogeneity between studies was identified. However it may also be that the relative impact of childhood SEP is contextual and varies by place and time.

Complementary to these meta-analyses are a series of in-depth analyses that have been undertaken in the NSHD [50,52–57]. At 53 years, there was evidence of associations between lower levels of indicators of SEP in both childhood and adulthood and poorer performance in chair rise and standing balance tests, but no evidence of associations with grip strength. When performance on the three tests were combined in a total score, higher maternal education was found to be

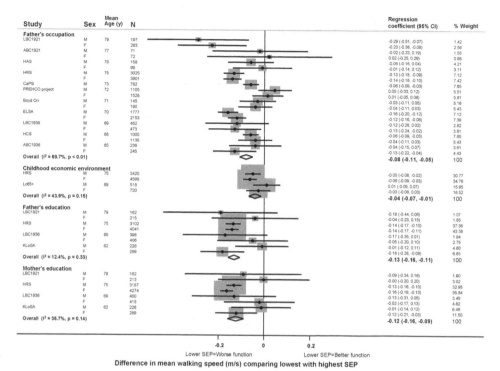

Figure 2.2 Results from meta-analyses of age-adjusted differences in mean walking speed (m/s) comparing lowest with highest childhood socioeconomic position [51].

associated with high levels of physical capability (i.e. total score in the top 10% of the distribution) whereas lower paternal occupational class was associated with low levels (i.e. total score in the bottom 10% of the distribution) [54]. Further analyses showed that maternal education was most strongly associated with standing balance performance whereas father's occupation was most strongly associated with chair rise times [50]. Associations of area-level socioeconomic characteristics across life with physical capability have also been explored in the NSHD [57] and further details of this work are described in Chapter 18.

Work on the NSHD and other studies [49] suggest that there are a range of different underlying pathways operating across life. Socioeconomic effects could act through their associations with factors including childhood infections, patterns of growth, early life nutrition, exposure to environmental hazards, cognition, health behaviours, obesity, and the development of chronic conditions. When factors representing pathways linked to childhood growth and neurodevelopment and adult SEP and lifestyle factors were taken into account, the associations found with balance and chair rise times in NSHD were only partially attenuated [50]. In none of these studies did adult SEP fully account for the effects of childhood SEP, indicating that continuity of socioeconomic circumstances is not the sole explanation. Instead results suggest that the effects of SEP may accumulate across life with poorer circumstances at any point in life likely to be detrimental for subsequent physical capability. Birnie et al. [58] tested this and found that an accumulation

ıost appropriately described most associations between SEP across life and physical capa-
ıserved in the Boyd Orr Cohort and Caerphilly Prospective studies.

ıı ᴜly one study of which we are aware, the Lothian Birth Cohort 1921, have indicators of SEP
in childhood been examined in relation to changes in physical capability, with the finding that
lower paternal education was associated with greater declines in grip strength in older age [59]. In
recent analyses in which associations of SEP in childhood and adulthood with physical capability
at 60–64 years in the NSHD were investigated, strikingly similar patterns of association between
father's occupational class and all four measures of physical capability assessed at this age were
found [56]. This included grip strength which was not associated with childhood SEP at 53 years,
suggesting that the effects of childhood SEP may change with age and be related to the rate of
functional decline.

2.4.2 Lifetime lifestyle

Understanding the lifetime patterns of association between lifestyle factors and physical capability
is important because they are potentially modifiable at a number of life stages. In addition, they
may explain lifetime socioeconomic gradients in physical capability. We begin with physical activity, where there has been most research in relation to physical capability. We then briefly discuss
smoking because even when assessed in later life it is a behaviour that is normally initiated in early
adulthood and so is likely to act through cumulative influences across adulthood. Diet, a third
modifiable lifestyle factor, is discussed in Chapter 16.

2.4.2.1 Physical activity

A comprehensive review of all published literature undertaken by the Physical Activity Guidelines
Advisory Committee in the US in 2008 summarized the evidence relating to the benefits of physical activity for health, including physical capability and the systems (including the musculoskeletal and cardiovascular systems) underlying this [60]. This found strong evidence that specific
exercise regimes are beneficial for muscle strength and other related characteristics of muscle at
all stages of life, with intervention studies that included children, adolescents or adults all demonstrating short-term beneficial effects of physical activity programmes, which usually included
a resistance training component, on muscle strength [60]. The benefits of physical activity for
other measures of physical capability across life have not been so clearly demonstrated. However,
evidence suggests that resistance and endurance exercises are beneficial from mid-adulthood
onwards [60,61].

In the US, this evidence has led to the initiation of one of the largest ever randomized controlled trials of physical activity and its impact on time to onset of major mobility disability (i.e.
inability to complete a 400 metre walk test within 15 minutes) and secondary outcomes including
physical capability. The Lifestyle Interventions and Independence for Elders (LIFE) study aims
to recruit 1600 sedentary adults at high risk of mobility disability aged 70–89. Participants are
being randomized to receive either a physical activity intervention or age-specific health information with differences in outcomes between the two arms of the trial assessed at baseline and
at regular follow-ups over an average of 2.7 years [62]. The pilot study (LIFE-P) has found that
administration of the physical activity intervention for 12 months led to improved physical performance (assessed using the SPPB and walking speed) in the intervention group after an average
of 1.2 years of follow-up [61].

Results from intervention studies suggest that there are beneficial effects of specific types of
short term physical activity programme on physical capability at any age, with results from the

LIFE-P study and other trials of older people [60,61] suggesting that it may never be too late in life to intervene and observe benefits. However, it is unclear whether these short-term activity programmes have long lasting effects on physical capability. It is also not clear from this evidence whether there are cumulative benefits of physical activity across life and whether the types and intensity of activity that people generally engage in as part of their everyday lives are sufficient for the benefits demonstrated in trials to be observed in the general population. Most observational studies have assessed physical activity at only one time point, generally finding that those who are physically active have higher levels of physical capability or experience slower declines in capability than those who are less active [40,63–67]. However, in older age these associations may be explained by reverse causality or residual confounding by health status. Such limitations are partially overcome in the few studies that have assessed the association of physical activity at more than one time point or at a time point earlier in adulthood than assessment of physical capability [68–71]. In a study of 229 older American women whose physical activity was assessed three times over a 14 year period, those women who were always active had faster walking speed and better total physical performance scores at follow-up than those who were consistently inactive, suggesting cumulative benefits of activity [68]. Results from the InChianti study in which the associations between retrospective self-reports of activity during three periods of adulthood (20–40 years; 40–60 years; in the past year) and the SPPB assessed at an average age of 74.8 years were examined suggested that being active earlier in adulthood was associated with better physical performance in later life [69]. In the NSHD, participation in leisure time physical activity prospectively assessed at three ages across adulthood was examined in relation to measures of physical capability at age 53. Cumulative benefits of activity across adulthood for chair rising and standing balance performance were observed even after adjustment for potential confounders with evidence that associations with physical activity earlier in adulthood were not solely explained by the tracking of physical activity across adulthood. However, leisure time physical activity was not associated with grip strength in women and in men, only contemporaneous physical activity levels were associated with strength [70]. This suggested that NSHD participants, especially the women, may not be engaging sufficiently often during their leisure time in the most appropriate type, intensity or frequency of activity across adulthood to beneficially impact on their upper body strength.

The changing pattern of physical activity with age is not well characterized or understood (Chapter 17) [72]. Using existing evidence it is therefore difficult to establish what impact these changes have on functional decline and the bi-directional nature of these relationships. It is also not clear whether the levels and types of activity required for benefits on physical capability are constant across life or change with age, making it difficult to establish specific recommendations for physical activity at different life stages. Most existing observational studies are limited by self-report of physical activity, which may be susceptible to reporting biases and usually results in a focus on specific forms of volitional physical activity undertaken in leisure time or during the working day. However, as instruments which objectively assess physical activity levels and total activity energy expenditure become more widely available and are used in a growing number of studies (Chapter 17), it will be possible to examine patterns of association using a wider range of parameters of physical activity, including non-volitional as well as volitional activity. This is important given a greater proportion of energy is expended in older age on non-volitional activity because of the increased amount of sedentary time and the decreased amount of volitional activity undertaken [73,74]. It will also be possible to examine whether intensities of activity within specific ranges, not accurately captured by self-report, are associated with physical capability and to establish whether for older people, higher levels of light activity in addition to moderate to vigorous activity are also beneficial for physical capability. It will also be useful to establish whether sedentary behaviour has an association with physical capability independent of physical activity levels across life similar to that observed for other health outcomes [75].

In addition to its direct beneficial effects on fitness and also cardiovascular, respiratory, musculoskeletal, and neurological structure and function, physical activity may also influence physical capability through its influence on other pathways. Physical activity is one of the key determinants of energy expenditure and therefore an important factor influencing energy balance. As energy balance influences body weight, physical activity may thus act on this pathway to influence subsequent capability. Other pathways related to energy require further research. For example, changes with age in the energy requirements of specific tasks and in the amount of energy available to perform these tasks may result in changes in physical capability with age; tasks which assess physical capability may be performed less well or more slowly as an adaptive method of conserving energy at older ages [76].

2.4.2.2 Smoking

Studies of the association between cigarette smoking and physical capability show consistent negative associations [77–81], most likely operating through the adverse cumulative effects of smoking across adulthood on respiratory function and other aspects of health. Evidence from longitudinal analyses in the NSHD supports a cumulative effect, with greater numbers of pack-years of smoking associated with poorer chair rising and standing balance performance at 53 years, even after adjustment for socioeconomic factors, lung function, and health status [79]. Smoking was not associated with grip strength in this cohort at midlife [79], but in other older study populations it was [77,78], suggesting that the association may emerge later in life. Lifetime patterns of smoking as well as current smoking behaviour were also found to be associated with physical capability in a large population of older American women [77]. Studies investigating smoking in relation to rate of decline have been inconsistent. Findings from the Health, Aging, and Body Composition (Health ABC) study demonstrated a negative effect of smoking on baseline levels of physical capability but not on subsequent decline over 7 years of follow-up, suggesting that smoking may be more likely to influence developmental pathways [80]. In contrast, in a study of 963 Finnish study participants, persistent smoking was associated with muscle strength decline over 22 years of follow-up [81].

2.4.3 Lifetime body size

In recent meta-analyses of cross-sectional results from eight HALCyon cohorts a negative impact of high body mass index (BMI) on walking speed, standing balance performance, and chair rise times in later life was found; these effects were stronger in women than men [82]. Higher BMI was associated with stronger grip in men only, and in both sexes, when BMI and grip strength were considered together it was found that those with weak strength and high BMI had the worst performance, and these effects were additive [82]. Work on body size and physical capability in later life undertaken across the HALCyon cohorts [82] and in other individual studies [83–85] has been extended in other studies to include an investigation of the influences of BMI across adulthood. In the Health ABC study, those participants who were overweight or obese from their twenties onwards, assessed using recalled data on heights and weights, had the poorest physical capability in later life [86]. Similarly, in the Health 2000 Survey in Finland which includes adults aged 55 and above with recalled data on weight in earlier adulthood, greater length of time exposed to obesity was associated with weaker grip strength [87]. However, this latter result is in contrast to some results, including those from HALCyon, reflecting the greater inconsistency of results in relation to weight across adulthood and grip strength than other physical capability measures. A limitation of these studies of weight history is their reliance on self-reported recalled data from earlier adulthood; further work is required to examine links between prospectively measured BMI/weight trajectories across adulthood and physical capability and to explore how these associations may change with age and differ by region and birth cohort, especially in light of differences between birth cohorts in the age at exposure to the obesity epidemic. Work in this area is also likely to be enhanced by the collection in a growing number of studies of more detailed measures of body composition by dual energy X-ray absorptiometry (DXA) or other similar methods. This is beginning to allow the links between direct measures of fat and muscle and the impact of interactions between these across adulthood on physical capability to be explored [88,89].

Associations between BMI across adulthood and physical capability could be explained by the adverse cumulative effects of high BMI, as a marker of higher fat mass, on a range of factors including chronic disease risk, fat infiltration of muscle, damage to joints, insulin resistance, and inflammation, which then impact on physical capability, or because of links to energy availability, or for biomechanical reasons.

Evidence also exists of links between growth and body size from the very earliest stages of life and physical capability. Results from a recent systematic review have shown consistent evidence of an association between lower birth weight and weaker grip strength, which is maintained after adjustment for age, gender, and height, in 19 studies published up to October 2011 [90]. These associations were observed in populations with average ages at time of strength assessment ranging from 9.3 to 67.5 years who were drawn from the UK, India, Sweden, Australia, the Philippines, Guatemala, Spain, Finland, Belgium, the Netherlands, and Canada. Fewer studies have examined the associations of birth weight with other measures of physical capability and these generally report small, inconsistent or null effects [55,91]. Similar differences in the patterns of association are also found in the few studies which have investigated the influence of growth in infancy (i.e. an association with grip strength, albeit often weaker than the association with prenatal growth, but little consistent evidence of association with other physical capability measures) [55,91–95].

In the NSHD, prospective measurement of height and weight at multiple time points has facilitated the study of patterns of growth across childhood and adolescence in relation to physical capability. Pre-pubertal growth (in weight or height gain) was positively associated with grip strength, chair rise times, and standing balance performance at 53 years, even after taking account of adult body size, chronic conditions, and lifestyle factors [52,55,92]. From puberty onwards, these positive associations remained for grip strength but weight gain started to adversely affect other physical capability measures, particularly in women, reflecting the initiation of associations which continue to be observed in later life. These patterns of growth accounted for the observed associations between age at puberty and midlife strength [92].

The associations of body size and growth in earlier life, from the prenatal period through to puberty, with physical capability in later life are likely to operate on different pathways to those that underlie associations found with BMI across adulthood. The greater consistency of associations of birth weight and infant growth with grip strength than other physical capability measures suggests that these associations are likely to be explained by influences of growth *in utero* and early postnatal life on the development of key characteristics of muscle that impact most directly on strength (including number and size of muscle cells and muscle fibre composition) [96,97], with genetic factors also implicated [97]. The positive associations between pre-pubertal growth and physical capability could reflect accrual of muscle mass or neurodevelopmental processes, with some evidence in support of the latter provided by findings that infant motor development and childhood cognitive ability are also associated with physical capability in adulthood [55,92,93,98].

2.5 **Future research directions and conclusions**

In this chapter we have presented evidence that factors across life influence physical capability levels later in life and discussed many potential pathways which are likely to explain these associations. As most studies identified have assessed physical capability only in later life, even where factors across life have been assessed in relation to these, it is often difficult to identify when in life these associations emerged, which stage/s of the life course trajectory they are influencing and hence to what extent they change with age. Further work in this area will be aided by the assessment of physical capability in populations at a wider range of different ages which will allow differences in association by age and birth cohort to be formally tested. However, if used in younger study populations it is necessary to bear in mind that some tests of physical capability, specifically those developed for use in older populations, may need to be adapted to provide meaningful variation.

Studies that have taken a life course approach to the study of physical capability tend to have examined factors associated with population level variation in physical capability at one particular point in time. This is because studies with data on longitudinal change in physical capability in later life are rarely the same studies that have data on potential explanatory factors from earlier in life. It is therefore going to be necessary to build on these two bodies of literature (one on life course factors associated with physical capability and the other on changes in physical capability in later life) to establish whether factors across life do influence timing of onset and rate of decline in physical capability.

In our review of the literature we considered each set of factors separately, as do many studies in this area. However, many health behaviours, other lifestyle factors (such as social networks) and body size tend to cluster and be socially patterned in a similar way and so future research should pay more attention to the joint lifetime effects of different but related factors on physical capability.

In this chapter we have tried to draw on all the relevant published literature. Reflecting the fact that there are a number of well-established longitudinal studies in the UK with data available from different stages of life to test life course hypotheses on ageing, much of the work we have identified is based on findings from this country. However, from a national and international policy perspective it is going to be important to perform cross-national comparisons to identify which life course associations are universal and which are contextual. The inclusion in meta-analyses of the associations between childhood SEP and physical capability of studies from a wide range of countries (Section 2.4.1), demonstrates the growing number of studies from different countries, not only of high income but also of middle and low income, with data from earlier in life that are also assessing physical capability later in life. This will make it possible to perform more cross-national comparisons in the future, which should prove to be illuminating.

Existing evidence from observational studies demonstrates that factors from early life onwards are associated with physical capability in later life and that the influence of many of these factors is cumulative. A priority of future work is to elucidate the specific underlying explanations of these associations, with investigations of potential mediating factors so far undertaken unable to fully explain associations observed, for example, between SEP and physical capability [43,46,50,99]. Despite this, existing work clearly demonstrates that factors from early life onwards play key roles in influencing physical capability in later life. This suggests that early intervention may be required to ensure that physical capability is maintained in later life and that people age healthily. While it is hoped that intervention studies such as LIFE will provide robust evidence on the benefits of intervention in later life in relation to physical capability we may also need to design novel intervention studies which allow us to test the life course effects of intervening earlier in life within a realistic timeframe.

References

1 **Cooper R, et al.** Objectively measured physical capability levels and mortality: systematic review and meta-analysis. *BMJ* 2010;**341**:c4467.

2 **Cooper R, et al.** Objective measures of physical capability and subsequent health: a systematic review. *Age Ageing* 2011;**40**:14–23.

3 **den Ouden MEM, et al.** Physical performance characteristics related to disability in older persons: a systematic review. *Maturitas* 2011;**69**:208–19.

4 **Depp CA, Jeste DV.** Definitions and predictors of successful aging: a comprehensive review of larger quantitative studies. *Am J Geriatr Psychiatry* 2006;**14**:6–20.

5 **Parsons S, et al.** Physical capability and the advantages and disadvantages of ageing: perceptions of older age by men and women in two British cohorts. *Ageing Soc.* In press. <http://dx.doi.org/10.1017/S0144686X12001067>

6 **Kuh D.** A life course approach to healthy aging, frailty, and capability. *J Gerontol A Biol Sci Med Sci* 2007;**62**:717–21.

7 **Guralnik JM, et al.** Physical performance measures in aging research. *J Gerontol Med Sci* 1989;**44**: M141–6.

8 **Guralnik JM, Ferrucci L.** Assessing the building blocks of function utilizing measures of functional limitation. *Am J Prev Med* 2003;**25**:112–21.

9 **Sternberg SA, et al.** The identification of frailty: a systematic literature review. *J Am Geriatr Soc* 2011;**59**: 2129–38.

10 **Roberts HC, et al.** A review of the measurement of grip strength in clinical and epidemiological studies: towards a standardised approach. *Age Ageing* 2011;**40**:423–9.

11 **Gill TM.** Assessment of function and disability in longitudinal studies. *J Am Geriatr Soc* 2010;**58**:S308–12.

12 **Cooper R, et al.** Age and gender differences in physical capability levels from mid-life onwards: the harmonisation and meta-analysis of data from eight UK cohort studies. *PLoS One* 2011;**6**:e27899.

13 **Freiberger E, et al.** Performance-based physical function in older community-dwelling persons: a systematic review of instruments. *Age Ageing* 2012;**41**:712–21.

14 **Guralnik JM, et al.** A short physical performance battery assessing lower extremity function: association with self-reported disability and prediction of mortality and nursing home admission. *J Gerontol* 1994;**49**:M85–94.

15 **Bohannon RW.** Is it legitimate to characterize muscle strength using a limited number of measures? *J Strength Cond Res* 2008;**22**:166–73.

16 **Manini TM, Clark BC.** Dynapenia and aging: an update. *J Gerontol A Biol Sci Med Sci* 2012;**67**:28–40.

17 **Molenaar HM, et al.** Growth diagrams for grip strength in children. *Clin Orthop Relat Res* 2010;**468**: 217–23.

18 **Silverman IW.** The secular trend for grip strength in Canada and the United States. *J Sports Sci* 2011;**29**: 599–606.

19 **Hager-Ross C, Rosblad B.** Norms for grip strength in children aged 4–16 years. *Acta Paediatr* 2002;**91**: 617–25.

20 **Kallman DA, et al.** The role of muscle loss in the age-related decline of grip strength—cross-sectional and longitudinal perspectives. *J Gerontol* 1990;**45**:M82–8.

21 **Metter EJ, et al.** Age-associated loss of power and strength in the upper extremities in women and men. *J Gerontol A Biol Sci Med Sci* 1997;**52**:B267–76.

22 **Nahhas RW, et al.** Bayesian longitudinal plateau model of adult grip strength. *Am J Hum Biol* 2010;**22**: 648–56.

23 **Frederiksen H, et al.** Age trajectories of grip strength: cross-sectional and longitudinal data among 8,342 Danes aged 46 to 102. *Ann Epidemiol* 2006;**16**:554–62.

24 **Rantanen T, et al.** Grip strength changes over 27 yr in Japanese-American men. *J Appl Physiol* 1998;**85**: 2047–53.

25 **Andersen-Ranberg K, et al.** Cross-national differences in grip strength among 50 + year-old Europeans: results from the SHARE study. *Eur J Ageing* 2009;**6**:227–36.

26 **Oksuzyan A, et al.** Cross-national comparison of sex differences in health and mortality in Denmark, Japan and the US. *Eur J Epidemiol* 2010;**25**:471–80.

27 **Goodpaster BH, et al.** The loss of skeletal muscle strength, mass, and quality in older adults: the health, aging and body composition study. *J Gerontol A Biol Sci Med Sci* 2006;**61**:1059–64.

28 **Samson MM, et al.** Relationships between physical performance measures, age, height and body weight in healthy adults. *Age Ageing* 2000;**29**:235–42.

29 **Bohannon RW.** Single limb stance times—a descriptive meta-analysis of data from individuals at least 60 years of age. *Top Geriatr Rehab* 2006;**22**:70–7.

30 **Bohannon RW.** Reference values for the timed up and go test: a descriptive meta-analysis. *J Geriatr Phys Ther* 2006;**29**:64–8.

31 **Bohannon RW.** Reference values for the five-repetition sit-to-stand test: a descriptive meta-analysis of data from elders. *Percept Mot Skills* 2006;**103**:215–22.

32 **Steffen TM, et al.** Age- and gender-related test performance in community-dwelling elderly people: Six-Minute Walk Test, Berg Balance Scale, Timed Up & Go Test, and gait speeds. *Phys Ther* 2002;**82**: 128–37.

33 **Butler AA, et al.** Age and gender differences in seven tests of functional mobility. *J Neuroeng Rehabil* 2009;**6**:31.

34 **Faulkner JA, et al.** Age-related changes in the structure and function of skeletal muscles. *Clin Exp Pharmacol Physiol* 2007;**34**:1091–6.

35 **Arden NK, Spector TD.** Genetic influences on muscle strength, lean body mass, and bone mineral density: a twin study. *J Bone Miner Res* 1997;**12**:2076–81.

36 **Reed T, et al.** Genetic influences and grip strength norms in the NHLBI twin study males aged 59–69. *Ann Hum Biol* 1991;**18**:425–32.

37 **Carmelli D, et al.** The contribution of genetic influences to measures of lower-extremity function in older male twins. *J Gerontol A Biol Sci Med Sci* 2000;**55**:B49–53.

38 **Pajala S, et al.** Contribution of genetic and environmental factors to individual differences in maximal walking speed with and without second task in older women. *J Gerontol A Biol Sci Med Sci* 2005;**60**: 1299–1303.

39 **Deeg DJH, et al.** Predictors of 10-year change in physical, cognitive and social function in Japanese elderly. *Arch Gerontol Geriatr* 1992;**15**:163–79.

40 **Rantanen T, et al.** Muscle strength according to level of physical exercise and educational-background in middle-aged women in Finland. *Eur J Appl Physiol Occup Physiol* 1992;**65**:507–12.

41 **Seeman TE, et al.** Predicting changes in physical performance in a high-functioning elderly cohort: MacArthur studies of successful aging. *J Gerontol* 1994;**49**:M97–108.

42 **Rautio N, et al.** Socio-economic position and its relationship to physical capacity among elderly people living in Jyvaskyla, Finland: five- and ten-year follow-up studies. *Soc Sci Med* 2005;**60**:2405–16.

43 **Coppin AK, et al.** Low socioeconomic status and disability in old age: evidence from the InChianti study for the mediating role of physiological impairments. *J Gerontol A Biol Sci Med Sci* 2006;**61**:86–91.

44 **Russo A, et al.** Lifetime occupation and physical function: a prospective cohort study on persons aged 80 years and older living in a community. *Occup Environ Med* 2006;**63**:438–42.

45 **Thorpe RJ, et al.** Relationship of race and poverty to lower extremity function and decline: findings from the women's health and aging study. *Soc Sci Med* 2008;**66**:811–21.

46 **Brunner E, et al.** Social inequality in walking speed in early old age in the Whitehall II study. *J Gerontol A Biol Sci Med Sci* 2009;**64**:1082–9.

47 **Hairi FM, et al.** Does socio-economic status predict grip strength in older Europeans? Results from the SHARE study in non-institutionalised men and women aged 50+. *J Epidemiol Community Health* 2010;**64**:829–37.

48 **Thorpe RJ, et al.** Race, socioeconomic resources, and late-life mobility and decline: findings from the Health, Aging, and Body Composition study. *J Gerontol A Biol Sci Med Sci* 2011;**66**:1114–23.

49 **Syddall H, et al.** Social inequalities in grip strength, physical function, and falls among community dwelling older men and women: findings from the Hertfordshire Cohort Study. *J Aging Health* 2009;**21**: 913–39.

50 **Strand BH, et al.** Lifelong socioeconomic position and physical performance in midlife: results from the British 1946 birth cohort. *Eur J Epidemiol* 2011;**26**:475–83.

51 **Birnie K, et al.** Childhood socioeconomic position and objectively measured physical capability levels in adulthood: a systematic review and meta-analysis. *PLoS One* 2011;**6**:e15564.

52 **Kuh D, et al.** Birth weight, childhood size, and muscle strength in adult life: evidence from a birth cohort study. *Am J Epidemiol* 2002;**156**:627–33.

53 **Kuh D, et al.** Grip strength, postural control, and functional leg power in a representative cohort of British men and women: associations with physical activity, health status, and socioeconomic conditions. *J Gerontol Med Sci* 2005;**60A**:224–31.

54 **Guralnik JM, et al.** Childhood socioeconomic status predicts physical functioning a half century later. *J Gerontol Med Sci* 2006;**61**:694–701.

55 **Kuh D, et al.** Developmental origins of midlife physical performance: evidence from a British birth cohort. *Am J Epidemiol* 2006;**164**:110–21.

56 **Hurst L, et al.** Lifetime socioeconomic inequalities in physical and cognitive aging. *Am J Public Health.* 2013;**103**:1641–8.

57 **Murray ET, et al.** Area deprivation across the life course and physical capability in midlife: findings from the 1946 British birth cohort. *Am J Epidemiol.* 2013;**178**:441–50.

58 **Birnie K, et al.** Socio-economic disadvantage from childhood to adulthood and locomotor function in old age: a lifecourse analysis of the Boyd Orr and Caerphilly prospective studies. *J Epidemiol Community Health* 2011;**65**:1014–23.

59 **Starr JM, Deary IJ.** Socio-economic position predicts grip strength and its decline between 79 and 87 years: the Lothian Birth Cohort 1921. *Age Ageing* 2011;**40**:749–52.

60 **Physical Activity Guidelines Advisory Committee.** Physical activity guidelines advisory committee report. Washington, DC: US Department of Health and Human Services; 2008

61 **Pahor M, et al.** Effects of a physical activity intervention on measures of physical performance: results of the Lifestyle Interventions and Independence for Elders Pilot (LIFE-P) study. *J Gerontol A Biol Sci Med Sci* 2006;**61**:1157–65.

62 **Fielding RA, et al.** The Lifestyle Interventions and Independence for Elders Study: design and methods. *J Gerontol A Biol Sci Med Sci* 2011;**66**:1226–37.

63 **Visser M, et al.** Physical activity as a determinant of change in mobility performance: the Longitudinal Aging Study Amsterdam. *J Am Geriatr Soc* 2002;**50**:1774–81.

64 **Brach JS, et al.** The association between physical function and lifestyle activity and exercise in the health, aging and body composition study. *J Am Geriatr Soc* 2004;**52**:502–9.

65 **Lang IA, et al.** Physical activity in middle-aged adults reduces risks of functional impairment independent of its effect on weight. *J Am Geriatr Soc* 2007;**55**:1836–41.

66 **Rantanen T, et al.** Disability, physical activity, and muscle strength in older women: the Women's Health and Aging Study. *Arch Phys Med Rehabil* 1999;**80**:130–5.

67 **Martin HJ, et al.** Relationship between customary physical activity, muscle strength and physical performance in older men and women: findings from the Hertfordshire Cohort Study. *Age Ageing* 2008;**37**:589–93.

68 Brach JS, et al. Physical activity and functional status in community-dwelling older women—a 14-year prospective study. *Arch Intern Med* 2003;**163**:2565–71.

69 Patel KV, et al. Midlife physical activity and mobility in older age—the InCHIANTI Study. *Am J Prev Med* 2006;**31**:217–24.

70 Cooper R, et al. Physical activity across adulthood and physical performance in midlife: findings from a British Birth Cohort. *Am J Prev Med* 2011;**41**:376–84.

71 Tikkanen P, et al. Physical activity at age of 20–64 years and mobility and muscle strength in old age: a community-based study. *J Gerontol A Biol Sci Med Sci* 2012;**67**:905–10.

72 Koeneman MA, et al. Determinants of physical activity and exercise in healthy older adults: a systematic review. *Int J Behav Nutr Phys Act* 2011;**8**:142.

73 Hughes JP, et al. Leisure-time physical activity among US adults 60 or more years of age: results from NHANES 1999–2004. *J Phys Act Health* 2008;**5**:347–58.

74 Manini TM, et al. Activity energy expenditure and mobility limitation in older adults: differential associations by sex. *Am J Epidemiol* 2009;**169**:1507–16.

75 Ford ES, Caspersen CJ. Sedentary behaviour and cardiovascular disease: a review of prospective studies. *Int J Epidemiol* 2012;**41**:1338–53.

76 Schrack JA, et al. The energetic pathway to mobility loss: an emerging new framework for longitudinal studies on aging. *J Am Geriatr Soc* 2010;**58**:S329–36.

77 Nelson HD, et al. Smoking, alcohol, and neuromuscular and physical function of older women. *JAMA* 1994;**272**:1825–31.

78 Rapuri PB, et al. Smoking is a risk factor for decreased physical performance in elderly women. *J Gerontol A Biol Sci Med Sci* 2007;**62**:93–100.

79 Strand BH, et al. Smoking history and physical performance in midlife: results from the British 1946 birth cohort. *J Gerontol Med Sci* 2011;**66A**:142–9.

80 van den Borst B, et al. Is age-related decline in lean mass and physical function accelerated by obstructive lung disease or smoking?*Thorax* 2011;**66**:961–9.

81 Stenholm S, et al. Long-term determinants of muscle strength decline: prospective evidence from the 22-Year Mini-Finland Follow-Up Survey. *J Am Geriatr Soc* 2012;**60**:77–85.

82 Hardy R, et al. Body mass index, muscle strength and physical performance in older adults from eight cohort studies: the HALCyon programme. *PLoS One* 2013;**8**:e56483.

83 Ferrucci L, et al. Characteristics of nondisabled older persons who perform poorly in objective tests of lower extremity function. *J Am Geriatr Soc* 2000;**48**:1102–10.

84 Woo J, et al. BMI, body composition, and physical functioning in older adults. *Obesity (Silver Spring)* 2007;**15**:1886–94.

85 Lang IA, et al. Obesity, physical function, and mortality in older adults. *J Am Geriatr Soc* 2008;**56**:1474–8.

86 Houston DK, et al. The association between weight history and physical performance in the Health, Aging and Body Composition study. *Int J Obes (Lond)* 2007;**31**:1680–7.

87 Stenholm S, et al. Association between obesity history and hand grip strength in older adults—exploring the roles of inflammation and insulin resistance as mediating factors. *J Gerontol A Biol Sci Med Sci* 2011;**66**:341–8.

88 Delmonico MJ, et al. Alternative definitions of sarcopenia, lower extremity performance, and functional impairment with aging in older men and women. *J Am Geriatr Soc* 2007;**55**:769–74.

89 Koster A, et al. Does the amount of fat mass predict age-related loss of lean mass, muscle strength, and muscle quality in older adults? *J Gerontol A Biol Sci Med Sci* 2011;**66**:888–95.

90 Dodds R, et al. Birth weight and muscle strength: a systematic review and meta-analysis. *J Nutr Health Aging* 2012;**16**:609–15.

91 Martin HJ, et al. Physical performance and physical activity in older people: are developmental influences important? *Gerontology* 2009;**55**:186–93.

92 **Kuh D, et al.** Developmental origins of midlife grip strength: findings from a birth cohort study. *J Gerontol Med Sci* 2006;**61**:702–6.

93 **Ridgway CL, et al.** Birth size, infant weight gain, and motor development influence adult physical performance. *Med Sci Sports Exerc* 2009;**41**:1212–21.

94 **Aihie Sayer A, et al.** Does sarcopenia originate in early life? Findings from the Hertfordshire cohort study. *J Gerontol A Biol Sci Med Sci* 2004;**59**:930–4.

95 **Kuzawa CW, et al.** Rapid weight gain after birth predicts life history and reproductive strategy in Filipino males. *Proc Natl Acad Sci USA* 2010;**107**:16800–5.

96 **Patel H, et al.** Developmental influences, muscle morphology, and sarcopenia in community-dwelling older men. *J Gerontol A Biol Sci Med Sci* 2012;**67**:82–7.

97 **Ridgway CL, et al.** The contribution of prenatal environment and genetic factors to the association between birth weight and adult grip strength. *PLoS One* 2011;**6**:e17955.

98 **Kuh D, et al.** Lifetime cognitive performance is associated with midlife physical performance in a prospective national birth cohort study. *Psychosom Med* 2009;**71**:38–48.

99 **Koster A, et al.** Is there a biomedical explanation for socioeconomic differences in incident mobility limitation? *J Gerontol A Biol Sci Med Sci* 2005;**60**:1022–7.

Chapter 3

A life course approach to cognitive capability

Marcus Richards and Ian J Deary

3.1 Introduction

Cognitive function is shaped by factors operating across the whole of life, with implications for the accumulation of cognitive reserve [1], and the development of mastery and wisdom [2]. These factors begin with genes but include the uterine environment and the highly malleable stage of infancy; they include experiences through the school years and during transition into the adult word of work and lifestyle choices; finally, there are factors still evident in later life, when the protective effects of healthy physical ageing on the brain are increasingly important.

Behind these influences, cognitive function itself tracks across life. Cognitive ability in childhood [3] and early adulthood [4] is correlated with cognition in midlife and old age, and childhood and midlife cognition are strongly intercorrelated even when the influence of educational attainment and parental and own socioeconomic position (SEP) are controlled [5]. It is less clear whether level of cognitive ability in childhood influences rate of cognitive decline in later life, or simply the level from which such decline begins [6]. Nevertheless, to the extent that cognition does track, it follows that influences on cognition at any life stage are capable of indirectly influencing cognitive functioning at subsequent stages. This chapter aims to offer the reader a broad overview of these processes with an emphasis on healthy cognitive ageing. We draw on a variety of sources, but will prioritize information gained from studies based on general population samples, preferably with longitudinal data.

3.2 Cognitive function, cognitive capability, and healthy cognitive ageing

Cognitive function encompasses the 'processing of information, applying knowledge, and developing and changing mental representations (or mental maps) based on experience' [7: p. 877]. In children, cognitive function is most commonly measured as general cognitive ability, often divided into two correlated factors: crystallized and fluid ability. The former refers to the acquisition and use of knowledge (as tested by, for example, vocabulary, pronunciation, and general knowledge), whereas the latter is concerned with reasoning and problem-solving in novel situations (for example, completing a logical sequence) [8]. Both sets of skills are also measured in adulthood; typically fluid ability declines with age and morbidity, whereas crystallized ability is well preserved, even in the face of mild dementia (Figure 3.1) [9], and can continue to improve in old age [10]. In the adult years other age-sensitive cognitive tests are also administered, mostly within the domains of memory, executive function, speed of processing, praxis, and visuospatial function. However, cognitive function incorporates more than can be captured by psychometric

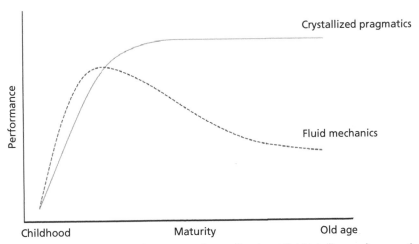

Figure 3.1 The different life course trajectories of crystallized and fluid intelligence ('pragmatics') [9].

Reprinted from *Trends in Cognitive Sciences*, Volume **10**, Issue 3, Craik FIM and Bialystok E, Cognition through the lifespan: mechanisms of change, pp. 131–8, Copyright © 2006, with permission from Elsevier.

test scores alone, and also includes functions referred to as 'everyday cognition', such as planning, communicating, managing day to day demands and circumstances, and the processing of information that has emotional valence [7]. In recognition of this broader context the US National Academies-based Committee on Future Directions for Cognitive Research on Aging adopted the term 'the aging mind', referring to how people adapt to bodily changes, and to changes in society, culture, and technology in order to perform skilled activities of daily living [11: p. 9]. This emphasis on functionality rather than process leads to the notion of cognitive capability, defined by the HALCyon research collaboration as the capacity to undertake the mental tasks of daily living.

The definition of healthy cognitive ageing is slightly more troublesome, because there is no clearly recognized entity that provides a positive mirror image of the clinical categories of mild cognitive impairment, and dementia. This is not to enter the argument about whether the latter classifications are clear cut, or represent specific diseases, or are just arbitrary marks on the population cognitive distribution [12]; only to acknowledge that there are no established equivalent ascertainment criteria for 'healthy cognitive ageing'. The term genius is suggested to apply to those with an IQ of at least 140, but by definition this would only include approximately 0.4% of the population—considerably less than the prevalence of Alzheimer's disease. In reality, longitudinal studies focusing on healthy cognitive ageing have emphasized absence of cognitive impairment or decline [13] rather than try to interpret the significance of the upper extreme of the cognitive distribution. This reflects the widely quoted general definition of healthy ageing by Rowe and Kahn (Chapter 1), who emphasized *absence* of disease, and engagement in life, and the *maintenance* of cognitive and physical function (our emphasis) [14]. A more interesting view, however, is to consider healthy cognitive ageing as a component of self-determined behaviour, with respect to the psychological needs of autonomy, competence, and relatedness, proposed by Deci and Ryan [15]. These represent positive aspects of function and mental state rather than just absence of impairment, aspects to which we will return (Sections 3.3.7–8). Following this, a stronger statement came from the UK Government's Foresight Project on Mental Capital and Wellbeing. Echoing the mental health spectrum of Keyes [16], and perhaps an older definition of healthy ageing as achieving maximum life satisfaction [17], this refers to the need for cognitive resources to be able to 'prosper and flourish' [18: p. 1057]. We argue that a life course approach provides a powerful way to understand how such flourishing develops, and can be maintained during ageing. Towards this understanding we first summarize some of the key positive influences on cognitive development and ageing across the life course.

3.3 Key stages of the life course and healthy cognitive ageing

3.3.1 Genetic and epigenetic influence

As O'Donovan and Owen note, 'with its role in human adaptability and survival, it would be remarkable if traits that result from variation in brain function were not influenced in part by genes' [19: p. 1]. Indeed, the heritability of general cognitive ability is approximately 30% in early childhood, rising to as much as 80% in older adults [20]. This increase may partly result from a gradual matching to environment, i.e. a reciprocal causation between cognitive ability and environment leading to gene-environment correlation [21]; and also from increasing genetic influence on neural processes with age [22]. Later still in life, the operation of neural defence and repair mechanisms, themselves under genetic control, may become important as the brain accumulates insults [20].

In parallel with heritability studies, a large genome-wide association study (GWAS), using novel analytical methods, showed that a substantial proportion of individual differences in general cognitive ability is due to genetic variation [23].

In addition to any effects of the DNA sequence, genetic influence on mental development also occurs through epigenetic alteration of gene expression during interaction with the environment (Chapter 15). In animal studies, offspring of high-nurturing mothers (in terms of licking or grooming) tend to have relatively low levels of anxiety [24]. They also show an attenuated hypothalamic-pituitary-adrenal (HPA) axis response to stress, and higher levels of glucocorticoid receptor gene expression in the hippocampus (with parallel implications for cognition), a difference in methylation that persists across life. This epigenetic alteration almost certainly occurs in humans, and information is accumulating about the way this affects risk of neurocognitive disorders [25].

3.3.2 Fetal growth and the uterine environment

The developmental origins theory of David Barker led to increasing interest in fetal growth as a determinant of mental function. In this context there is a clear consensus that birth weight across the full population range, which reflects rate of fetal growth and duration of pregnancy, is associated with cognitive development in childhood, independently of social origins [26]. This association is biologically plausible, and is almost certainly due to common physiological cause, such as insulin-like growth factors, which influence skeletal growth while also targeting brain regions (including the hippocampus) responsible for learning and memory. However, it is important to place these findings into epidemiological perspective. Effect sizes are modest [26], there is no evidence that they have long-term impact on cognitive ageing [27], and effects may be substantially confounded by maternal cognitive ability [28]. Indeed, many apparent protective effects on fetal growth and pregnancy duration, such as maternal wellbeing, healthy maternal diet, and avoidance of teratogenic agents, are themselves confounded by maternal cognitive ability [29] and genetic common cause; and many of these factors persist into postnatal life, so isolating sensitive periods for these exposures is not always easy [30]. On the other hand, positive associations between fetal growth and cognitive development are shown to be independent of postnatal skeletal growth [31].

3.3.3 **Early childhood**

Although the most rapid neural development occurs during fetal growth, this is still substantial during the first 5 years of postnatal life. Early cognitive development may be an effective marker of 'system integrity', defined as 'a body that is generally "well wired", and that responds more efficiently to environmental challenges or "allostatic load"' [32: p. 675]. Consistent with this, a range of maturational and health-related variables are positively associated with cognitive development, including postnatal somatic growth (independently of birth weight) [31], motor development [33], and exposure to important micronutrients [34]. As with prenatal exposures, however, confounding by maternal cognitive ability, for example in regard to putative effects of long-chain fatty acids in breast milk [35], is a serious analytic consideration.

If the effects of social origin on the developing fetal brain are difficult to disentangle (Section 3.3.2), then evidence for the emergence of social inequalities in cognition in childhood is clearer [2], particularly when focused on the role of poverty, which can also negatively affect cognitive ageing if this becomes prolonged over life [36]. Mechanisms responsible include exposure to chronic stressors, physical ill-health at birth and in childhood, low cognitive stimulation and affection from parents, and poor material environmental conditions [2,37]. The latter includes the neighbourhood, which plays a role in maintaining social inequalities in cognitive function independently of individual and family-level characteristics (Chapter 18). Potential mechanisms include quality of services, control of noxious or hazardous exposures, and more subtle factors such as community responsibility for individuals [38].

We previously mentioned parenting, but it is also important to emphasize the positive role of the caregiver in cognitive development. The security of the mother–infant attachment in early life requires intense reciprocal regulation, and organization [39], manifested, for example, in games such as peek-a-boo and hide-and-seek, which help to provide a 'scaffold' for language structure and function [40]. In the present context it is worth noting that the authoritative parenting style suggested by Baumrind [41] (high expectation of compliance with rules, open dialogue, and a child-centred approach characterized by warmth and involvement) is most associated with the development of competence and adjustment, where autonomy-granting is particularly important [42].

3.3.4 **The development of self-regulation**

Consideration of positive parenting and autonomy-granting raises the important issue of emotional wellbeing (Chapter 4). There is little doubt that cognition and socio-emotional function are intertwined across life, and it has been argued that these gradually fuse to form skills for life [2]. The latter, originally described as 'non-cognitive skills' [43], have gained currency in other disciplines, particularly economics [44], and they are equally familiar today through the concept of self-regulation or self-organization [45]. This has important implications for healthy cognitive ageing through the emergence of mastery and wisdom, expressed in many ways across life, including achievements in education and work, and successful self-management of health. Indeed, one definition of self-regulation–'self-generated thoughts, feelings, and actions that are planned and cyclically adapted to the attainment of personal goals' [46: p. 14] resonates with the cognitive construct of executive function, i.e. specific skills, such as response initiation and inhibition, underlying goal-oriented behaviour. Yet it also involves interpersonal feeling and functions, such as belonging, social engagement, and respect for others, that arise from socio-emotional development and underpin psychological wellbeing [45]. As framed by Schunk and Ertmer, self-regulated learning involves 'setting goals for learning . . . using effective strategies to organise, code and rehearse information to be remembered . . . monitoring performance . . . seeking assistance when needed . . . *and experiencing pride and satisfactions with one's efforts*' (our emphasis) [47: p. 631]. Underlying the importance of parenting in this context, a recent study found that parental warmth was associated with better self-regulation in adulthood [48].

3.3.5 **Education, work, and retirement**

The topic of self-regulated learning leads logically to that of education. Cognition is an important determinant of educational achievement [49], yet education is capable of augmenting cognitive skills net of this [5,50,51], even allowing for genetic common cause [52]. Effects have been observed for adult education as well as formal schooling [53], and can rapidly respond to policy changes, such as raising the minimum school leaving age [54]. Far less clear, however, is the question of whether level of education influences rate of cognitive decline, or merely the level at which such decline begins [55]. Nevertheless, there are plausible reasons for the benefit of education to cognition. Schooling teaches specific knowledge, teaches practical skills for the workplace, refines other cognitive skills, socializes the individual for success, and shapes confidence and motivation [56]. Education also provides a readily identifiable credential that selects the individual into the workforce [57]. Both of these processes may explain why education is also capable of maintaining social inequalities in cognitive capability, which are particularly evident in the context of ethnicity. For example quality of schooling is suggested to be poorer for African American children [58], and mean income returns to a bachelor's degree are nearly 30% lower for African American and Hispanic males than those for Whites [59].

If schooling teaches specific knowledge and skills, and socializes the individual for success, then these processes are likely to continue in the world of work. At the broadest level, a clue that this is the case comes from studying occupational mobility. In the MRC National Survey of Health and Development (NSHD), also known as the British 1946 birth cohort study, those who entered the workforce at a manual occupational level yet gained non-manual status by midlife had higher verbal ability than those who did not achieve such upward mobility, allowing for prior cognition, formal schooling, and any adult education or job training that might have led to this mobility [53]. This is consistent with the seminal studies of Kohn and Schooler, which show that while cognitive ability is a determinant of intellectually demanding work, work complexity is also beneficial to cognitive function [60]. Importantly, this is observed when adolescent cognitive ability is controlled [61]. The effect of work complexity appears to be greater for older compared to younger workers, possibly because of the reduction in routine, and the growing reliance on occupational self-direction with age and experience [62]. In regard to underlying mechanisms, a striking example of how occupational skill can directly alter brain structures supporting cognition comes from the 'taxi driver' study. Qualifying as a licensed London cab driver requires passing a test on the layout of all 25,000 or so streets in the city, which takes an average of 3–4 years to learn. Neuroimaging revealed a shift in the hippocampus from anterior to posterior in drivers compared to controls, which favours visuospatial learning, the extent of which was correlated with time spent in the job [63].

Since work activities help to support cognition, it follows that loss of work through long-term unemployment or retirement may be a risk factor for accelerated cognitive decline, unless compensatory activities are taken up. This is the disuse or *'use it or lose it'* hypothesis [64], although the same effect has also been hypothesized to result from reduced incentives to invest in older workers who are expected to retire at an early age [65]. Research in this area is hampered by lack of longitudinal cognitive data spanning the retirement transition, although results from the Whitehall II study, which has such information, tentatively support the disuse hypothesis in regard to cognitive ageing [66]. Further studies, representing those of lower SEP as well as white collar workers, are urgently required now that extending working age has become a policy issue following the global economic downturn and the ageing of the population.

3.3.6 **Cognitive engagement: use it or lose it?**

The disuse hypothesis plausibly applies to the workplace, but it is more commonly identified with advice to keep mentally active during ageing. In this context it was noted many years ago that, although cell activation in most organs leads to 'wear and tear' (for example from increased free radical formation), activation of nerve cells within the physiological range seems to be neuroprotective [67]. Again there is evidence from Schooler and his colleagues of a recursive process where initially high levels of cognitive functioning lead to high levels of complex leisure time engagement, which in turn raise levels of cognitive functioning, albeit modestly [68]. Since then there have been attempts to estimate retrospectively levels of cognitive engagement across life, which show positive associations with cognitive function in later life [69], independently of education.

This raises the controversial issue of cognitive training. There is little question that performance specific to a cognitive training task will improve with practice; less clear is whether there are 'transfer effects' to more general tests of cognitive function when these are given subsequently to this training. A large online experiment failed to provide such evidence [70], although criticism has arisen from sample selection and the relatively young mean age of participants. Somewhat more encouraging has been a recent trial of training on a 'Space Fortress' game, given to 54 community-dwelling older adults free of cognitive impairment or dementia. This game exercises divided attention, multi-tasking, visual scanning, working memory, long-term memory, and motor control. After a 3 month training phase, offline testing of executive control showed modest improvement in one out of three measures (letter–number sequencing) [71]. As the authors of this study themselves acknowledge, however, more work in this area needs to be conducted before robust conclusions about the efficacy of executive training can be drawn. Neural mechanisms of skill learning are gradually being elucidated, with evidence consistently pointing to the role of the dorsolateral prefrontal cortex and posterior parietal cortex in coordinating retrieval, and use of information from content-specific regions of the brain; and in reorganizing information into structures ('chunking') that can improve memory performance in expert tasks [72].

3.3.7 **Mastery and wisdom**

We began this chapter by hinting that a life course approach to cognition could enhance our understanding of mastery and wisdom, both of which are implicitly regarded as quintessential manifestations of healthy cognitive ageing. In fact the principal authors of these constructs have themselves emphasized life course approaches [73–75]. The construct of mastery refers to the ability to manage life circumstances, and to control those circumstances, that significantly impact the individual. It can develop relatively early in life through achievement, effective management of challenges, and successful coping with stressors, all of which confer a sense of control and self-direction [73,74]. This clearly recapitulates the notion of self-regulated learning discussed in Section 3.3.4, and therefore the interrelationship between cognition and emotional wellbeing established earlier in life. Thus mastery binds cognition and emotion into a tool for developing goals, accepting and organizing the information we need for these goals, establishing and protecting the right setting for their achievement, and experiencing self-esteem when they are achieved [47].

Continuing this theme, a related expression of healthy cognitive ageing may be found in wisdom. This has various definitions, but a common theme is the integration of specific expertise with more subtle skills such as ability to advise and manage others, to see things in context, to tolerate uncertainty (including the limits of our own knowledge), and to engage in spiritual reflection [75–77]. This too is a *'fine tuned coordination of cognition, motivation, and emotion'* [75: p. 77]; it too has a life course perspective, involving the integration of past, present, and future in life planning, management, and review, that appears to be shaped by experience. For example, in a test requiring the solution to two life-planning tasks (see Supplementary web material Box 3.1 at www.halcyon.ac.uk) given to a highly educated sample, professional training and practice accounted for a significantly larger proportion of test variance than personality variables and general cognitive ability [78].

We should note some awkward caveats to this apparently rather neat narrative. Mastery and wisdom can both be impaired by difficult conditions that are resistant to personal control, for example job loss through bankruptcy of an employer, or demands from a family member with severe illness [74]. Importantly, although mastery and wisdom appear to have universal underlying meaning, the criteria by which they are valued can vary widely. For example, the skills that are necessary for a person on a low income to survive are very different to those deployed by individuals with a high income to signal status [79]. We cannot even take for granted that mastery and wisdom are *sine qua non* of ageing. As Sternberg and Lubart tartly observe, 'People become wiser at a given age with respect to the problems that confront them at that point in their lives' [80: p. 504].

3.3.8 Cognitive ageing and health literacy

We might also add that the concepts of mastery and wisdom are at risk of over-abstraction, but it is not hard to see how they lead to practical life skills. Imperative among these for healthy ageing is good 'health literacy', i.e. the degree to which individuals have the capacity to obtain, process, and understand basic health information and services needed to make basic health decisions [81]. We mentioned wisdom in relation to planning, which is an important part of this decision-making; for example in the wider sense of preparing for financial security after retirement, and arranging advance directives, such as granting lasting power of attorney for health and financial decisions. A skilled approach to this is needed because such planning is vulnerable in later life, since brain circuitry that underpins the recall of detailed information (particularly the medial temporal lobe) also recombines these memories for imagining the future [82]; and because cognitive resources are increasingly channeled away from achieving new material goals in ageing, towards maintaining emotional stability [83]. These two factors in combination can lead to a future that seems 'bright but blurry' [82].

Another important aspect of health literacy in regard to cognitive ageing is self-management of health in general. There is no doubt that many chronic physical diseases of ageing are associated with cognitive decline, above all those which increase risk of cerebrovascular disease [84]. Thus awareness of prevention and management possibilities for conditions such as hypertension, type II diabetes, hypercholesterolaemia, and chronic kidney disease, are vital for healthy cognitive ageing. Indeed, low functional literacy can be literally fatal; in the English Longitudinal Study of Ageing (ELSA), participants who made more than one error in comprehending a fictitious medicine label had a 40% increased risk of all-cause mortality, after adjusting for cognitive function, education, SEP, baseline health, and health behaviours [85]. With regard to the life course approach, however, careful attention should be paid to age-specific effects. Risk from midlife hypertension accumulates over decades, yet hypotension becomes a risk for dementia in later life, possibly suggesting that older people need higher blood pressure to maintain cerebral perfusion [86]. Similar inversions appear with other cardiovascular risk factors. For example high midlife serum total cholesterol (TC) is a risk factor for dementia, but decreasing serum TC after midlife may represent a risk marker for this outcome [87]; midlife obesity is widely regarded as a risk factor for dementia (although the evidence for this is actually unclear), yet recent evidence from the NSHD suggests that weight gain beginning in late midlife may become protective of cognitive function [88]. A second caution is over the possibility of reverse causation, i.e. that these associations are explained by factors associated with prior cognition. For example a study using the Lothian 1932 birth cohort found that an association between chronic kidney disease and poorer cognition was explained by childhood cognition, which (in men) was in turn mediated by vascular risk factors [89]. This does not rule out the possibility of recursive effects of physical disease on cognition, but does suggest that estimates of the latter may be inflated if such reverse causality is not controlled.

An equally important aspect of health self-management is health-related behaviour. It is impossible here to summarize adequately the huge body of contemporary research on cognition in relation to health behaviours. However, systematic reviews and meta-analyses of prospective studies show that physical activity [90], light to moderate alcohol consumption [91], and avoidance of smoking [92], are protective of cognitive function at older ages. Biological mechanisms responsible include neurogenesis with physical activity, and reduction of inflammation and oxidative stress with moderate alcohol consumption and avoidance of smoking. The topic of diet in relation to cognitive capability is addressed in Chapter 16. In an investigation of the specificity of these behaviours in the NSHD, healthy diet was associated with slower memory decline between ages 43 and 60–64, and physical activity was associated with slower decline in processing speed, even when these behaviours were mutually adjusted, and adjustment was also made for smoking, childhood cognition, childhood and adult SEP, education, and affective symptoms [93].

3.4 **Cognitive reserve and the ageing brain**

An account of healthy cognitive ageing that does not embody the concept of 'reserve' may seem like a production of Don Giovanni without the nobleman; however, the cue is now out for his entry. The constructs of brain and cognitive reserve were formulated in a clinical context, to elucidate why some people with classical neuropathological features of Alzheimer's disease were cognitively spared at death. It became increasingly clear that aspects of brain structure and function in these individuals could buffer against the effects of this neuropathology, such that the greater this 'reserve', the more severe must be the neuropathology to cause clinical expression of dementia. This reserve is structural, in terms of neuronal density and degree of synaptic connectivity (brain reserve); and also functional, in regard to efficiency of neural networks and recruitment of alternative neural pathways following brain damage (cognitive reserve) [94]. Importantly, both kinds of reserve act to maintain healthy cognitive ageing in addition to shielding the effects of neurological disease. For example Stern proposed that the active model of cognitive reserve applies as a normal process in healthy people when coping with cognitively challenging task demands as well as a process of compensation for brain damage [95]. In considering the life course determinants of cognitive reserve we have argued that this is also viable as a life course model of cognitive development and ageing [1], as summarized in Figure 3.2. Historically, the principal determinant has been education, but we also suggested—as indeed we hope is clear from this chapter—that these determinants range across the life course, from genes to lifetime lifestyle [1].

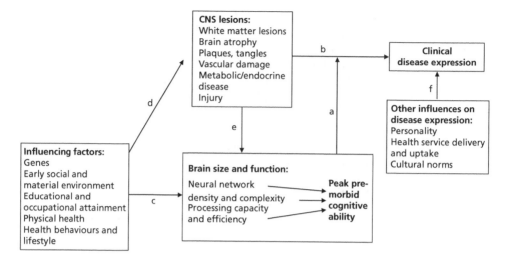

a. Cognitive reserve is represented by peak pre-morbid cognitive ability.
b. This modifies the clinical expression of CNS lesions.
c. Cognitive reserve is influenced by many factors across the life course.
d. These same factors influence the accumulation of CNS lesions.
e. CNS lesions in turn damage brain size and function.
f. There are also factors other than CNS lesions that affect disease (especially dementia) expression.

Figure 3.2 A life course model of cognitive reserve [1].

One of the most persistent and challenging criticisms of the reserve construct has been vagueness over the nature of its neurological substrate. However, progress is gradually being made in this area. On the structural side, Park and colleagues proposed a model of neurocognitive 'scaffolding', where age-associated functional deterioration in neural regions important for cognition, such as the hippocampus and mediotemporal areas, is compensated for by the 'scaffolding' of increased prefrontal activation [96]. Significantly, and consistent not only with the concept of active cognitive reserve but also with our own life course approach, development of this scaffolding represents a dynamic process of honing and refining frontal circuitry through experience, resulting in increased interconnectivity for efficient processing and storage; this experience, in turn, is proposed to arise from many of the life course factors for healthy cognitive ageing reviewed above: physical activity, cognitive engagement, and cognitive training. As ageing proceeds, however, the ability of the brain to nurture this scaffolding eventually declines, exposing the previously protected neurodegeneration and resulting in functionally significant cognitive decline.

More generally, a comprehensive review of brain structural correlates of healthy cognitive ageing was recently conducted [97]. Although there were notable discrepancies across 39 cross-sectional and 11 longitudinal studies, this review found a general consensus that is consistent with the scaffolding model above: that positive associations were repeatedly observed between hippocampal-formation size and memory and global cognitive function, and between frontal measures and executive functions. These associations have particular relevance for self-regulation and mastery. Executive function is a complex cognitive construct, involving diverse mental operations such as response inhibition, set-shifting, and spatial and temporal sequencing. In addition, executive tasks often involve what Hofman and colleagues refer to as 'updating' of relevant information, which closely connects with working memory [98]. This is defined by these authors as 'the ability to keep information in an active, quickly retrievable state, and shield this information from distraction' (p. 174), and thus lies at the boundary between memory and executive function. Accordingly, a connection between self-organization and working memory arises because the former involves, among other processes, top-down control of attention toward goal-relevant information, and away from attention-grabbing material, ruminative thoughts, and competing affect [98].

3.5 Conclusions

Rowe and Kahn famously listed six myths of ageing, one of which is that 'you can't teach an old dog new tricks' [99]. In fact people continue to learn across life, and to develop a rich set of cognitive skills [100]. Of course age-associated cognitive decline occurs, particularly in the intentional recall of information bound to time and place, and in the level of information processing necessary for complex multi-tasking. However, older people can maintain everyday skills such as driving, particularly when based on expertise or supported by routine and familiarity; may actually be better at understanding the gist of a topic than younger people; and can master, albeit more slowly, complex skills that seem to epitomize the challenge of ageing in the modern world, such as those required to use information technology [100]. In trying to understand the origins of this we have seen that cognitive function has a life course story, with clear implications for healthy cognitive ageing. The accumulation of cognitive reserve is an investment, beginning with an endowment (genetic), which can accrue across life and can be drawn against in times of emergency (brain disease and injury), although it can also be depleted. Thus we leave the last word to Foresight: 'A range of skills and behaviours is crucial in empowering people to develop and maintain their mental capital and well-being. These include executive function (self-regulation) skills; an eagerness to learn, train and re-train throughout life; the resilience to cope with stress and life events; and behaviours that can promote a healthy lifestyle and protect against decline in old age' [18: p. 1060]. We can only fully agree.

References

1 **Richards M, Deary IJ.** A life course approach to cognitive reserve: a model for cognitive aging and development? *Ann Neurol* 2005;**58**:617–22.

2 **Richards M, Hatch, SL.** A life course approach to the development of mental skills. *J Gerontol B Psychol Sci* 2011;**66**:i26–35.

3 **Deary IJ, et al.** The stability of individual differences in mental ability from childhood to old age: follow-up of the 1932 Scottish Mental Survey. *Intelligence* 2000;**28**:49–55.

4 **Gold DP, et al.** Structural equation model of intellectual change and continuity and predictors of intelligence in older men. *Psychol Aging* 1995;**10**:294–303.

5 **Richards M, Sacker A.** Lifetime antecedents of cognitive reserve. *J Clin Exp Neuropsychol* 2003;**25**: 614–24.

6 **Gow A, et al.** Is age any kinder to the initially more able? Yes and no. *Intelligence* 2012;**40**:49–59.

7 **Fiocco AJ, Yaffe K.** Defining successful aging. The importance of including cognitive function over time. *Arch Neurol* 2010;**67**:876–80.

8 **Horn JL, Cattell RB.** Refinement and test of the theory of fluid and crystallised general intelligences. *J Educ Psychol* 1966;**57**:253–70.

9 **Craik FI, Bialystok E.** Cognition through the lifespan: mechanisms of change. *Trends Cogn Sci* 2006;**10**:131–8.

10 **Rabbitt P.** Does it all go together when it goes? The nineteenth Bartlett memorial Lecture. *Q J Exp Psychol A* 1993;**6**:385–434.

11 **National Research Council.** The Aging Mind. Washington DC: National Academy Press; 2000.

12 **Brayne C.** The elephant in the room: healthy brains in later life, epidemiology and public health. *Nature Neurosci* 2007;**8**:233–9.

13 **Yaffe K, et al.** The effect of maintaining cognition on risk of disability and death. *J Am Geriatr Soc* 2010;**58**:889–94.

14 **Rowe JW, Kahn RL.** Human aging: usual and successful. *Science* 1987;**4811**:143–9.

15 **Deci EL, Ryan RM.** The 'what' and 'why' of goal pursuits: human needs and the self-determination of behavior. *Psychol Enq* 2000;**11**:227–68.

16 **Keyes CLM.** The mental health continuum: from languishing to flourishing in life. *J Health Soc Res* 2002;**43**:207–22.

17 **Havinghurst R.** Successful aging. *Gerontologist* 1961;**1**:4–7.

18 **Beddington J, et al.** The mental wealth of nations. *Nature* 2008;**455**:1057–60.

19 **O'Donovan MC, Owen MJ.** Genetics and the brain: many pathways to enlightenment. *Hum Genet* 2009;**126**:1–2.

20 **Deary IJ, et al.** Genetic foundations of human intelligence. *Hum Genet* 2009;**126**:215–232.

21 **Dickens WT, Flynn JR.** Heritability estimates versus large environmental effects: the IQ paradox resolved. *Psychol Rev* 2001;**108**:346–69.

22 **Lenroot RK, et al.** Differences in genetic and environmental influences on the human cerebral cortex associated with development during childhood and adolescence. *Hum Brain Mapp* 2009;**30**:163–74.

23 **Davies G, et al.** Genome-wide association studies establish that human intelligence is highly heritable and polygenic. *Mol Psychiatry* 2011;**16**:996–1005.

24 **Meaney MJ, Szyf M.** Environmental programming of stress responses through DNA methylation: life at the interface between a dynamic environment and a fixed genome. *Dialogues Clin Neurosci* 2005;**7**:103–23.

25 **Chouliaras L, et al.** Epigenetic regulation in the pathophysiology of Alzheimer's disease. *Prog Neurobiol* 2010;**90**:498–510.

26 **Shenkin SD, et al.** Birth weight and cognitive ability in childhood: a systematic review. *Psychol Bull* 2004;**130**:989–1013.

27 **Richards M, et al.** Birthweight and cognitive function in the British 1946 birth cohort. *BMJ* 2001;**322**: 199–202.

28 **Deary IJ, et al.** Does mother's IQ explain the association between birth weight and cognitive ability in childhood? *Intelligence* 2005;**33**:445–54.

29 **Batty GD, et al.** Effect of maternal smoking during pregnancy on offspring's cognitive ability: empirical evidence for complete confounding in the US national longitudinal survey of youth. *Pediatrics* 2006;**118**:943–50.

30 **Thapar A, Rutter M.** Do prenatal factors cause psychiatric disorder? Be wary of causal claims. *Br J Psychiatry* 2009;**195**:100–1.

31 **Richards M, et al.** Postnatal growth and cognitive function in a national UK birth cohort. *Int J Epidemiol* 2002;**31**:342–8.

32 **Gale CR, et al.** Psychomotor co-ordination and intelligence in childhood and health in adulthood: testing the system integrity hypothesis. *Psychosom Med* 2009;**71**:675–81.

33 **Murray GK, et al.** Infant developmental milestones and subsequent cognitive function. *Ann Neurol* 2007;**62**:128–36.

34 **Richards M, et al.** Infant feeding, mental development, and mental ageing. In: Wyness L, et al., editors. Nutrition and Development: Long and Short Term Consequences for Health. A report of the British Nutrition Foundation Task Force. Chichester: Wiley Blackwell; 2013:206–215.

35 **Der G, et al.** Effect of breast feeding on intelligence in children: prospective study, sibling pairs analysis, and meta-analysis. *BMJ* 2006;**333**:929–30.

36 **Lynch JW, et al.** Cumulative impact of sustained hardship on physical, cognitive, psychological, and social functioning. *N Engl J Med* 1997;**337**:1889–95.

37 **Guo G, Harris KM.** The mechanisms mediating the effects of poverty on children's intellectual development. *Demography* 2000;**37**:431–47.

38 **Evans GW.** Child development and the physical environment. *Annu Rev Psychol* 2006;**57**:423–51.

39 **Cairns RB, Cairns BD.** The making of developmental psychology. In Lerner RM, editor. Handbook of Child Psychology. Vol. 1, 6th ed. Hoboken, NJ: John Wiley & Sons; 2006:89–165.

40 **Ratner N, Bruner J.** Games, social exchange and the acquisition of language. *J Child Lang* 1978;**5**:391–401.

41 **Baumrind D.** The influence of parenting style on adolescent competence and substance use. *J Early Adolesc* 1991;**11**:56–95.

42 **McLeod BD, et al.** Examining the association between parenting and childhood anxiety: a meta-analysis. *Clin Psychol Rev* 2007;**27**:155–72.

43 **Bowles S, Gintis H.** Schooling in Capitalist America. New York: Basic Books; 1976.

44 **Heckman JJ, Rubenstein Y.** The importance of noncognitive skills: lessons from the GED testing program. *Am Econ Rev* 2001;**91**:145–9.

45 **Duckworth K, et al.** (2009). Self-regulated learning: a literature review. Available at: <http://www.learningbenefits.net/Publications/ResRepIntros/ResRep33intro.htm>

46 **Zimmerman B.** Attaining self-regulation: a social cognitive perspective. In Boekaerts M et al, editors. Handbook of Self-Regulation. Burlington, MA: Elsevier Academic Press; 2000:13–39.

47 **Schunk D, Ertmer P.** Self-regulation and academic learning: self-efficacy enhancing interventions. In Boekaerts M, et al., editors. Handbook of Self-Regulation. Burlington, MA: Elsevier Academic Press; 2000:631–49.

48 **Baker CN, Hoerger M.** Parental child-rearing strategies influence self-regulation, socio-emotional adjustment, and psychopathology in early adulthood: evidence from a retrospective cohort study. *Pers Individ Dif* 2012;**52**:800–5.

49 **Deary IJ, et al.** Intelligence and educational achievement. *Intelligence* 2006;**35**:13–21.

50 **Lager ACJ, et al.** Social origin, schooling and individual change in intelligence during childhood influence long-term mortality: a 68-year follow-up study. *Int J Epidemiol* 2012;**41**:398–404.

51 **Clouston S, et al.** Benefits of educational attainment on adult fluid cognition: international evidence from three birth cohorts. *Int J Epidemiol* 2012;**41**:1729–36.

52 **Richards M, Sacker A.** Is education causal? Yes. *Int J Epidemiol* 2011;**40**:516–8.

53 **Hatch SL, et al.** The continuing benefits of education: adult education and midlife cognitive ability in the British 1946 birth cohort. *J Gerontol B Psychol Sci Soc Sci* 2007;**62**:S404–14.

54 **Richards M, et al.** Paths to literacy and numeracy problems: evidence from two British birth cohorts. *J Epidemiol Community Health* 2009;**63**:239–44.

55 **Piccinin AM, et al.** Coordinated analysis of age, sex, and education effects on change in MMSE scores. *J Gerontol B Psychol Sci Soc Sci* 2013;**68**:374–90.

56 **Kohn M, Slomcznski KM.** Social Structure and Self-Direction. A Comparative Analysis of the United States and Poland. Cambridge, MA: Blackwell; 1993.

57 **Collins R.** The Credential Society: An Historical Sociology of Education and Stratification. New York: Academic Press; 1979.

58 **Glymour MM, Manly JJ.** Lifecourse social conditions and racial and ethnic patterns of cognitive aging. *Neuropsychol Rev* 2008;**18**:223–54.

59 **Williams DR, et al.** Race, socioeconomic status, and health: complexities, ongoing challenges, and research opportunities. *Ann N Y Acad Sci* 2010;**1186**:69–101.

60 **Kohn M, Schooler** C. Work and Personality: an Enquiry into the Impact of Social Stratification. Norwood, NJ: Ablex; 1983.

61 **Hauser RM, Roan CL** (2007). Work complexity and cognitive functioning at midlife: Cross-validating the Kohn-Schooler hypothesis in an American cohort (CDE Working Paper No. 2007–08). Madison: University of Wisconsin, Center for Demography and Ecology.

62 **Schooler C, et al.** The continuing effects of substantively complex work on the intellectual functioning of older workers. *Psychol Aging* 1999;**14**:483–506.

63 **Maguire EA, et al.** Navigation-related structural change in the hippocampi of taxi drivers. *Proc Natl Acad Sci USA* 2000;**97**:4398–403.

64 **Hultsch DF, et al.** Use it or lose it: engaged lifestyle as a buffer of cognitive decline in aging? *Psychol Aging* 1999;**14**:245–63.

65 **Rohwedder S, Willis RJ.** Mental retirement. *J Econ Perspect* 2010;**24**:119–38.

66 **Roberts BA, et al.** Does retirement influence cognitive performance? The Whitehall II Study. *J Epidemiol Community Health* 2011;**65**:958–63.

67 **Swaab DF.** Brain aging and Alzheimer's disease, 'wear and tear' versus 'use it or lose it'. *Neurobiol Aging* 1991;**12**:317–24.

68 **Schooler C, Mulatu MS.** The reciprocal effects of leisure time activities and intellectual functioning in older people: a longitudinal analysis. *Psychol Aging* 2001;**16**:466–82.

69 **Wilson RS, et al.** Assessment of lifetime participation in cognitively stimulating activities. *J Clin Exp Neuropsychol* 2003;**25**:634–42.

70 **Owen AM, et al.** Putting brain training to the test. *Nature* 2010;**465**:775–8.

71 **Stern Y, et al.** Space Fortress game training and executive control in older adults: a pilot intervention. *Neuropsychol Dev Cogn B Aging Neuropsychol Cogn* 2011;**18**:653–77.

72 **Bor D, Owen A.** Cognitive training: neural correlates of expert skill. *Curr Biol* 2007;**17**:R95–7.

73 **Pearlin, LI, Schooler** C. The structure of coping. *J Health Soc Behav* 1978;**22**:337–56.

74 **Pearlin LI, et al.** The life-course origins of mastery among older people. *J Health Soc Behav* 2007;**48**: 164–79.

75 **Baltes PB, Staudinger UM.** The search for a psychology of wisdom. *Curr Dir Psychol Sci* 1993;**2**:75–80.

76 **Kramer DA.** Conceptualizing wisdom: the primacy of affect-cognition relations. In: Sternberg RJ, editor. Wisdom: Its Nature, Origins and Development. New York: Cambridge University Press; 1990: 279–313.

77 **Coleman PG, O'Hanlon A.** Ageing and Development: Theories and Research. Arnold, London; 2004.

78 **Staudinger UM, et al.** What predicts wisdom-related performance? A first look at personality, intelligence, and facilitative experiential contexts. *Eur J Person* 1998;**12**:1–17.

79 **Farkas G.** Cognitive skills and noncognitive traits and behaviors in stratification processes. *Annu Rev Sociol* 2003;**29**:541–62.

80 **Sternberg RJ, Lubart TI.** Wisdom and creativity. In: Birren JE, Schaie KW, editors. Handbook of the Psychology of Aging. San Diego, CA: Academic Press; 2001: 500–22.

81 **Ratzan SC, Parker R.** Introduction. National Library of Medicine Current Bibliographies in Medicine: Health Literacy. Bethesda, Maryland: National Institutes of Health; 2000.

82 **Weierich MR, et al.** Older and wiser? An affective science perspective on age-related challenges in financial decision making. *Soc Cogn Affect Neurosci* 2011;**6**:195–206.

83 **Nielsen L, Mather M.** Emerging perspectives in social neuroscience and neuroeconomics of aging. *Soc Cogn Affect Neurosci* 2011;**6**:149–64.

84 Warsch JRL, Wright CB. The aging mind: vascular health in normal cognitive aging. *J Am Geriatr Soc* 2010;**58**:S319–24.

85 Bostock S, Steptoe A. Association between low functional health literacy and mortality in older adults: longitudinal cohort study. *BMJ* 2012;**344**:e1602.

86 Qiu C, et al. The age-dependent relation of blood pressure to cognitive function and dementia. *Lancet Neurol* 2005;**4**:487–99.

87 Solomon A, et al. Serum cholesterol changes after midlife and late-life cognition. *Neurology* 2007;**68**: 751–6.

88 Albanese E, et al. No association between gain in body mass index across the life course and midlife cognitive function and cognitive reserve—the 1946 British birth cohort study. *Alzheimers Dement* 2012;**8**:470–82.

89 Munang L, et al. Renal function and cognition in the 1932 Scottish mental Survey Lothian cohort. *Age Ageing* 2007;**36**:323–5.

90 Hamer M, Chida Y. Physical activity and risk of neurodegenerative disease: a systematic review of prospective evidence. *Psychol Med* 2009;**39**:3–11.

91 Anstey KJ, et al. Alcohol consumption as a risk factor for dementia and cognitive decline: meta-analysis of prospective studies. *Am J Geriatr Psychiatry* 2009;**17**:542–55.

92 Peters R, et al. Smoking, dementia and cognitive decline in the elderly, a systematic review. *BMC Geriatr* 2008;**8**:36.

93 Cadar D, et al. The role of lifestyle behaviours on 20-year cognitive decline. *J Aging Res* 2012;**2012**: 304014

94 Stern Y. Cognitive reserve. *Neuropsychologia* 2009;**47**:2015–28.

95 Stern Y. The concept of cognitive reserve: a catalyst for research. *J Clin Exp Neuropsychol* 2003;**25**: 589–93.

96 Park DC, Reuter-Lorenz P. The adaptive brain: aging and neurocognitive scaffolding. *Annu Rev Psychol* 2009;**60**:173–96.

97 Kaup AR, et al. A review of the brain structure correlates of successful cognitive aging. *J Neuropsychiatry Clin Neurosci* 2011;**23**:6–15.

98 Hofmann W, et al. Executive functions and self-regulation. *Trends Cogn Sci* 2012;**16**:174–80.

99 Rowe JW, Kahn RL, editors. Chapter 1: Breaking down the myths of aging. In: Successful Aging. New York: Pantheon Press; 1998.

100 Richards M, Hatch SL. Good news about the ageing brain. *BMJ* 2011;**343**:882–3.

Chapter 4

A life course approach to psychological and social wellbeing

Catharine R Gale, Ian J Deary, and Mai Stafford

4.1 Introduction

There is increasing recognition among governments that whereas economic indicators provide one measure of a country's welfare, such indicators do not adequately reflect levels of psychological wellbeing among their citizens. A striking example of this is the fact that although gross domestic product per capita has risen over the past 50 years in most developed countries, people's level of satisfaction with their lives is almost unchanged [1]. There is now considerable support for suggestions that wellbeing should be an end goal of public policy, not just from policymakers and researchers but also from the public [2]. Wellbeing is highly rated by young and old alike. When over 7000 young adults from 42 countries were asked to rate the importance of money and happiness, only 6% rated money as more important than happiness, and 69% rated happiness at the top of the importance scale [3]. In a qualitative study of people aged 85 and over, being happy and socially engaged was valued more highly than physical and cognitive capability [4]. Yet, whereas there is widespread agreement that wellbeing is an important end in itself, there remains a lack of consensus among researchers about how wellbeing should be defined and measured [2].

In this chapter we first examine how wellbeing has been conceptualized. We consider whether wellbeing changes with increasing age and assess the evidence on the early life determinants of wellbeing. We review evidence from longitudinal studies on the relations between physical or cognitive capability, physical activity, diet, or health in later life and subsequent wellbeing, consider the evidence that wellbeing itself may influence these factors, and examine potential mechanisms that might underlie these latter findings.

4.2 Conceptualizing wellbeing

Many researchers now agree that wellbeing is best thought of as a multi-faceted construct [5] although opinion remains divided as to which components should be part of this construct [2].

Much of the research on wellbeing to date has concentrated on what is often called 'subjective wellbeing', or in colloquial terms 'happiness'. Subjective wellbeing refers to how people think and feel about their lives. This has been conceptualized in terms of four main components: life satisfaction (global cognitive evaluations of one's life), satisfaction with important domains (e.g. work, health, marriage), positive affect (experiencing many pleasant emotions and moods), and low levels of negative affect (experiencing few unpleasant emotions and moods) [3]. According to Diener [5], these components of wellbeing are moderately correlated with each other, yet each provides unique information about the subjective quality of an individual's life.

Others have conceptualized wellbeing as being not just about experiencing pleasant emotions or making positive judgements about how life is going, but also about positive functioning and realization of potential. Autonomy (feeling free to do what one wants), competence (feeling a sense of accomplishment), engagement (feeling absorbed in what one does), and meaning and purpose (feeling what one does is worthwhile and valued) have been proposed as important facets of wellbeing and policymakers are being urged to include these dimensions in national measures of wellbeing [6].

Differences in how wellbeing is conceptualized are largely driven by the fact that most of the research in this field has been informed by two distinct perspectives [7]. The hedonic perspective focuses on happiness or pleasure and defines wellbeing largely in terms of a preponderance of positive emotions over negative emotions. The eudaimonic perspective—based on Aristotle's view that true happiness comes from doing what is worth doing—focuses on meaning and self-realization, and defines wellbeing largely in terms of ways of thought and behaviour that provide fulfilment. One uniting factor in both these approaches to wellbeing is an emphasis on positive mental health, rather than disorder and dysfunction. Indeed, recent years have seen a growing interest in positive psychology [8], along with increasing awareness that wellbeing is far more than just the absence of mental illness.

One factor that helps determine how people evaluate the quality of their lives is their relationships with others. Social connections and the sense of reciprocity and trust that can accompany them are associated with higher levels of subjective wellbeing [1]. As a consequence, many large scale surveys on wellbeing include items to assess what is often called 'social wellbeing' – how one feels or functions in relation to other people, in terms of closeness to others, sense of trust, or social engagement [6]. Indeed, some researchers now take the view that having supportive and satisfying social relationships is a component of wellbeing. When the Warwick-Edinburgh Mental Wellbeing Scale (WEMWBS) was developed with the aim of capturing a wide conception of wellbeing, its 14 items included four on social functioning along with others on both hedonic and eudaimonic facets of wellbeing. Confirmatory factor analysis supported the hypothesis that the scale was measuring a single construct [9], suggesting that all these facets of wellbeing are closely related.

4.3 Age-related changes in wellbeing

Psychological wellbeing may be conceived of as a cumulative outcome reflecting one's traits, dispositions, circumstances, and experiences so far. It involves cognitive processing and encapsulates the level of satisfaction with life in general or constituent domains. Wellbeing may also be conceived as a response reflecting current experiences, capturing transient emotions or affect [10]. There are likely to be different age-related changes in these different elements of wellbeing, since cognitive and affective elements are satisfied by different social needs [11]. The time frame used to assess wellbeing is also important. For example, life satisfaction among centenarians has been found to be higher when they were asked to consider their whole life span than when asked to consider only present circumstances [12].

4.3.1 Stable or varying with age?

Early studies of wellbeing took the perspective that demographic and socioeconomic structural factors were key determinants (known as the 'social indicators perspective' or 'bottom-up' approach). These factors were thought to differentiate access to physical, material, and social resources that affect wellbeing [13]. According to this theory, the age-related change in combinations of these resources might be expected to underlie any age-related changes in wellbeing. An alternative perspective is the 'top-down' approach which assumes that an individual's stable personality traits primarily define whether they will experience and evaluate life in a positive or negative way [14]. In addition, humans tend to get used to changes in circumstances. This psychological adaptation has been referred to as the 'hedonic treadmill' since our expectations rise in parallel with our improved circumstances [15]. On this basis, changes in circumstances lead to only temporary changes in wellbeing and we would not expect to see consistent age-related change.

Whilst twin studies indicate a strong genetic component to life satisfaction and considerable stability in life satisfaction has been demonstrated empirically, it is now evident that set points in wellbeing can change under some conditions and that individuals differ in their psychological adaptation to events [16,17]. Longitudinal data enabling description of wellbeing across life are not available and methods to pool shorter run trajectories over cohorts capturing different sections of the life course have not yet been applied in HALCyon or other inter-cohort studies. Several studies have compared levels of wellbeing across age groups based on cross-sectional data and some have utilized longitudinal data over short time periods. These have been frequently reviewed elsewhere although the picture remains somewhat unclear given differences in the age ranges of the samples and wellbeing indicators examined [13,18–20]. Two recent, large studies based on representative samples from the US [21] and several European and developing nations [22] have concluded that life satisfaction and happiness decline through adulthood to around age 50, increase until the mid 70s, and from the mid 70s onwards subsequently level off or decline again, as illustrated in Figure 4.1, though methodological challenges in describing the relationship between happiness and age continue to be debated.

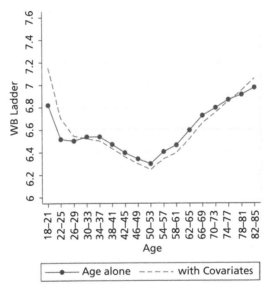

Figure 4.1 Mean global wellbeing (range 0–10) by 4-year age groups based on 340,847 individuals [21]. The connected line represents unadjusted data and dashed lines represent data adjusted for unemployment, marital status, and children living at home. Based on Gallup Organization and Healthways Corporation telephone survey conducted in 50 US states in 2008.

Reproduced from Stone AA, et al., A snapshot of the age distribution of psychological well-being in the United States. *Proceedings of the National Academy of Sciences of the United States of America*, Volume **107**, pp. 9985–90, Copyright © 2010, with permission from PNAS.

Based on the large, repeat cross-sectional data from the US mentioned above, the age-related change in positive affect appears to show the same pattern as life satisfaction [21]. Longitudinal analysis of four generations of adults followed up for 23 years revealed that levels of positive affect are similar and stable in young and middle-aged adults but are lower and decline over time among older adults [23].

As affect captures current emotional experience, it is of interest to consider not only the average level of affect but also the extent to which a person's affect varies—that is, how emotionally reactive a person is. Daily diary designs show that there is considerable variation in positive and negative affect across the day [24,25]. However, variation in affect occurs at the between-person level as well as within-person level. In other words, emotional reactivity to everyday events and stressors has a stable trait component [26]. The stability of positive emotions appears to be somewhat greater in older compared with younger people [25].

In summary, whereas longitudinal data are needed to document the nature of age-related change in wellbeing more accurately, the literature indicates that the life course trajectory of wellbeing is non-linear and does not follow the trajectory of physical or cognitive capability.

4.3.2 Social wellbeing and age

Social network composition and contact change with age. The number of and time spent with friends, neighbours and extended family is smaller in older age, whilst contact with intimate family is higher in older old compared with younger old people [27]. The people nominated as close and important changes over the life course (mother, father, siblings in childhood; mother, spouse in early adulthood; spouse in midlife; and spouse, children, and grandchildren in older age) [28]. The link between social connections and psychological wellbeing may also change with age. Older people's positive affect has been shown to benefit more than does younger people's when interacting with family members, whereas younger people appear to benefit more than older people from interaction with new friends [29]. Older people have more positive and fewer negative exchanges with their social network than do younger people, especially with their children and other family [30].

There are several explanations for improvements in wellbeing from midlife to at least early old age. A large divergence between aspirations and achievements contributes to lower wellbeing and this gap has been shown to be smaller in older compared with younger adults, though it is not clear whether this is because of higher achievements or lower aspirations in older people [31]. Priorities may also be altered in later life. At progressively older ages, according to socioemotional selectivity theory [32,33], awareness of the limited time left in life motivates people to regulate their social activities to maximize positive social interactions and emotional fulfilment thus contributing to better emotional regulation and higher wellbeing. The relative importance of the domains which contribute to overall life satisfaction may also change with age. Indeed, one study showed a substantial contribution to wellbeing of health factors in younger old age contrasted with a stronger contribution of social relationships in the oldest old [34] and suggested this was indicative of psychological adaptation. Across a wider age range, Beutel and colleagues found that satisfaction with health was more important among older compared with younger men [35].

4.4 Early life determinants of wellbeing

As long ago as 1984, Diener noted that a review of the determinants of wellbeing was too large for a single article and the field has expanded rapidly since then [19]. Here we focus on longitudinal research that has examined factors in childhood and early adulthood that may relate to wellbeing in later life.

4.4.1 **Personality traits**

Personality traits are key determinants of wellbeing. Greater levels of extraversion, agreeableness and conscientiousness and lower levels of neuroticism are strongly associated with higher levels of wellbeing cross-sectionally and prospectively [36,37]. Recent studies have considered simultaneous effects of these sometimes correlated personality traits and taken account of potential confounding and mediating factors [38,39]. Higher levels of extraversion in adolescence and early adulthood were associated with higher scores on the Ryff psychological wellbeing scales in middle-aged women and this was not explained by levels of psychological distress in adulthood [39]. In one of the longest follow-up studies to date, higher extraversion in youth was found to be directly associated with higher scores on the Warwick-Edinburgh Mental Wellbeing Scale and the Diener Satisfaction with Life Scale in men and women at age 60–64 years, whereas the links between neuroticism and wellbeing appeared to operate largely through psychological distress and physical health [38].

There are several possible explanations for the links between personality and wellbeing. One partial explanation might be that they are influenced by shared genetic factors. In a representative sample of 973 twin pairs the genetic variance underlying individual differences in wellbeing was also responsible for individual differences in neuroticism and extraversion [40]. At least some of the association between personality and subjective wellbeing may be due to overlap in the measures used to capture these constructs; both tend to be assessed using self-report scales, and it is probably difficult for people fully to separate states from traits in their reports [7]. Biobehavioural systems which regulate emotional and behavioural reactions to rewards and punishments may also underlie the close association [36]. Personality may also be causally linked to wellbeing through its impact on experiences including events and behaviours [41,42].

4.4.2 **Socioeconomic circumstances**

Socioeconomic circumstances also contribute to wellbeing. On the basis of findings from a meta-analysis, Heller and colleagues concluded that personality factors place limits on the range of life satisfaction that an individual can experience but that social circumstances can additionally affect life satisfaction [36]. More disadvantaged socioeconomic circumstances in childhood have been linked to lower wellbeing and poorer psychological function in later life with some evidence of contribution independently of adult socioeconomic factors. [43–45]. Meta-analysis of over 205 studies revealed a positive though fairly weak correlation between socioeconomic position (SEP) in adulthood and life satisfaction, with effect sizes being very similar for education and income [46]. Although data from older populations predominated in this meta-analysis, some studies included adults aged 18 and upwards and longitudinal versus cross-sectional studies were not distinguished. SEP was more highly correlated with wellbeing among men than it was among women, whereas social contact was more highly correlated with wellbeing among women. Higher SEP may influence wellbeing in several ways. It provides greater access to material resources—being employed rather than unemployed and not being work-disabled, for example, are correlated with wellbeing [47]. Higher status occupations afford greater prestige and being productively engaged in fulfilling work enhances satisfaction [48]. The more socioeconomically advantaged tend to have a greater sense of control over their home and working lives [49,50] and are likely to be better able to cope with hassles and life events as well as benefiting from other psychosocial factors including more supportive social connections [51].

It may be relative rather than absolute SEP that is most important for wellbeing. Wellbeing might be expected to be higher for those who make downward rather than upward social comparisons. Social comparison may also contribute to explaining the higher levels of wellbeing in older compared with younger people since older people tend to make more downward comparisons than their younger counterparts [31]. Experiences earlier in life may also alter one's expectations [52] so the cross-sectional association between concurrent circumstances and wellbeing needs to be interpreted in the light of previous circumstances.

4.4.3 Social relationships

As noted earlier, social connections are integral to understanding wellbeing. Interest in the long-term implications of poor quality parent-child relationships for psychological ill health is long-standing [43,53–55]. Recent evidence has emerged that parenting styles are related to positive wellbeing in later life independently of psychological distress [56–58]; and that different attachment styles are associated with emotions such as joy and sadness [59]. Good quality childhood relationships with siblings and parents also distinguish people who are flourishing psychologically (based on a composite of life satisfaction, happiness, and self-efficacy at age 33) from those who are languishing [60]. Relationships provide the context for development of interpersonal feelings and functions and self-regulation (Chapter 3).

4.4.4 Early life determinants of social wellbeing

Factors in early life are also relevant for social wellbeing in older age. Positive social interactions in older age depend strongly on social relationships throughout life beginning with early attachment and carrying through to family formation and dissolution and the quality and diversity of social networks throughout adulthood [61]. Recalled total childhood adversity (including emotional neglect but also financial need) has been associated with smaller social network size and perceived isolation in a small sample of older people [62] but we are not aware that this has been studied with prospective data to older age. Social and economic factors impact social relationships at all points across life, for example childhood socioeconomic disadvantage has, in some though not all studies, been associated with less positive parenting [63]. Women report a larger number of intimate relationships than men [28] and men and women differ in the support they give and receive [64] though gender differences in relationships vary across life [28].

4.4.5 Multiple and multilevel determinants of wellbeing

Social determinants of health and wellbeing have been described as operating at the individual, meso and macro levels [65]. Meso-level determinants may operate within neighbourhoods, schools, or other local settings. Early social relationships within the family could be considered as meso-level determinants but aside from this we are not aware that there has been any examination of meso-level exposures operating in childhood and early adulthood that plausibly influence later life wellbeing. For example, the early educational environment may be linked to subsequent wellbeing through its impact on self-efficacy and ambition [66,67]. Growing up in a neighbourhood or school rich in social capital—one characterized by high levels of trust, reciprocity, and civic engagement—could have long-term benefits for social wellbeing (Chapter 18). A link between democratic school environment and greater likelihood of membership in associations and clubs in adolescence has been documented cross-sectionally [68]. Neighbours may constitute a relevant reference group for the social comparison element of wellbeing. For example, more advantaged residents living in more deprived neighbourhoods rated themselves as higher up the ladder of society than their counterparts in less deprived neighbourhoods [69] though whether the reference group for comparison is stable across life is not known.

Although repeat measures of wellbeing across life are not available, the MRC National Survey of Health and Development has captured positive adolescent temperament (assessed by the teacher) and examined its association with adult indicators of wellbeing. The findings demonstrate continuity of wellbeing over several years, through several of the pathways described above. Positive children were less likely to experience lifetime emotional problems and more likely to have high satisfaction with work, a high frequency of contact with friends or family and engagement in social activities in midlife [70].

Exposures related to wellbeing are typically considered in isolation rather than in combination. Recursive partitioning is an approach which considers multiple factors integratively rather than independently. It is used to classify individuals into groups on the basis of multiple (categorical) characteristics, and to identify groups that have a high or low probability of the outcome of interest. It has been used to show that low neuroticism, high extraversion, and high financial control were associated with positive affect in early adulthood, midlife and older age [14]. In this study the lowest level of positive affect was found in the group with high neuroticism and low financial control. The highest positive affect was found in the group with low neuroticism and high extraversion. Relationship quality was additionally associated but only for middle-aged adults. In contrast, marital status was only important for older adults. Those who were not married and had high levels of neuroticism had the lowest wellbeing. This approach allows exploration of multiple interactions between personality and economic and social factors and is particularly relevant for understanding life course determinants.

4.5 **Wellbeing in relation to later life determinants or outcomes**

Studies that have repeated measures of wellbeing over several years suggest that wellbeing tends to decline slightly in people aged around 70 and over [23,71,72]. Given that this is a period in life when impairments in physical and cognitive capability or chronic disease are more likely to constrain an individual's ability to manage some routine aspects of life, it might be expected that these factors would have an adverse effect on the trajectory of wellbeing, although the existing evidence base is limited. There is rather more evidence to suggest that wellbeing may itself affect capability and health, particularly in the case of mortality. Establishing the true direction of effect in studies of outcomes other than mortality can be difficult because measures of wellbeing and physical and cognitive capability track over time, raising the possibility that in some such studies the apparent direction of the association may be an artefact.

4.5.1 **Physical capability**

Evidence as to whether poorer physical capability has a detrimental effect on wellbeing is sparse. In a meta-analysis of data from five cohorts in the HALCyon programme, stronger grip and faster walking, timed get up and go, and chair rise speeds were all associated with slightly higher scores on the Warwick-Edinburgh Mental Wellbeing Scale a few years later [73]. However, so far as we are aware, there has been no longitudinal investigation of whether poorer physical capability *per se* leads to a decline in wellbeing. There is some evidence that when physical capability deteriorates sufficiently to cause functional limitations these may result in decline in wellbeing. In one longitudinal study of people aged 70 and over who were free of disability at baseline, worsening scores at performing instrumental activities of daily living was associated with a small decline in positive affect 4.5 years later [74]. In the Berlin Ageing Study, those who had more functional constraints on a composite measure of mobility, vision, and hearing at baseline were more likely to experience a decline in positive affect over the 4 year follow-up [75].

All existing evidence on the relation between wellbeing and subsequent physical capability supports the hypothesis that greater wellbeing might have a protective effect. In a cohort of Mexican-Americans aged 65 or over, those with high positive affect had a reduced risk of having slow walking speed or of becoming disabled as regards activities of daily living (ADL) 2 years later [76]. Older people with a stronger sense of mastery—the feeling that one has control over life circumstances—experienced a less steep decline in lower extremity physical performance over a 6 year period in the Invecchiare in Chianti Study [77]. In the Rush Memory and Aging Project, being more socially engaged or having a stronger sense of purpose in life was associated with slower subsequent decline in motor performance and a lower risk of incident disability as regards ADL, instrumental activities of daily living (IADL) and mobility [78–80]. One study in Taiwan found that in people with no mobility limitations those who reported greater satisfaction with life developed fewer mobility problems over an 8 year period [81]. In all these studies the association between facets of wellbeing and physical capability or disability persisted after adjustment for negative affect so cannot be due just to the absence of symptoms of depression.

A few other longitudinal studies have examined the relation between social engagement and different types of functional limitations. Their results have been mixed, with some reporting an apparently protective effect [82], others finding that associations varied by age or sex, but very few of these studies examined incident disability. It may be that wellbeing is a less important predictor of functional status in samples of people where disabilities are already present. In two studies that examined whether baseline positive affect or life satisfaction were predictive of change in functional status in older people who already had some degree of disability, there were no significant associations after adjustment for potential confounding factors [81,83]. One of these studies found that increase in positive affect over a 6 year period was linked with less decline in functional status over the same period, but the extent to which this was due to the effect of wellbeing on functional status or *vice versa* is uncertain [83].

4.5.2 Cognitive capability

Only a few studies have examined whether poorer cognitive ability in later life is linked with a decline in wellbeing. One study of people aged 70 and over found no evidence that increases in cognitive limitations, as measured by the Mini Mental State Examination, over a 54 month period influenced the trajectory of positive affect [74]. Similarly, in the Berlin Ageing Study when wellbeing was assessed using a measure that reflected satisfaction with life, satisfaction with ageing and level of anxiety, no association was found between decline in perceptual speed and trajectory of wellbeing over a 13 year period [71]. In an analysis of data on people aged 50 to 90 years in the English Longitudinal Study of Ageing (ELSA), where wellbeing was assessed using a measure that covered both hedonic and eudaimonic aspects, we found that in general, differences between individuals in cognitive ability were not predictive of levels of wellbeing. [72]. There is slightly stronger evidence that poorer cognition in later life may have an impact on social wellbeing, as measured by social engagement. Examination of several waves of data from the Victoria Longitudinal Study showed that decline in memory performance led to people becoming less socially active [84]. This is perhaps unsurprising as being socially engaged necessitates complex cognitive functioning.

In the HALCyon programme, we lacked the data to examine whether cognitive capability was associated with changes in wellbeing. In a meta-analysis of data from four cohorts aged 50 to 87 we found that people who had greater cognitive ability in childhood or whose later life cognitive ability was better than expected given their cognition in childhood had very slightly higher scores on the Warwick-Edinburgh Mental Wellbeing Scale, but these differences were attenuated and no longer significant after adjustment for the personality traits neuroticism and extraversion [85]. With the possible exception of social wellbeing as indicated by social engagement, it seems that cognitive capability is not a strong predictor of wellbeing in older people [86].

Almost all of the longitudinal research to date into the potential influence of how older people feel on change in cognitive capability has concentrated on depressive symptoms rather than wellbeing. Results have been inconsistent. In ELSA, we found that being more depressed was associated with a slightly faster rate of cognitive decline but this was only statistically significant in people aged 60 to 80 years [87]. Whether higher levels of positive emotions might be a protective factor for cognitive decline, independent of depressive symptoms, is largely unknown. We referred earlier to two studies that had examined whether cognitive decline predicted levels of wellbeing; these studies also examined whether there was an effect in the reverse direction. Their results provide partial support for the notion that wellbeing might be protective. In the Berlin Aging Study people with higher levels of wellbeing experienced a slower rate of decline in perceptual speed over a 13 year period, after adjustment for depression [71]. In ELSA, people with greater wellbeing tended to have better cognition, whether assessed as executive function, processing speed or memory, after adjustment for depression and other risk factors, but there was no evidence that for an individual, improving wellbeing would necessarily lead to better cognitive performance [72].

One facet of wellbeing which has fairly consistently been linked with risk of cognitive decline in a number of longitudinal studies is lack of social engagement. People who are more socially engaged have been found to have a slower rate of decline in perceptual speed [88], a lower risk of cognitive decline [89], and may be less likely to develop dementia [90]. Social engagement requires complex cognitive functioning. As yet, very few studies have examined the long-term relation between changes in social engagement and changes in cognitive function in older people and the temporal order in which they occur. Analysis of 12 years of data from the Victoria Longitudinal study provided support for the hypothesis that being more socially engaged may help maintain cognitive function with advancing age, but also suggested that this relation may vary depending on the cognitive domain assessed. Greater social activity was associated with less decline in verbal speed, and vice versa, but it had no protective effect on episodic or semantic memory; instead, poorer memory performance led to people becoming less socially active [84].

4.5.3 Physical activity and diet

Cross-sectional evidence from the Whitehall II study shows that higher levels of life satisfaction at a mean age of 50 years are associated with healthier behaviours, including taking more exercise and eating more fruit and vegetables [91]. Whether happier people are more likely to behave in a healthier fashion or whether such behaviours increase wellbeing is unclear. A systematic review of randomized controlled trials in older people found that being more physically active had a small beneficial effect on wellbeing, particularly in those who are usually sedentary [92], but little is known about the potential impact of diet on wellbeing in later life.

4.5.4 **Chronic illness**

In two longitudinal studies of older people where wellbeing was assessed regularly over periods of between 4.5 and 6 years using a measure of positive affect or a measure covering both hedonic and eudaimonic aspects of wellbeing, there was no association in either study between the number of doctor-diagnosed chronic illnesses reported at baseline and change in wellbeing over the follow-up period [72,74]. In both these studies poorer health was associated with lower wellbeing cross-sectionally but, this could be because people with lower wellbeing may be more susceptible to poorer health [91].

4.5.5 **Mortality**

Perhaps the strongest evidence for the importance of wellbeing for healthy ageing comes from studies that show that people with greater wellbeing have lower mortality. In 2008, Chida and Steptoe carried out a meta-analysis of some of these studies to gauge the overall relation between psychological wellbeing—defined here as positive affect, life satisfaction or related trait-like constructs such as optimism and cheerfulness—and mortality [93]. Greater psychological wellbeing was associated with a significantly reduced rate of death regardless of whether the participants were healthy or had a specific established illness at baseline. The effect was stronger in the healthy population (adjusted hazard ratio (HR) 0.82, 95% confidence interval 0.76, 0.89, p<0.001) than in those with existing illness (HR 0.98, 95% confidence interval 0.95, 1.00, p = 0.03). Separate analysis of healthy populations aged over 60 showed that the link between greater wellbeing and lower mortality was even stronger at older ages (HR 0.74, 95% confidence interval 0.64, 0.84, p<0.001). There were too few studies of older populations with established disease at baseline for separate analysis so it was not possible to tell whether a similar protective effect was apparent in this group. A report from the Rotterdam study found that greater positive affect was associated with lower mortality in people aged 60 to 79 independently of illness at baseline. In those aged 80 and over the relation disappeared after taking account of baseline health. It is possible that, in this age group, perception of wellbeing is more strongly influenced by health problems than at younger ages [94].

The other facet of wellbeing which appears to be a powerful predictor of mortality is social engagement. The relationship between social relationships and survival has been a topic of increasing interest to researchers since the late 1980s. House and colleagues carried out a review of five prospective studies and proposed that a lack of social relationships was 'a major risk factor for health—rivaling the effect of well-established health risk factors such as cigarette smoking, blood pressure, blood lipids, obesity, and physical activity' [95: p. 541]. A recent meta-analysis of 148 such studies found that, of various aspects of social relationships, the strongest predictor of mortality was lack of social engagement. Its effect on survival was comparable in size to that of well-established risk factors and differed little by age or by initial state of health [96].

4.6 **Mechanisms underlying associations between wellbeing and healthy biological ageing**

The pathways through which wellbeing might influence how people age in terms of their physical and cognitive capability and how long they survive are not fully understood. One possible explanation is that people who are high in wellbeing have more favourable health behaviours than those who are low in wellbeing [91]. Yet it is noteworthy that several of the prospective studies of wellbeing in relation to physical capability, functional disability or mortality adjusted for at least some health behaviours, primarily physical activity and smoking, and the protective effect of greater wellbeing remained.

It may be that direct psychobiological mechanisms underline the links between wellbeing and healthier ageing. Higher levels of positive affect have been associated cross-sectionally with lower levels of cortisol and inflammatory factors and with more favourable levels of blood pressure and heart rate, and importantly, these links appear to be independent of depressive symptoms [97]. More recently, Steptoe and colleagues examined cross-sectional relationships between a wide range of biological measures and two aspects of wellbeing, eudaimonic wellbeing (sense of autonomy and purposeful engagement in life) and hedonic wellbeing (happiness and pleasure) in ELSA. Higher levels of both aspects of wellbeing were linked with less central obesity, better lung function, lower concentrations of inflammatory factors and triglycerides and higher concentrations of high-density lipoprotein cholesterol, after adjustment for depressive symptoms, smoking, and other potential confounders, with evidence of sex differences in some of these associations [98]. Prospective studies are needed to investigate whether biological correlates such as these help explain associations between facets of wellbeing and healthy ageing.

4.7 **Conclusions**

Most researchers now accept that wellbeing is best thought of as a multi-faceted construct, although it remains a matter of debate as to which components should be part of this construct. Some experts think that research into wellbeing is being hampered by the common practice of distinguishing between hedonic and eudaimonic wellbeing and by the fact that eudaimonia is not consistently defined or measured. Others have recommended a 'dashboard approach' to measurement whereby information is collected on a variety of facets of wellbeing [2]. As yet there are too few data from longitudinal and life course studies to establish whether individual facets of wellbeing vary in their antecedents or trajectories; the 'dashboard approach' to wellbeing measurement may be the best way to throw light on this in future studies.

There is growing evidence to suggest that wellbeing may be a protective factor for healthy biological ageing, but there are still uncertainties about this relationship. There is a need for more long-term studies that have repeated detailed measurements of cognitive and physical capability and different facets of wellbeing over many years to help elucidate the temporal order in which changes occur, how those changes relate to each other, and to investigate whether any protective effect of wellbeing varies depending on the domain of cognition or physical capability assessed. We also need prospective studies with detailed biological and lifestyle data in order to investigate the extent to which such factors mediate any relationship between facets of wellbeing and indicators of healthier ageing.

In 2008 the UK Government's Foresight Review on Mental Capital and Wellbeing concluded that government policies need to 'nurture the mental capital and wellbeing in the wider population so everyone can flourish in their lives' [99: p. 10]. First results on levels of national wellbeing in the UK were published in 2012 [47] enabling the government to start incorporating findings on wellbeing into the policymaking process. There has been considerable scientific pessimism as to whether it is possible to effect sustainable increases in wellbeing [100]. Lyubomirsky and colleagues suggest that of the three main factors that determine an individual's wellbeing, their set point for happiness, their life circumstances, and their intentional activities, the latter may offer most scope for developing interventions [100]. Understanding the mechanisms through which such interventions might operate and their potential long-term effects may be possible in randomized controlled trials though may be more practically addressed through analysis of longitudinal data from observational studies.

References

1 Helliwell JF, Putnam RD. The social context of wellbeing. In Huppert FA, et al., editors. The Science of Wellbeing. Oxford: Oxford University Press; 2005: 436–59.

2 Forgeard MJ, et al. Doing the right thing: measuring wellbeing for public policy. *Int J Wellbeing* 2011;**1**:79–106.

3 Diener E. Subjective well-being—the science of happiness and a proposal for a national index. *Am Psychol* 2000;**55**:34–43.

4 von Faber M, et al. Successful aging in the oldest old—who can be characterized as successfully aged? *Arch Int Med* 2001;**161**:2694–700.

5 Diener E. The evolving concept of subjective well-being: the multifaceted nature of happiness. *Adv Cell Aging Gerontol* 2003;**15**:187–219.

6 Michaelson J, et al. National Accounts of Well-being: Bringing Real Wealth onto the Balance Sheet. London: New Economics Foundation; 2009.

7 Ryan RM, Deci EL. On happiness and human potentials: a review of research on hedonic and eudaimonic well-being. *Annu Rev Psychol* 2001;**52**:141–66.

8 Seligman MEP, Csikszentmihalyi M. Positive psychology—an introduction. *Am Psychol* 2000;**55**: 5–14.

9 Tennant R, et al. The Warwick-Edinburgh Mental Well-being Scale (WEMWBS): development and UK validation. *Health Qual Life Outcomes* 2007;**5**:63.

10 Kahn RL, Juster FT. Well-being: concepts and measures. *J Soc Issues* 2002;**58**:627–44.

11 Steverink N, Lindenberg S. Which social needs are important for subjective well-being? what happens to them with aging? *Psychol Aging* 2006;**21**:281–90.

12 Samuelsson SM, et al. The Swedish centenarian study: a multidisciplinary study of five consecutive cohorts at the age of 100. *Int J Aging Hum Dev* 1997;**45**:223–53.

13 Mroczek DK, Kolarz CM. The effect of age on positive and negative affect: a developmental perspective on happiness. *J Pers Soc Psychol* 1998;**75**:1333–49.

14 Gruenewald TL, et al. Diverse pathways to positive and negative affect in adulthood and later life: an integrative approach using recursive partitioning. *Dev Psychol* 2008;**44**:330–43.

15 Brickman P, et al. Lottery winners and accident victims—is happiness relative. *J Pers Soc Psychol* 1978;**36**:917–27.

16 Fujita F, Diener E. Life satisfaction set point: stability and change. *J Pers Soc Psychol* 2005;**88**:158–64.

17 Diener E, et al. Beyond the hedonic treadmill—revising the adaptation theory of well-being. *Am Psychol* 2006;**61**:305–14.

18 Pinquart M. Correlates of subjective health in older adults: a meta-analysis. *Psychol Aging* 2001;**16**: 414–26.

19 Diener E. Subjective Well-Being. *Psychol Bull* 1984;**95**:542–75.

20 Charles ST, Carstensen LL. Social and emotional aging. *Annu Rev Psychol* 2010;**61**:383–409.

21 Stone AA, et al. A snapshot of the age distribution of psychological well-being in the United States. *Proc Natl Acad Sci USA* 2010;**107**:9985–90.

22 Blanchflower DG, Oswald AJ. Is well-being U-shaped over the life cycle? *Soc Sci Med* 2008;**66**: 1733–49.

23 Charles ST, et al. Age-related differences and change in positive and negative affect over 23 years. *J Pers Soc Psychol* 2001;**80**:136–51.

24 Kolanowski A, et al. Concordance of self-report and informant assessment of emotional well-being in nursing home residents with dementia. *J Gerontol B Psychol Sci Soc Sci* 2007;**62**:P20–7.

25 Carstensen LL, et al. Emotional experience in everyday life across the adult life span. *J Pers Soc Psychol* 2000;**79**:644–55.

26 **Sliwinski MJ, et al.** Intraindividual change and variability in daily stress processes: findings from two measurement-burst diary studies. *Psychol Aging* 2009;**24**:828–40.

27 **Fung HH, et al.** Age-related patterns in social networks among European Americans and African Americans: implications for socioemotional selectivity across the life span. *Int J Aging Hum Dev* 2001;**52**:185–206.

28 **Antonucci TC, et al.** Attachment and close relationships across the life span. *Attachment Hum Dev* 2004;**6**:353–70.

29 **Charles ST, Piazza JR.** Memories of social interactions: age differences in emotional intensity. *Psychol Aging* 2007;**22**:300–9.

30 **Stafford M, et al.** Positive and negative exchanges in social relationships as predictors of depression: evidence from the English Longitudinal Study of Aging. *J Aging Health* 2011;**23**:607–28.

31 **George LK.** Still happy after all these years: research frontiers on subjective well-being in later life. *J Gerontol B Psychol Sci Soc Sci* 2010;**65**:331–9.

32 **Carstensen LL.** Social and emotional patterns in adulthood—support for socioemotional selectivity theory. *Psychol Aging* 1992;**7**:331–8.

33 **Carstensen LL, et al.** Taking time seriously—a theory of socioemotional selectivity. *Am Psychol* 1999;**54**:165–81.

34 **Jopp D, et al.** Valuation of life in old and very old age: the role of sociodemographic, social, and health resources for positive adaptation. *Gerontologist* 2008;**48**:646–58.

35 **Beutel ME, et al.** Life satisfaction, anxiety, depression and resilience across the life span of men. *Aging Male* 2010;**13**:32–9.

36 **Heller D, et al.** The role of person versus situation in life satisfaction: a critical examination. *Psychol Bull* 2004;**130**:574–600.

37 **Steel P, et al.** Refining the relationship between personality and subjective well-being. *Psychol Bull* 2008;**134**:138–61.

38 **Gale CR, et al.** Neuroticism and extraversion in youth predict mental wellbeing and life satisfaction 40 years later. *J Res Personality.* In press. <http://www.sciencedirect.com/science/article/pii/S0092656613000901>

39 **Abbott RA, et al.** The relationship between early personality and midlife psychological well-being: evidence from a UK birth cohort study. *Soc Psychiatry Psychiatr Epidemiol* 2008;**43**:679–87.

40 **Weiss A, et al.** Happiness is a personal(ity) thing: the genetics of personality and well-being in a representative sample. *Psychol Sci* 2008;**19**:205–10.

41 **Gomez V, et al.** The influence of personality and life events on subjective well-being from a life span perspective. *J Res Pers* 2009;**43**:345–54.

42 **Headey BW, Wearing AJ.** Personality, life events and subjective well-being. Toward a dynamic equilibrium model. *J Pers Soc Psychol* 1989;**57**:731–9.

43 **Kuh D, et al.** Lifetime risk factors for women's psychological distress in midlife. *Soc Sci Med* 2002;**55**:1957–73.

44 **Stansfeld SA, et al.** Repeated exposure to socioeconomic disadvantage and health selection as life course pathways to mid-life depressive and anxiety disorders. *Soc Psychiatry Psychiatr Epidemiol* 2011;**46**:549–58.

45 **Niedwiedz CL, Katikireddi SV, Pell JP, Mitchell R.** Life course socio-economic position and quality of life in adulthood: a systematic review of life course models. *BMC Public Health* 2012;**12**:628.

46 **Pinquart M, Sorensen S.** Influences of socioeconomic status, social network, and competence on subjective well-being in later life: a meta-analysis. *Psychol Aging* 2000;**15**:187–224.

47 **Office for National Statistics.** First ONS annual experimental subjective well-being results. Available at <http://www.ons.gov.uk/ons/dcp171766_272294.pdf> (accessed 17 July 2013).

48 **Myers DG, Diener E.** Who is happy. *Psychol Sci* 1995;**6**:10–9.

49 Chandola T, et al. The effect of control at home on CHD events in the Whitehall II study: gender differences in psychosocial domestic pathways to social inequalities in CHD. *Soc Sci Med* 2004;**58**:1501–9.

50 Marmot MG, et al. Contribution of job control and other risk factors to social variations in coronary
heart disease incidence. *Lancet* 1997;**350**:235–9.

51 Stansfeld SA, et al. Psychosocial work characteristics and social support as predictors of SF-36 health
functioning: the Whitehall II study. *Psychosom Med* 1998;**60**:247–55.

52 Crosnoe R, Elder GH. Successful adaptation in the later years: a life course approach to aging. *Soc
Psychol Quart* 2002;**65**:309–28.

53 Maughan B, McCarthy G. Childhood adversities and psychosocial disorders. *Br Med Bull* 1997;**53**:
156–69.

54 McLaren L, et al. Postnatal depression and the original mother-child relationship: a prospective cohort
study. *J Affect Disord* 2007;**100**:211–9.

55 Rodgers B. Reported parental behaviour and adult affective symptoms. 1. Associations and moderating factors. *Psychol Med* 1996;**26**:51–61.

56 Huppert FA, et al. Parental practices predict psychological well-being in midlife: life-course associations among women in the 1946 British birth cohort. *Psychol Med* 2010;**40**:1507–18.

57 Rothrauff TC, et al. Remembered parenting styles and adjustment in middle and late adulthood.
J Gerontol B Psychol Sci Soc Sci 2009;**64**:137–46.

58 Stafford M, et al. (2013). Childhood material and psychosocial circumstances predict midlife subjective wellbeing. In preparation.

59 Consedine NS, Magai C. Attachment and emotion experience in later life: the view from emotions
theory. *Attachment Hum Dev* 2003;**5**:165–87.

60 Hatch SL, et al. A developmental-contextual approach to understanding mental health and well-being
in early adulthood. *Soc Sci Med* 2010;**70**:261–8.

61 Marks NF, Ashleman K. Life course influences on women's social relationships at midlife. In: Kuh D,
Hardy R, editors. A Life Course Approach to Women's Health. Oxford: Oxford University Press; 2002.

62 Wilson RS, et al. Childhood adversity and psychosocial adjustment in old age. *Am J Geriatr Psychiatry*
2006;**14**:307–15.

63 Kiernan KE, Mensah FK. Poverty, family resources and children's early educational attainment: the
mediating role of parenting. *Br Educ Res J* 2011;**37**:317–36.

64 Kessler RC, Mcleod JD. Sex-differences in vulnerability to undesirable life events. *Am Sociol Rev*
1984;**49**:620–31.

65 Berkman LF, et al. From social integration to health: Durkheim in the new millennium. *Soc Sci Med*
2000;**51**:843–57.

66 Ryff CD. In the eye of the beholder—views of psychological well-being among middle-aged and older
adults. *Psychol Aging* 1989;**4**:195–210.

67 Deci EL, Ryan RM. The 'what' and 'why' of goal pursuits: human needs and the self-determination of
behavior. *Psychol Inq* 2000;**11**:227–68.

68 Lenzi M, et al. Family affluence, school and neighborhood contexts and adolescents' civic engagement:
a cross-national study. *Am J Community Psychol* 2012;**50**:197–210.

69 Stafford M, Marmot M. Neighbourhood deprivation and health: does it affect us all equally? *Int
J Epidemiol* 2003;**32**:357–66.

70 Richards M, Huppert FA. Do positive children become positive adults? Evidence from a longitudinal
birth cohort study. *J Positive Psychol* 2011;**6**:75–87.

71 Gerstorf D, et al. Well-being affects changes in perceptual speed in advanced old age: longitudinal evidence for a dynamic link. *Dev Psychol* 2007;**43**:705–18.

72 Allerhand M, et al. The dynamic relationship between cognitive function and positive wellbeing in
older people: a prospective study using the English Longitudinal Study of Ageing. *Psychol Aging*. In press.

73 **Cooper R, et al.** Physical capability and subsequent positive mental wellbeing in older people: findings from five HALCyon cohorts. *Age.* In press.

74 **Kurland BF, et al.** Longitudinal change in positive affect in community-dwelling older persons. *J Am Geriatr Soc* 2006;**54**:1846–53.

75 **Kunzmann U, et al.** Is age-related stability of subjective well-being a paradox? Cross-sectional and longitudinal evidence from the Berlin Aging Study. *Psychol Aging* 2000;**15**:511–26.

76 **Ostir GV, et al.** Emotional well-being predicts subsequent functional independence and survival. *J Am Geriatr Soc* 2000;**48**:473–8.

77 **Milaneschi Y, et al.** Personal mastery and lower body mobility in community-dwelling older persons: the Invecchiare in Chianti Study. *J Am Geriatr Soc* 2010;**58**:98–103.

78 **Boyle PA, et al.** Purpose in life is associated with a reduced risk of incident disability among community-dwelling older persons. *Am J Geriatr Psychiatry* 2010;**18**:1093–102.

79 **James BD, et al.** Relation of late-life social activity with incident disability among community-dwelling older adults. *J Gerontol A Biol Sci Med Sci* 2011;**66**:467–73.

80 **Buchman AS, et al.** Association between late-life social activity and motor decline in older adults. *Arch Int Med* 2009;**169**:1139–46.

81 **Collins AL, et al.** Is positive well-being protective of mobility limitations among older adults? *J Gerontol B Psychol Sci Soc Sci* 2008;**63**:321–7.

82 **Unger JB, et al.** Functional decline in the elderly: evidence for direct and stress-buffering protective effects of social interactions and physical activity. *Ann Behav Med* 1997;**19**:152–60.

83 **Brummett BH, et al.** Positive emotion is associated with 6-year change in functional status in individuals aged 60 and older. *J Positive Psychol* 2011;**6**:216–23.

84 **Small BJ, et al.** Do changes in lifestyle engagement moderate cognitive decline in normal aging? Evidence From the Victoria Longitudinal Study. *Neuropsychol* 2012;**26**:144–55.

85 **Gale CR, et al.** Cognitive function in childhood and lifetime cognitive change in relation to mental wellbeing in four cohorts of older people. *PLoS One* 2012;**7**:e44860.

86 **Gow AJ, et al.** Lifetime intellectual function and satisfaction with life in old age: longitudinal cohort study. *BMJ* 2005;**331**:141–2.

87 **Gale CR, et al.** Is there a bidirectional relationship between depressive symptoms and cognitive ability in older people? A prospective study using the English Longitudinal Study of Ageing. *Psychol Med* 2012;**42**:2057–69.

88 **Lovden M, et al.** Social participation attenuates decline in perceptual speed in old and very old age. *Psychol Aging* 2005;**20**:423–34.

89 **Bassuk SS, et al.** Social disengagement and incident cognitive decline in community-dwelling elderly persons. *Ann Intern Med* 1999;**131**:165–73.

90 **Fratiglioni L, et al.** An active and socially integrated lifestyle in late life might protect against dementia. *Lancet Neurol* 2004;**3**:343–53.

91 **Boehm JK, et al.** Heart health when life is satisfying: evidence from the Whitehall II cohort study. *Eur Heart J* 2011;**32**:2672–7.

92 **Netz Y, et al.** Physical activity and psychological well-being in advanced age: a meta-analysis of intervention studies. *Psychol Aging* 2005;**20**:272–84.

93 **Chida Y, Steptoe A.** Positive psychological well-being and mortality: a quantitative review of prospective observational studies. *Psychosom Med* 2008;**70**:741–56.

94 **Krijthe BP, et al.** Is positive affect associated with survival? A population-based study of elderly persons. *Am J Epidemiol* 2011;**173**:1298–307.

95 **House JS, et al.** Social relationships and health. *Science* 1988;**241**:540–5.

96 **Holt-Lunstad J, et al.** Social relationships and mortality risk: a meta-analytic review. *PLoS Med* 2010;**7**:e1000316.

97 **Steptoe A, et al.** Positive affect and psychobiological processes relevant to health. *J Pers* 2009;**77**: 1747–76.

98 **Steptoe A, et al.** Distinctive biological correlates of positive psychological well-being in older men and women. *Psychosom Med* 2012;**74**:501–8.

99 **Foresight Mental Capital and Wellbeing Project.** Final project report. London: The Government Office for Science; 2008.

100 **Lyubomirsky S, et al.** Pursuing happiness: the architecture of sustainable change. *Rev Gen Psychol* 2005;**9**:111–31.

Part II

Methods for studying ageing from a life course and interdisciplinary perspective

Chapter 5

Design of life course studies of healthy ageing

Rebecca Hardy, Graciela Muniz-Terrera, and Scott Hofer

5.1 Introduction

The design of life course studies is vital to the delivery of good quality research on healthy ageing. The design of a study not only determines the research questions that can be addressed, but also many sources of error and bias. Many life course hypotheses can only be examined through observational studies following the same individuals over time, as randomized controlled trials will often not be possible or ethical. Appropriate statistical analyses of the collected data are also necessary to avoid bias, but analysis methods cannot ever entirely make up for inadequacies in study design. Replication is the basis of scientific discovery and carrying out analyses across multiple cohorts means findings are likely to be more robust. Caution is required in comparing across studies to ensure they are addressing exactly the same question. However, different study designs can usefully provide complementary information while addressing the same general scientific question.

The production of high quality data on large samples of individuals over time in long running longitudinal studies requires strategic planning and study management, and dedication of researchers and study participants. Participants recruited into life course studies of healthy ageing give a long-term, in some cases lifelong, commitment to a study. Thus cooperation and engagement of study members is vital to the success of such studies. Through in-depth interview and written memories, participants in the oldest British birth cohort study who were born in 1946—the Medical Research Council (MRC) National Survey of Health and Development (NSHD)—highlight the importance of a sense of study identity, their pride at being in the study, and the knowledge that the data they provide is benefitting society:

> 'I've always been proud to say I was part of it, yes. As a child I was not at all happy about being part of this cohort, but now feel it has been a privilege to be a part of it.'
>
> 'The National Survey has never gone away. Like a lifetime friend, it's always been in touch. I really hope the data continue to benefit all.'
>
> 'In short a privilege to belong to this group of people . . . I hope and know some good will have come from being a member of a band of people born in March 1946.'

In this chapter, we provide examples of the design of existing studies of healthy ageing, explore practical issues in the design and implementation of such studies. Finally, we briefly introduce analytical challenges in life course studies and across studies.

5.2 **Longitudinal and life course studies of ageing**

A life course study has been described as a cohort study that has information from at least one stage of development (gestation, childhood or adolescence) and in adult life [1]; this distinguishes it from a general cohort or longitudinal study, where individuals may be followed up repeatedly but over a shorter period of life. The study of age-related change in function across the whole of life within individuals, a central concept of a life course approach to healthy ageing (Chapter 1), requires repeated measures on the same individuals over time. To date cross-sectional studies which record the same measurement on an age-heterogeneous sample are most common in investigations of age-related changes [2]. Although such studies have the advantage that measurements are generally recorded at the same time using the same protocol, the serious disadvantage is that analyses of between-person age differences are confounded with cohort effects [3].

The vast majority of existing studies of ageing have begun in later age, recruiting participants aged over 50, or often over 65, years [4,5]. Most of these longitudinal studies of ageing are currently in westernized industrial nations, although studies in low and middle income countries (LMICs) are increasingly being initiated. Cohort studies set up to study the adult risk factors of specific diseases, in particular heart disease and cancer, have generally begun in midlife, but have now continued into older age thus providing the opportunity to study ageing in relation to midlife risk factors. Historical cohorts, such as those included in the Healthy Ageing Across the Life Course (HALCyon) Research Collaboration have linked individuals' birth records [6,7] or other early life data [8,9] with their later life health, but have gaps in information during adolescence and earlier adulthood. The ideal study design for research taking a life course approach to healthy ageing is a birth cohort, which follows the same individuals from birth (or pregnancy or even pre-conception). The oldest such cohorts are only just entering older age; the MRC NSHD being the oldest where participants turned 65 in 2011 [10,11]. Birth cohorts in LMICs, such as those in the COHORTS consortium [12], are still young.

5.3 **Data collection**

In this section we focus on challenges related to the quantitative measurement of healthy ageing and age-related change.

5.3.1 **Capturing healthy ageing**

As highlighted in Chapter 1, this book focusses on optimal functioning as the primary aspect of healthy ageing, and less on longevity and delaying the onset of age-related disease and disability. Specific measures of function are discussed in relevant chapters, so here we focus on general issues relating to the capture of healthy ageing and particularly longitudinal profiles of ageing. There has been little consensus in how to measure healthy ageing (Chapter 1), but it is generally agreed that objective measures of function should be part of the assessment; although even in this case multiple protocols for the measurement of the same function often exist. Moving forward, the National Institutes of Health (NIH) toolbox <http://www.nihtoolbox.org> may be useful in this respect. The validity and reliability of tests and instruments and the psychometric properties of scales are important, and in particular whether they have been tested in the appropriate age group. In order to study the full spectrum of ageing, normally distributed continuous measures which discriminate across the whole range of function and structure are beneficial. Categorization of continuous measurements, although possibly useful from a clinical perspective, results in a loss of information; from a life course perspective studying the pattern of change in health is of particular interest, and continuous measures also capture change more accurately.

Ideally when studying change, exactly the same measurement procedure would be used at every time point. Measurement of some aspects of function must, however, change over time as the tests need to be age appropriate. Tests of physical performance are required to get easier as participants age. For example, in a cohort in their 50s, ten chair rises are required to discriminate adequately between those with high functioning and those with moderate functioning, while fewer rises are needed in older age. When assessing cognitive development, tests need to become increasingly challenging as children get older. There is debate as to whether scales such as the Short-Form-36 (SF-36) health status questionnaire, which measures health related quality of life, are valid in older people. Investigation in the HALCyon cohorts showed the SF-36 to behave well, except for certain scales not being appropriate in those over 70 years [13]. Other quality of life scales have been specifically developed for older populations; the CASP-19 is based on theories of need satisfaction and self-actualization and measures the domains of control (C), autonomy (A), self-realization (S) and pleasure (P) [14]. It has acceptable psychometric properties [14–16], although it performed less well in an ethnically diverse cohort of older people in one study [16]. Technological advances mean that methods of measurement of the same function may improve over the lifetime of long running studies. For example, many studies have changed the instruments used to measure blood pressure (BP); from the old manual random zero sphygmomanometers to automated devices. Research suggests that conversion equations are required to make the measurements from the different machines equivalent [17] and the impact of failing to take account of such changes in longitudinal analysis of BP change has been demonstrated [18]. When investigating change, we assume that the observed differences reflect true change in the constructs being measured. Hence, whatever the reason for measurement change, evidence for the equivalence, and thus comparability, of measurements across age and time should be obtained whenever possible [19].

Scientific discovery also leads to the development of completely novel measures during the lifetime of a study. The first ultrasound assessment of cardiac anatomy was not made until 1954 by Edler and Hertz in Sweden [20] and it was not until the 1970s that it was routinely adopted in clinical practice. Although BP was first measured in the middle of the eighteenth century [21], it was not until the 1960s when the Framingham Heart Study linked high BP with coronary heart disease (CHD) [22] that it began commonly being measured in cohort studies. Objective assessments of physical capability were not introduced widely until the 1980s (Chapter 2). Hence, many measures of function have not yet been collected on the same group of individuals over the life course, as older studies do not have measurements at younger ages, while studies in which development and peak function have been captured with modern methodology must wait years to study age-related change. Perhaps the best evidence for life course trajectories to date comes from the integration of multiple longitudinal studies of different but overlapping ages [18], although cohort effects have to be considered. Within individual studies, it is necessary to balance collection of innovative new measures with continuity of measures already collected to maximize the scientific impact.

Generally, studies to date have attempted to capture a 'normal' or 'average' level of function at any given age. Hence, multiple measure of BP, lung function or physical performance are recorded and the average or maximum used in analyses. However, measurement of, for example cortisol, requires the daily pattern to be measured in order to capture potentially important patterns relevant to health (Chapter 10). There is increasing interest in the health implications of variability and short-term fluctuations in function (e.g. heart rate, BP, cognition). For example, both daily variability [23] and follow-up visit to visit variability (BP was measured approximately every

4–6 months) in BP [24] have been shown to be independent predictors of adverse outcomes, over and above mean BP. There are different timescales over which to assess relevant variability, which may be seconds, minutes, hours, days or weeks depending on the measure. Variability of the same measure over multiple timescales may also be important. The development of technology means that increasingly clinical indicators, such as BP, can be assessed over longer periods of time with study participants wearing monitors. Daily diaries or innovative modes of data collection such as mobile phone or computer-based technologies can be used to capture variations and patterns of self-reported aspects of health and lifestyle.

5.3.2 Mode of data collection

For many aspects of the study of ageing, objective assessment is the gold standard. This necessitates either that participants attend designated clinic facilities or that interviewers or research nurses visit participants' homes. Home visits mean that the type of measures that can be collected will be more restricted, although rapidly developing technology makes it possible to include more clinical and biological measures in the home setting. All measurements require a standardized protocol and central training of the researchers carrying out the data collection, and often equipment calibration. A single clinic and fewer observers results in easier standardization of measurement, but may be impractical when the sample is geographically dispersed.

Face to face visits are expensive and thus many studies collect measures of health and risk factors through the administration of questionnaires. However, self-reported measures may be biased. For example, a systematic review of studies comparing self-reported body size and measured body size showed trends toward an under-reporting for weight and body mass index (BMI) and an over-reporting for height [25], with variation according to the characteristics of the study samples. Of course, many measures of body function or structure cannot be directly self-reported and hence subjective measures are collected instead. Assessment of physical capability based on self-reports of functional limitations and performance of activities of daily living has been widely used, but these can be influenced by factors such as cognitive function. Caution is required in using performance on objective tests to make inferences about individuals' abilities to undertake the tasks of daily living [26] and the subjective and objective measures can be seen as complementary rather than equivalent alternatives. Aspects of lifestyle important for healthy ageing, such as physical activity and diet have been traditionally collected through questionnaires, and are extremely challenging to assess accurately, especially in older adults (Chapters 16 and 17). A number of questionnaires have been validated to assess physical activity in older adults, but all have limitations [27,28]. More recently it has become possible to measure activity using heart rate and movement monitors, and development of devices and algorithms to automatically interpret the data is ongoing [29]. A study in older people comparing physical activity levels using questionnaire with accelerometers and pedometers found that although objective measures of physical activity showed strong associations with health and anthropometric and psychological variables, the questionnaire score was not significantly related to most health or anthropometric measures but was associated with psychological variables [27]. Physical activity questionnaires, however, can provide information about activity type which currently objective monitoring cannot. Biological assays which require blood generally require contact with a nurse, but biological measures which can be obtained from urine or saliva samples may be collected remotely and the development of dried blood spot technology raises the possibility of also collecting blood samples remotely [30].

Some important aspects of healthy ageing such as wellbeing and quality of life cannot be measured objectively and are captured by validated scales. These may be administered at face to face interviews, telephone interviews, via postal questionnaires or, increasingly, web-based question-naires. Even in this instance, the mode of collection can have an impact on response. In a rand-omized cross-over study comparing self-completion with interviewer assessment, scores on the SF-36 were consistently lower using self-assessment than at the clinic based interviews [31]. A similar study showed that on average, reported mental status score (using the SF-12 score) was lower on the self-administered questionnaire compared to a telephone interview [32]. There will be increasing need to assess the validity of responses obtained using innovative methods of data collection such as web-based, mobile phone-based and interactive computer-based technolo-gies. A review of innovative technologies for measuring diet in nutritional epidemiology, while acknowledging the potential to provide cost- and time-effective data collection and higher par-ticipant acceptance rates, concluded that the inherent bias related to self-reported dietary intake will not be resolved and that more research is crucial [33].

Record linkage, for mortality, cancer registrations, hospital admissions and general practi-tioner (GP) records also provides vital data for many studies. Some countries, such as those in Scandinavia, are currently better able to easily link multiple sources of registry data [34]. Increasingly, studies may be based on record linkage information from multiple sources of records [35,36] with the possibility of the construction of longitudinal cohorts; although work is still required on the errors in data linkage and the impact that this has on data analysis [37]. Alternatively, medical records must be recovered individually from health care institutions by the researcher. Studies comparing self-reports of CHD and myocardial infarction with medi-cal records generally report good or moderate agreement [38–40], although variation has been observed according to sociodemographic characteristics [39].

In some studies of ageing which began in later life, earlier life information has been collected retrospectively, with the possibility of recall bias. There have been multiple studies comparing recall of earlier life characteristics with records or prospective reports. Studies generally report moderate to good agreement, but both random and systematic errors in reporting do occur and the level of agreement may vary according to study participant characteristics such as level of education [41]. The important question, however, is whether the error in a recalled risk factor has an important effect on the estimate of its relationship with the later health outcome. One study suggested that despite the moderate to good validity of recall, the associations of birthweight with childhood and adult BMI were attenuated when birthweight reported in midlife was used, hence, limiting its utility for detecting modest associations with health in later life periods [42]. Another study found substantial attenuation of the disease-exposure relationship due to reporting errors in birthweight and also age at menarche [43]. Even in birth cohort studies, a fundamental chal-lenge is that data collected can only be representative of the science of the time [44]. For example, information on parental smoking was not collected in the MRC NSHD as the link with disease was not established until the publication of the ground breaking study of British doctors by Doll and Hill in 1956 linking cigarette smoking with lung cancer [45]. Such omissions can be remedied by retrospective data collection, but are then subject to recall bias in the same way as data from studies starting later in life.

We have so far assumed that the study members themselves provide the responses to a questionnaire or interview, but this is not always the case. In birth cohort studies, the parent is often a respondent for the child study member. Of particular relevance to ageing is where the participant is unable to respond due to cognitive or other impairment. Tomkins provided a review of the literature on the validity and reliability of data from proxy respondents [46]. This review concluded that, from the evidence available, the main factors increasing validity and reliability of proxy responses are a focus on directly observable characteristics, questions requiring a binary response, use of face to face interviews, and the spouse/partner being the selected proxy.

5.3.3 Frequency of data collection

Practical and financial considerations can inevitably determine timing of data collections over and above the scientific arguments discussed here, and the burden on participants of repeated and long-term testing is also a consideration. From a scientific perspective, some ageing processes change rapidly with age and others slowly, with some changing more rapidly at certain points in life. The timing of measurement in life course research may thus need to reflect the velocity of change in the phenomena under study [47]. More regular assessment during development and age-related decline may be more helpful than during the midlife peak or plateau. Consideration should also be given to capturing key life events, which influence trajectories, such as the life transitions of marriage, job change, retirement, and biological transitions such as menopause, and clinical events, such as disease diagnosis. More detailed assessment around these events may be justified to capture their impact on trajectories. Closely spaced repeated measurements allow for non-linear changes and possible change points to be modelled (Chapter 6), while with fewer widely spaced measurements it may only be possible to model a linear rate of change. Intensive measurement designs, where repeated measurements are taken over a short period of time, can be embedded within long-term longitudinal designs [48] and thus permit the evaluation of short-term fluctuation, as well as long-term change. The required sample size to detect influences of change in longitudinal studies is dependent on the number of measurement occasions and the spacing of the measurements. Most widely spaced longitudinal designs with four (and many with three) occasions have substantial power to detect both variances and covariances among rates of change in a variety of cognitive, physical functioning, and mental health outcomes [49].

Repeated exposure to some forms of assessments, particularly tests of cognitive functioning, but also measures of physical functioning such as strength and lung function, can in itself produce change in performance. Such effects due to repeated testing are generally referred to as reactivity and can be due to warm-up effects (i.e. underperformance at baseline testing related possibly to anxiety and novelty of test conditions) and retest or practice effects (i.e. learning gains in performance due to familiarity, content learning, or strategy use). Practice effects related to content learning can be minimized by having more than one version of the same test which is then rotated at each contact, but this approach does not minimize other forms of reactivity and the use of the different forms of the test can itself introduce bias. Statistical procedures have been proposed to directly model retest effects, but these require strong and untenable assumptions because test exposure and within-person age changes are directly confounded in most longitudinal studies [50]. Measurement intensive designs have been used to model retest effects at the individual level over the short-term with changes observed over longer periods based on maximal performance [51].

5.4 Study management

Good study management is required for studies to run successfully over long periods of time. Long running studies will have gone through various different ways of collecting and storing data with changes from pen and paper based questionnaires and tests to rapidly evolving electronic and web-based systems. Computer systems and methods for storing and archiving data and documents change over the life of studies. Therefore, documentation in long term studies of ageing is of paramount importance [52] to ensure that data remain easily accessible to future researchers.

Data sharing systems, including development of systems for storing variables and classifying metadata, are evolving to meet the needs of both biomedical and social scientists and to ensure data security and participant confidentiality [1]. Ethical requirements for research change over time. For example, there have been changes in the requirements to obtain informed consent, and of particular relevance for studies of ageing, for informed consent in situations where the cohort member no longer has the capacity to give consent themselves. Issues surrounding duty of care and disclosure of results to study participants are particularly complex and much debated, most recently in the context of genetic information [53,54]. Difficult decisions have to be made, as the clinical relevance of more novel measurements remains equivocal, while it also remains questionable whether diagnoses of conditions without an effective treatment should be fed back to an apparently healthy study participant. In the NSHD, for example, ethically approved strategies detail how clinically relevant results are fed back to the cohort members directly or via their general practitioner, and immediate action is taken where necessary. Other cohorts provide no feedback on the grounds that the measurements taken are for research purposes and cannot be considered as a health screening.

Although the impact of missing data can be addressed through statistical techniques (Chapter 6), strategies for maintaining high response rates remain a priority. Loss through mortality which must be considered in analyses, is unavoidable, whereas drop out and loss of contact are avoidable. An initial step to maintaining response rates is to maintain up to date contact information for study participants. A recent experimental study using the British Household Panel Survey found that the most effective method was to mail a change of address card with an incentive conditional on return if a move occurs [55]. This study suggested that asking all study members, irrespective of whether they had moved or not, to confirm their address was not an efficient strategy. However, the amount of the incentive made no difference leading to the conclusion that the strategy rather than the value of the incentive was more important. Systematic reviews have suggested that monetary incentives, repeat mailing strategies and/or telephone reminders may improve response to one-off postal questionnaires [56,57]. However, effective strategies for retaining response rates in long running longitudinal studies remain less clear due to the difficulty in obtaining experimental evidence. The British Birth Cohorts send birthday cards to cohort members every year, also providing feedback of study findings. Qualitative work in the National Child Development Study (NCDS), the 1958 British Birth Cohort Study, found that 'feedback' was the topic most often raised by respondents when asked what would improve the experience of being part of NCDS [58]. Tailoring respondent feedback reports to the particular group could be a successful strategy. A trial suggested that tailored materials increased the overall rate of response among 'busy people' and the face to face response in 'young people' [55]. Very few NCDS participants raised payment in relation to improving experience and maximizing future participation. In line with other research, participation was influenced by the belief that their time and contribution are valued and worthwhile [59,60], and they expressed their reasons for participation in terms of 'personal fulfilment', the 'greater good' and 'obligation' [58]. Developing and maintaining relationships with participants and creating a study identity have been identified as crucial to ensuring highly motivated participants [60,61]. Response rates may vary depending on the mode of data collection. Participation rates may be lower in more impersonal communications such as telephone, postal or web-based surveys. The study members' experience of an interview is likely to influence their future participation, with the convenience of the scheduling and location of interview, the length of interview and the personal nature of questions having been highlighted as potentially important in this respect [61,62]. The characteristics and behaviour of the interviewer may also have a strong influence on participants' willingness to continue in a study [58,63,64], emphasizing the need for good interviewer training which should include equipping them with adequate information about the study.

A systematic review of drop out in studies in the over 65s identified only cognitive impairment and advancing age as predictors of attrition [65]. Lower cognitive scores in childhood have also been associated with non-response 40 to 60 years later for both postal questionnaires and face to face contacts [66,67]. The importance of offering both a home visit in older samples in addition to a clinic visit is highlighted by studies which have shown that those attending clinic are more healthy than those having home visits [67,68]. Paradata, that is data which contain information about the way in which data were collected such as the number of attempts made to contact a participant or reasons for refusal to participate, are being increasingly collected. It may be used, among other things, to identify reasons for non-response, to explore whether non-response bias is possible, and even to adjust for bias [69].

5.5 Overview of statistical methods in life course research

The statistical analysis of life course data is complex and challenging as it aims to study how risk factors from across the whole of life jointly influence later health or function and their age-related trajectories. By their very nature therefore, life course analyses will need to deal with repeated outcome variables or repeated exposure variables or both. In terms of the modelling of repeated outcome data, the statistical methods are well developed; for example, random effects models are in widespread use. Methodology is less standard when attempting to relate one time-varying measure to another and the method depends on the research question. The modelling of longitudinal outcomes is discussed in Chapter 6, as are methods for dealing with missing data; in life course research, and particularly in ageing research, the potential bias induced by high mortality rates and the increased likelihood of missing data being non-ignorable must be considered. Most explanatory variables being studied will be correlated because of common underlying pathways or because they are actually repeated measures of the same risk factor at different ages. The theoretical life course models (critical/sensitive period and accumulation) outlined in Chapter 1 have been operationalized [70], but distinguishing between these different models is challenging. When considering a continuous repeated exposure such as body size, a multitude of different approaches have been proposed. The approaches range from simpler methods based on multivariable regression [71], through two stage processes where firstly either characteristics of the growth curves [72,73], or latent classes [74,75], are extracted and then related to the outcome, to full multivariate models [76]. Chapter 7 provides further discussion of many of these models and illustration through a worked example.

5.5.1 Beyond associations to causality

One recent methodological focus in life course epidemiology is how observational studies can be used to go beyond simply demonstrating associations and help determine causality. Comparing relationships within and between family members—between generations or siblings or twins for example—can help to clarify the mechanisms underlying associations in life course studies and help to determine causality [77]. Prenatal influences can be studied by comparing the relationship between the exposure experienced by the mother during pregnancy and outcome in the offspring with that between the experience of the father to the same exposure and offspring outcome [78]. Investigating the associations between the number of children and health in men as well as women can help distinguish a biological effect of pregnancy from a social and behavioural impact of childrearing [79,80]. The fact that confounding structures vary in different populations has been used to beneficial effect to strengthen claims of causality. For example, breastfeeding was associated with lower childhood BP and BMI and higher cognition in a UK cohort (Avon Longitudinal Study of Parents and Children (ALSPAC)), but was only associated with higher cognition in studies from LMICs making up the COHORTS consortium [81]. In the COHORTS studies breastfeeding was not related to socioeconomic position as it is in the UK. Thus it can be concluded that associations of breastfeeding with child BP and BMI found in the UK and other developed countries are likely to reflect residual confounding, while breastfeeding may have causal effects on cognitive function, which is supported by findings from randomized controlled trials of breastfeeding.

Another increasingly popular approach is the use of instrumental variables such as the use of offspring BMI as an indicator of own BMI in analysis relating BMI and mortality to avoid reverse causation [82]. To date genetic instrumental variables have most commonly been used with this technique being termed Mendelian Randomization (MR) [83]. Because the genetic instrumental variable is related to the outcome only through the exposure, and is unrelated to any confounders of exposure and outcome, the relationships between instrument and outcome and between instrument and exposure can be used to derive an unconfounded estimate of the causal effect of exposure on outcome. For example, although greater adiposity was associated with increased odds of psychological distress, MR analysis using genetic variants robustly associated with adiposity suggested an inverse association [84]. In contrast MR confirmed a causal link between BMI and ischaemic heart disease [85]. A two-step epigenetic MR method has recently been proposed which may help establish the causal role of epigenetic processes in pathways to disease, since like any molecular biomarker, epigenetic markers are prone to confounding and reverse causality [86]. In addition to the instrumental variables approach, there are broadly three other causal analysis approaches [87,88]; graphical causal models [89] including the application of the theory of directed acyclic graphs (DAGs), structural equation models [90] (Chapter 6), and potential outcome or counterfactual models which include marginal structural means modelling [91] and propensity scores [92]. Propensity scores are discussed in detail in Chapter 8.

5.5.2 **Cross cohort analysis**

There is increasing awareness of the benefits of collaboration across cohort studies. Genome-wide association studies including multiple cohorts and hundreds of investigators have been at the forefront of pushing forward large consortia, but largely non-genetic groups such as HALCyon and IALSA (Integrative Analysis of Longitudinal Studies of Aging) also exist. Collaborations allow immediate replication of findings, increase the statistical power and improve the precision of estimates if meta-analysis or pooled analysis can be achieved, which may be particularly relevant for the precise estimation of null effects. Differences in findings across time and place can reveal important mechanisms and different confounding structures can be used to provide evidence of causality as illustrated in Section 5.5.1.

In order to achieve comparison, and certainly to carry out meta-analysis or pooled analysis, harmonization of data is required. The level of harmonization can vary depending on the scientific question under consideration, whether the variable to be harmonized is an outcome, the main explanatory variable or a potential confounder, and on the method of analysis. Again, genetics has been at the forefront of data harmonization infrastructure and has developed platforms and software for this purpose [93]. Addressing life course studies across cohorts is more complicated than studying genetics. There is a need to balance the additional variation due to the differences in measures with increased power of including more studies, and the need to keep a balance between the richness of data within individual studies and increasing comparability by harmonizing to the lowest common denominator. In HALCyon, measures of physical and cognitive capability have been harmonized to the extent that a meta-analysis could be used to combine results from individual studies [94]. Sensitivity analyses are important to assess the robustness of findings to the decisions made, while it is possible to allow differences in confounding variables in each study to reduce confounding as much as possible within each study. IALSA has used an integrated analysis approach where harmonized statistical methods are used across multiple studies, but no attempt is made to combine results [5,95] Collaboration between studies can also facilitate prospective harmonization of data. This is not to imply, however, that there should be total harmonization of data across similar studies. Each study has to have aspects which are unique, not least to attract funding, but also because the value of some measures collected may only become apparent much later in the lifetime of a study. Hence, studies need to be able to collect different measures of particular interest to maximize the possibilities of scientific discovery in the future.

5.6 **Conclusions**

The study of healthy ageing across the life course is a remarkable endeavour, requiring long-term commitment by both researchers and study members in order to collect quality data which can be analysed to address appropriate and important policy relevant research questions. Innovations in data collection technology and record linkage are allowing more detailed data to be collected on larger samples and on more frequent schedules of assessment. The current resource of studies available provides great opportunities for the replication and generalizability of life course hypotheses relating risk factors to function in later life and age-related change in function. Comparison across countries and across cohorts born at different times provide opportunities to assess policy implications and, in some cases, help determine causal effects. The resource can also provide the opportunity to piece together different parts of the life course story using complementary studies with different strengths and weaknesses.

References

1 Hardy R, Kuh D. Discussant chapter—the practicalities of undertaking family-based studies. In: Lawlor DA, Mishra GD, editors. Family Matters. Oxford: Oxford University Press; 2009.

2 Hofer SM, Sliwinski MJ. Design and analysis of longitudinal studies of aging. In: Birren JE, Schaie KW, editors. Handbook of the Psychology of Aging. 6th ed. San Diego: Academic Press; 2006:15–37.

3 Schaie KW. Historical processes and patterns of cognitive aging. In: Hofer SM, Alwin DF, editors. Handbook of Cognitive Aging: Interdisciplinary Perspectives. Thousand Oaks: Sage; 2008:368–83.

4 Erten-Lyons D, et al. Review of selected databases of longitudinal aging studies. *Alzheimers Dement* 2012;**8**:584–9.

5 Piccinin AM, Hofer SM. Integrative analysis of longitudinal studies on aging: Collaborative research networks, meta-analysis, and optimizing future studies. In: Hofer SM, Alwin DF, editors. Handbook on Cognitive Aging: Interdisciplinary Perspectives. Thousand Oaks: Sage Publications; 2008:446–76.

6 Syddall HE, et al. Cohort profile: the Hertfordshire cohort study. *Int J Epidemiol* 2005;**34**:1234–42.

7 Syddall HE, et al. Cohort profile: The Hertfordshire Ageing Study HAS). *Int J Epidemiol* 2010;**39**:36–43.

8 Deary IJ, et al. Cohort profile: the Lothian birth cohorts of 1921 and 1936. *Int J Epidemiol* 2012;**41**: 1576–84.

9 Martin RM, et al. Cohort profile: The Boyd Orr cohort—an historical cohort study based on the 65 year follow-up of the Carnegie Survey of Diet and Health (1937–39). *Int J Epidemiol* 2005;**34**:742–9.

10 Kuh D, et al. Cohort profile: updating the cohort profile for the MRC National Survey of Health and Development: a new clinic-based data collection for ageing research. *Int J Epidemiol* 2011;**40**:e1–e9.

11 **Pearson H.** Study of a lifetime. *Nature* 2011;**471**:20–4.

12 **Richter LM, et al.** Cohort profile: the consortium of health-orientated research in transitioning societies. *Int J Epidemiol* 2012;**41**:621–6.

13 **Mishra GD, et al.** How useful are the SF-36 sub-scales in older people? Mokken scaling of data from the HALCyon programme. *Qual Life Res* 2011;**20**:1005–10.

14 **Hyde M, et al.** A measure of quality of life in early old age: the theory, development and properties of a needs satisfaction model (CASP-19). *Aging Ment Health* 2003;**7**:186–94.

15 **Wiggins RD, et al.** The evaluation of a self-enumerated scale of quality of life (CASP-19) in the context of research on ageing: a combination of exploratory and confirmatory approaches. *Social Indicators Research* 2008;**89**:61–77.

16 **Bowling A.** The psychometric properties of the older people's quality of life questionnaire, compared with the CASP-19 and the WHOQOL-OLD. *Curr Gerontol Geriatr Res* 2009;**2009**:298950.

17 **Stang A, et al.** Algorithms for converting random-zero to automated oscillometric blood pressure values, and vice versa. *Am J Epidemiol* 2006;**164**:85–94.

18 **Wills AK, et al.** Life course trajectories of systolic blood pressure using longitudinal data from UK cohorts. *PLoS Med* 2011;**8**:e1000440.

19 **Bontempo DE, Hofer SM.** Assessing factorial invariance in cross-sectional and longitudinal studies. In: Ong AD, van Dulmen M, editors. Handbook of Methods in Positive Psychology. Oxford: Oxford University Press; 2007:153–75.

20 **Edler I, Hertz CH.** The early work of ultrasound in medicine at the University of Lund. *J Clin Ultrasound* 1977;**5**:352–6.

21 **Booth J.** A short history of blood pressure measurement. *Proc R Soc Med* 1977;**70**:793–9.

22 **Kannel WB, et al.** Factors of risk in the development of coronary heart disease—six year follow-up experience. The Framingham Study. *Ann Intern Med* 1961;**55**:33–50.

23 **Johansson JK, et al.** Prognostic value of the variability of home-measured blood pressure and heart rate: the Finn-Home Study. *Hypertension* 2012;**59**:212–8.

24 **Rothwell PM, et al.** Prognostic significance of visit-to-visit variability, maximum systolic blood pressure, and episodic hypertension. *Lancet* 2010;**375**:895–905.

25 **Connor Gorber S, et al.** A comparison of direct vs. self-report measures for assessing height, weight and body mass index: a systematic review. *Obes Rev* 2007;**8**:307–26.

26 **Guralnik JM, et al.** Physical performance measures in aging research. *J Gerontol Med Sci* 1989;**44**: M141–6.

27 **Harris TJ, et al.** A comparison of questionnaire, accelerometer, and pedometer: measures in older people. *Med Sci Sports Exerc* 2009;**41**:1392–402.

28 **Stel VS, et al.** International physical activity questionnaire: 12-country reliability and validity. Comparison of the LASA Physical Activity Questionnaire with a 7-day diary and pedometer. *J Clin Epidemiol* 2004;**57**:252–8.

29 **Warren JM, et al.** Assessment of physical activity—a review of methodologies with reference to epidemiological research: a report of the exercise physiology section of the European Association of Cardiovascular Prevention and Rehabilitation. *Eur J Cardiovasc Prev Rehabil* 2010;**17**:127–39.

30 **Gallacher J, Hofer SM.** Generating large-scale longitudinal data resources for aging research. *J Gerontol Psych Sci* 2011;**66**:i172–9.

31 **Lyons RA, et al.** SF-36 scores vary by method of administration: implications for study design. *J Public Health Med* 1999;**21**:41–5.

32 **Lungenhausen M, et al.** Randomised controlled comparison of the Health Survey Short Form (SF-12) and the Graded Chronic Pain Scale (GCPS) in telephone interviews versus self-administered questionnaires. *BMC Med Res Methodol* 2007;**7**:50.

33 **Illner A-K, et al.** Review and evaluation of innovative technologies for measuring diet in nutritional epidemiology. *Int J Epidemiol* 2012;**41**:1187–203.

34 **Naess O, et al.** Life-course influences on mortality at older ages: evidence from the Oslo Mortality Study. *Soc Sci Med* 2006;**62**:329–36.

35 **Denaxas SC, et al.** Data Resource Profile: cardiovascular disease research using linked bespoke studies and electronic health records (CALIBER). *Int J Epidemiol* 2012;**41**:1625–38.

36 **Moe JO, et al.** Trends in educational inequalities in old age mortality in Norway 1961–2009: a prospective register based population study. *BMC Public Health* 2012;**12**:911.

37 **Goldstein H, et al.** The analysis of record-linked data using multiple imputation with data value priors. *Stat Med* 2012;**31**:3481–93.

38 **Lampe FC, et al.** Validity of a self-reported history of doctor-diagnosed angina. *J Clin Epidemiol* 1999; **52**:73–81.

39 **Okura Y, et al.** Agreement between self-report questionnaires and medical record data was substantial for diabetes, hypertension, myocardial infarction and stroke but not for heart failure. *J Clin Epidemiol* 2004;**57**:1096–103.

40 **Barr EL, et al.** Validity of self-reported cardiovascular disease events in comparison to medical record adjudication and a statewide hospital morbidity database: the AusDiab study. *Intern Med J* 2009;**39**:49–53.

41 **Cooper R, et al.** Validity of age at menarche self-reported in adulthood. *J Epidemiol Community Health* 2006;**60**:993–7.

42 **Tehranifar P, et al.** Validity of self-reported birth weight by adult women: sociodemographic influences and implications for life-course studies. *Am J Epidemiol* 2009;**170**:910–7.

43 **Cairns BJ, et al.** Lifetime body size and reproductive factors: comparisons of data recorded prospectively and self reports in middle age. *BMC Med Res Methodol* 2011;**11**:7.

44 **Hardy R, Wadsworth M.** The British Birth Cohort studies: childhood influences on adult life. *American Statistical Associations 2000 Proceedings of the Section of Government Statistics and Section of Social Statistics.* Alexandria, Virginia: American Statistical Association; 2001:28–34.

45 **Doll R, Hill AB.** Lung cancer and other causes of death in relation to smoking; a second report on the mortality of British doctors. *BMJ* 1956;**2**:1071–81.

46 **Tomkins S.** Using available family members as proxies to provide information on other family members who are difficult to reach. In: Lawlor DA, Mishra GD, editors. Family Matters. Oxford: Oxford University Press; 2009.

47 Carolina Consortium on Human Development. Developmental science: a collaborative statement. In: Cairns RB, Elder GH Jr, Costello EJ, editors. Developmental Science. New York: Cambridge University Press; 1996:1–6.

48 **Walls TA, et al.** Timescale dependent longitudinal designs. In: Laursen B, et al., editors. Handbook of Developmental Research Methods. New York: Guilford Press; 2011.

49 **Rast P, Hofer SM.** Substantial power to detect variance and covariance among rates of change: simulation results based on current longitudinal studies. *Psychol Methods.* In press.

50 **Hoffman L, et al.** On the confounds among retest gains and age-cohort differences in the estimation of within-person change in longitudinal studies: A simulation study. *Psychol Aging* 2011;**26**:778–91.

51 **Sliwinski MJ, et al.** Evaluating convergence of within-person change and between-person age differences in age-heterogeneous longitudinal studies. *Res Hum Dev* 2010;**7**:45–60.

52 **Nybo Andersen A-M, et al.** Birth cohorts: a resource for life course studies. In: Lawlor DA, Mishra GD, editors. Family Matters. Oxford: Oxford University Press; 2009.

53 **Schalowitz DI, Miller FG.** Disclosing individual results of clinical research, implications of respect for participants. *JAMA* 2005;**294**:737–40.

54 **Forsberg JS, et al.** Changing perspectives in biobank research: from individual rights to concerns about public health regarding the return of results. *Eur J Hum Genet* 2009;**17**:1544–9.

55 **Fumagalli L, et al.** Experiments with methods to reduce attrition in longitudinal surveys. *J R Stat Soc A* 2013;**176**:499–519.

56 **Edwards PJ, et al.** Methods to increase response to postal and electronic questionnaires. *Cochrane Database Syst Rev* 2009;**8**:MR000008.

57 **Nakash RA, et al.** Maximising response to postal questionnaires—a systematic review of randomised trials in health research. *BMC Med Res Methodol* 2006;**23**:5.

58 **Parsons S.** Understanding participation: being part of the 1958 National Child Development Study from birth to age 50. CLS Working Paper. London: Centre for Longitudinal Studies; 2010.

59 **Cotter RB, et al.** Innovative retention methods in longitudinal research: a case study of the developmental trends study. *J Child Fam Stud* 2002;**11**:485–98.

60 **Adamson L, Chojenta C.** Developing relationships and retaining participants in a longitudinal study. *Int J Mult Res Approaches* 2007;**1**:137–46.

61 **Hunt JR, White E.** Retaining and tracking cohort study members. *Epidemiol Rev* 1998;**20**:57–70.

62 **Stouthamer-Loeber M, et al.** The nuts and bolts of implementing large-scale longitudinal studies. *Violence Vict* 1992;**71**:63–78.

63 **Blohm M, et al.** The influence of interviewers' contact behavior on the contact and cooperation rate in face-to-face household surveys. *Int J Publ Opin Res* 2007;**19**:97–111.

64 **Davis RE, et al.** Interviewer effects in public health surveys. *Health Educ Res* 2010;**25**:14–26.

65 **Chatfield MD, et al.** A systematic literature review of attrition between waves in longitudinal studies in the elderly shows a consistent pattern of dropout between differing studies. *J Clin Epidemiol* 2005;**58**:13–19.

66 **Nishiwaki Y, et al.** Early life factors, childhood cognition and postal questionnaire response rate in middle age: the Aberdeen Children of the 1950s study. *BMC Med Res Methodol* 2005;**5**:16.

67 **Stafford M, et al.** Using a birth cohort to study ageing: representativeness and response rates in the National Survey of Health and Development. *Eur J Ageing* 2013;**10**:145–57.

68 **Kearney PM, et al.** Comparison of centre and home-based health assessments: early experience from the Irish Longitudinal Study on Ageing (TILDA). *Age Ageing* 2011;**40**:85–90.

69 **Stoop I, et al.** Paradata in the European Social Survey: studying nonresponse and adjusting for bias. *Proceedings of the Survey Research Methods Section.* Alexandria, Virginia: American Statistical Association; 2010:407–21.

70 **Mishra GD, et al.** A structured approach to modelling the effects of binary exposure variables across the life course. *Int J Epidemiol* 2009;**38**:528–37.

71 **Cole TJ.** The life course plot in life course analysis. In: Pickles A, Maughan B, Wadsworth MEJ, editors. Epidemiological Methods in Life Course Research. Oxford: Oxford University Press; 2007: 137–55.

72 **Tilling K, et al.** Associations of growth trajectories in infancy and early childhood with later childhood outcomes. *Am J Clin Nutr* 2011;**94**:1808S–13S.

73 **Sandhu J, et al.** Timing of puberty determines serum insulin-like growth factor-I in late adulthood. *J Clin Endocrinol Metab* 2006;**91**:3150–7.

74 **Wills AK, et al.** Population heterogeneity in trajectories of midlife blood pressure: the 1946 British birth cohort study. *Epidemiology* 2012;**23**:203–11.

75 **Silverwood RJ, et al.** Early-life overweight trajectory and CKD in the 1946 British birth cohort study. *Am J Kidney Dis* 2013. Epub ahead of print May 25. doi: pii: S0272-6386(13)00777-4. 10.1053/j.ajkd. 2013.03.032.

76 **De Stavola B, et al.** Statistical issues in life course epidemiology. *Am J Epidemiol* 2006;**163**:84–96.

77 **Lawlor DA, Mishra GD.** Why family matters: an introduction. In: Lawlor DA, Mishra GDeditors, Family Matters. Oxford: Oxford University Press; 2009.

78 **Davey Smith G, et al.** Challenges and novel approaches in the epidemiological study of early life influences on later disease. *Advances in Experimental and Medical Biology* 2009;**646**:1–14.

79 **Hardy R, et al.** Number of children and cardiovascular risk factors at age 53 years in men and women. *BJOG* 2007;**114**:721–30.

80 **Lawlor DA, et al.** Is the association between parity and coronary heart disease due to biological effects of pregnancy or adverse lifestyle risk factors associated with child-rearing? Findings from the British Women's Heart and Health Study and the British Regional Heart Study. *Circulation* 2003;**107**:1260–4.

81 **Brion MJ, et al.** What are the causal effects of breastfeeding on IQ, obesity and blood pressure? Evidence from comparing high-income with middle-income cohorts. *Int J Epidemiol* 2011;**40**:670–80.

82 **Davey Smith G, et al.** The association between BMI and mortality using offspring BMI as an indicator of own BMI: large intergenerational mortality study. *BMJ* 2009;**339**:b5043.

83 **Davey Smith G, Ebrahim S.** What can Mendelian randomisation tell us about modifiable behavioural and environmental exposures? *BMJ* 2005;**330**:1076–9.

84 **Lawlor DA, et al.** Using genetic loci to understand the relationship between adiposity and psychological distress: a Mendelian randomization study in the Copenhagen General Population Study of 53,221 adults. *J Intern Med* 2011;**269**:525–37.

85 **Nordestgaard BG, et al.** The effect of elevated body mass index on ischemic heart disease risk: causal estimates from a Mendelian randomisation approach. *PLoS Med* 2012;**9**:e1001212.

86 **Relton CL, Davey Smith G.** Two-step epigenetic Mendelian randomization: a strategy for establishing the causal role of epigenetic processes in pathways to disease. *Int J Epidemiol* 2012;**41**:161–76.

87 **Greenland S, Brumback B.** An overview of relations among causal modelling methods. *Int J Epidemiol* 2002;**31**:1030–7.

88 **Pickles A, De Stavola B.** An overview of models and methods for life course analysis. In: Pickles A, Maughan B, Wadsworth M, editors. Epidemiological Methods in Life Course Research. Oxford: Oxford University Press; 2007.

89 **Robins JM.** Data, design, and background knowledge in etiologic inference. *Epidemiology* 2001;**10**: 37–41.

90 **Bollen KA.** Structural equations with latent variables. New York: Wiley; 1989.

91 **Robins JM, et al.** Marginal structural models and causal inference in epidemiology. *Epidemiology* 2000;**11**:550–60.

92 **Rosenbaum PR, Rubin DB.** The central role of the propensity score in observational studies for causal effects. *Biometrika* 1993;**70**:41–55.

93 **Fortier I, et al.** Quality, quantity and harmony: the DataSHaPER approach to integrating data across bioclinical studies. *Int J Epidemiol* 2010;**39**:1383–93.

94 **Cooper R, et al.** Age and gender differences in physical capability levels from mid-life onwards: the harmonisation of data from eight UK cohort studies. *PLoS ONE* 2011;**6**:e27899.

95 **Hofer SM, Piccinin AM.** Integrative data analysis through coordination of measurement and analysis protocol across independent longitudinal studies. *Psychol Methods* 2009;**14**:150–64.

Chapter 6

Longitudinal data analysis in studies of healthy ageing

Graciela Muniz-Terrera and Rebecca Hardy

6.1 Introduction

As discussed in Chapter 1, life course functional trajectories are a dynamic way of studying life-time influences on health and ageing. Gaining a better understanding of trajectories of physical and cognitive capability, and of the physiological systems on which they depend, permit the identification of critical or sensitive periods of development and decline, and of the relative impact of early and later life exposures on these changes.

Longitudinal study designs are necessary to describe functional trajectories. In addition to the study design and data collection strategies discussed in Chapter 5, there is a need to consider the analytical method best suited to address any proposed research question. A range of analytical tools are available. The choice of analytical method has to be based on a match between the method and the question asked, and the decision should be made in the context of study design, the nature of the outcome variable to be modelled, features of the exposure, and the extent of missing observations.

In this chapter we present a series of statistical models that have been proposed to evaluate specific questions regarding change in single and multiple outcomes; we discuss considerations that may affect inferences that can be made when these methods are employed. Taking the perspective of a researcher who is interested in identifying the most appropriate method to address a specific hypothesis, we formulate a series of questions and suggest models that can be considered to elucidate each question. As missing data are likely to be present in longitudinal studies and may have a serious impact on model estimates and inferences, we conclude with a brief description of statistical techniques that can be used to minimize the effect of missing data on model estimates.

6.2 Modelling functional trajectories: discrete versus continuous change

When modelling functional trajectories over the life course, an initial step is to conceptualize whether change will be regarded as occurring in discrete states or along a continuum. Multistate models (MSMs) are used to analyse a stochastic process that, at any moment in time, occupies one of a series of discrete states. MSMs permit the estimation of transition rates between the discrete states and the identification of factors that are relevant for these transitions. For a discussion of MSMs and their applications in epidemiology, see Commenges [1]. MSMs are not suitable for the examination of trajectories of change, as implicitly, a trajectory implies that change is conceptualized on a continuum.

When the outcome of interest is measured on only two occasions, difference (change) scores are often used to quantify change, although they have several limitations [2]. For instance, difference scores can only be calculated for individuals with complete data, which may result in a significant bias of estimates of change, are likely to be affected by regression to the mean, and may reflect measurement error rather than true change [3,4]. Change in a construct can only be modelled reliably when at least three repeated measures of the outcome of interest are available. The chapter therefore focuses on continuous change where three or more repeated outcome measurements are available.

Several statistical models describe change as a continuous process. Generalized estimating equation (GEE) models [5], for instance, are an extension of general linear models that take into account the correlated nature of the repeated measures on the same individuals. GEE models describe marginal or mean change, permit the inclusion of covariates and the use of all available data, though under assumptions that might not be realistic (Section 6.7). Although GEE models inform us about mean change, we are interested in understanding variation between individuals and in identifying possible sources of divergence between individual ageing trajectories. Mean change is a form of data aggregation that does not inform about these and therefore the utility of GEE models in the presence of heterogeneity across individual trajectories is rather limited.

Random effects (RE) models [6], also known as multilevel or mixed effects models, permit the description of a population mean trajectory while also providing information about the heterogeneity of individuals' trajectories around this population mean. Time invariant and time varying covariates can be easily incorporated into RE models. Because of this flexibility a simple RE model could be considered, for instance, to test hypotheses about the effect of early life exposures on later life ageing processes. RE models are almost equivalent to latent growth models (LGMs), which are models for repeated measures formulated within a structural equation modelling (SEM) approach.

6.3 Random effects and latent growth models

For simplicity, we present the mathematical representation of a RE model that describes change in the outcome as occurring at a constant rate, although extensions to models describing non-linear change are straightforward.

RE models are often formulated using a set of equations that represent change at the individual level (level 1) and differences between individuals (level 2).

Let Y be a continuous variable observed in $i = 1, \ldots, N$ individuals at occasions $t = 1, \ldots T_{n_i}$ (note that the number of observations may vary by individual). The level 1 equation describing change in individual i can be written as:

$$Y_{it} = \beta_{0i} + \beta_{1i} T_{it} + \varepsilon_{it} \tag{1}$$

where β_{0i} represents the intercept (or level) of Y for individual i at time 0 (time 0 to be defined by the researcher, as discussed in Section 6.4), and β_{1i} represents the rate of change in outcome Y per unit of change in time T. The error term, ε_{it} is assumed to be normally distributed with mean zero and variance σ^2. Individual level parameters (level β_{0i} and rate of change β_{1i}) are modelled as a function of population mean parameters and covariates of interest in level 2 equations as follows:

$$\begin{cases} \beta_{0i} = \beta_{00} + \gamma_0 X_0 + \upsilon_{0i} \\ \beta_{1i} = \beta_{11} + \gamma_1 X_1 + \upsilon_{1i} \end{cases} \tag{2}$$

Here, parameters β_{00} and β_{11} represent mean level and rate of change for an individual with values of zero in time invariant covariates X_0 and X_1 (both covariates measured at study entry or before). Coefficients γ_0 and γ_1 represent the effect of covariate X_0 on the level of Y at the set origin (time = 0) and the effect of X_1 on rate of change, respectively. Residuals v_{0i} and v_{1i} are assumed to be normally distributed, with mean zero and covariance matrix Σ and independent of the error term ε_{it}. Textbooks describing different technical and more applied aspects and applications of random effects models abound in the statistical and applied literature [7,8].

As standard RE models have strict distributional assumptions, data transformations have been suggested when these assumptions are not fulfilled. However, results obtained from models fitted to transformed variables can be difficult to interpret. Alternative approaches exist, which can all be implemented in the RE framework, particularly when dealing with skewed data, or with data affected by ceiling and floor effects. Tobit models have been shown to deal adequately with both ceiling and floor effects [9]. Other models, used in the context of cognitive tests, relax the assumption of normality for the conditional distribution of the outcome variable, and propose the consideration of alternative distributions to account for non-standard features of the outcome variable [10].

Latent growth models are formulated within an SEM framework to describe change over time in a variable measured repeatedly in a sample of individuals [11]. A mathematical representation of the LGM is similar to the RE model. One difference between LGM and random effects models is that in LGM it is not assumed that the level 1 and level 2 residuals are always normally distributed and homoscedastic. To obtain full equivalence between models, the further assumption of Var (ε_{it}) = constant for all t is required in the LGM [8,11].

SEM models are often represented using diagrams where observed variables are represented within squares, latent variables within ellipses, covariances with curved arrows and other associations (for example regressions) with straight arrows. Following these conventions, Figure 6.1 provides a graphical representation of an LGM equivalent to the RE model defined by equations 1 and 2 above. For simplicity we assume here that the outcome variable Y was measured on four occasions and we consider a common set of covariates X that impact the level and rate of change of variable Y.

Models can be easily extended in a SEM framework. For example, growth mixture models (GMMs) extend LGMs by relaxing the assumption that all individuals belong to the same population defined by their trajectory. GMMs identify groups (subpopulations) of individuals with similar trajectories, and have been applied to identify groups of individuals with similar trajectories

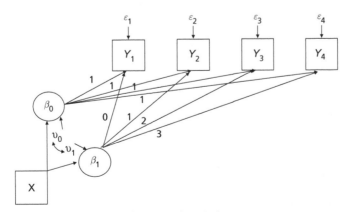

Figure 6.1 SEM diagram of a LGM that describes change that occurs at constant rate.

of cognitive function [12] and of blood pressure (BP) [13]. These models are used in Chapter 7 to link subgroups of body size trajectories with subsequent BP.

6.4 Separation of between-person and within-person effects

To obtain accurate estimates of change at the person level when analysing data from studies where the sample is age heterogenous at study entry (that is, when the study is not a birth cohort), it is necessary to separate the information provided by between-person differences from differences provided by each individual's own data (within-person differences). In age-based models fitted to age heterogeneous samples, estimates of level and rate of change will convey information that combines within-person and between-person effects and thus have no clear interpretation [14], unless separated explicitly. Results of models which do not separate within- and between-person information will only be valid under the age convergence hypothesis, which states that a measurement should only depend on the age at which the particular observation was made and not on when the individual was that particular age. For example, the inclusion of baseline age as a model covariate will inform us about how different an individual who joins the study at any given age is from an individual who reaches that same age during the study.

6.5 Matching research questions and methods

We first present a series of questions regarding change in a single outcome with time independent and time dependent covariates and then discuss questions regarding change in multiple outcomes. When we refer to 'baseline', we mean the point in a study at which the first of the repeated measurements was made. This may be entry into a study, but in a life course study this will not necessarily be the case.

6.5.1 Modelling change in single outcomes

Q1. What is the effect of a time independent covariate measured before or at baseline on level and rate of change? For example, what is the effect of adolescent body mass index (BMI) on the level and rate of change in mid to later life BP?

A classical RE model as represented in equations 1 and 2 or, equivalently, by the LGM model in Figure 6.1, can be employed to address this question. The inclusion of the time independent covariate (adolescent BMI, which is measured before baseline) on both level 2 equations permits the evaluation of whether the covariate is associated with level and rate of change.

Estimates obtained for parameters β_{00} and β_{11} are conditional on model covariates, that is, they represent level and rate of change for an individual with a value of zero in the covariate (to facilitate interpretation and estimation, covariates are usually centred at the sample mean, although they can be centred at other relevant values). Interpretation of parameters γ_0 and γ_1 is as in linear regression models. For instance, if γ_0 is estimated as a positive quantity, it will represent the amount by which the outcome (BP) level at $t = 0$ increases per one unit change in the covariate (BMI). If the estimate is negative, it represents the decrease in BP per one unit change in BMI. Although often not reported, random effects variance estimates provide relevant information regarding how much between-individual variance remains unexplained after adjustment for the variation explained by covariates included in the model.

Q2. What changes can be expected in an outcome once we partial out the effect of a time varying covariate? For example, what is the pattern of BP change once the effect of repeated measures of BMI on BP is removed?

A simple extension of the basic RE or LGM model can help answer this question. The level 1 equation (equation 1) is extended to include a time varying covariate TV_{it}, as follows:

$$Y_{it} = \beta_{0i} + \beta_{1i}T_{it} + \gamma_t TV_{it} + \varepsilon_{it}. \tag{3}$$

A simplified version (not showing errors and covariances between latent factors) of an LGM diagram including a time varying covariate (TVC) is shown in Figure 6.2(a), where the TVC is assumed to have a contemporaneous effect on the outcome. As before, in Figure 6.2(a) the TVC, X, is included at the level and rate of change of the outcome variable Y. Lindwall and colleagues [15], for instance, considered this modelling approach to describe associations over time between physical activity and cognitive change in older adults.

Although it is often assumed that the TVC has a constant effect on the outcome over time (γ_t = constant for every t), this assumption can be relaxed. LGM with TVCs have been discussed thoroughly in several textbooks [11,16]. For instance, Bollen and Curran [11] in an informative presentation of the interpretation of results of LGM with TVCs emphasize that when including a TVC, the growth process is estimated on the adjusted measure of the outcome.

TVCs, similar to outcome measures in age heterogeneous samples, are also composed of two sources of information: between- and within-individual. Hoffman and Stawski [17] suggested the disaggregation of between- from within-person information in the TVC by applying different centring techniques to the TVC. For example, when the TVC is grand-mean centred (that is, a constant is subtracted from the TVC), the level 1 effect of the TVC represents a weighted combination of both between- and within-person effects when included by itself. However, when the person-mean of the TVC is also included in the level 1 equation, then the level 1 TVC effect represents the within-person effect. But if person-mean centring (where the person-mean is subtracted from each value of the TVC) is used then the level 1 effect of the TVC only contains information about within-person variation, regardless of whether the person-mean predictor is included or not.

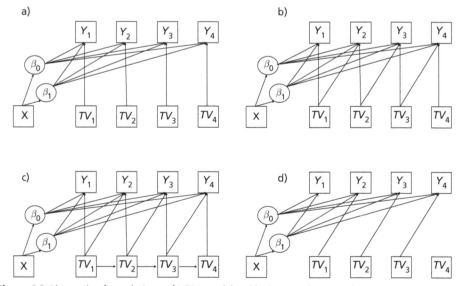

Figure 6.2 Alternative formulations of LGM models with time varying covariates.

Figures 6.2(b) to 6.2(d) depict three other possible formulations of growth models with TVCs. Figure 6.2(b) depicts a LGM where the TVC has a lagged effect on the outcome variable Y, Figure 6.2(c) shows simultaneous, contemporaneous and lagged effects of the TVC, and Figure 6.2(d) shows a model allowing for associations between consecutive measures of the TVC, in addition to contemporaneous and lagged effects of the TVC. The assumption of a contemporaneous effect of the TVC on the outcome may not be realistic in certain situations, and missing observations of the TVC may affect model results unless handled adequately with statistical techniques (Section 6.7).

Q3. How do changes in a TVC impact changes in the outcome? For example, how does BP change once we take into account changes in BMI?

Now, instead of being interested in BP change net of the effect of BMI on BP measures as in question 2, we aim to describe BP trajectories after removal of the effect of change in BMI.

A simple approach to understand the effect of changes in a TVC on the outcome Y, would be to calculate difference or change scores of the TVC and include these change scores in a growth model fitted to the outcome in ways similar to those described under question 2. Alternative versions of difference scores can be calculated depending on whether we are interested in assessing change in the TVC from the initial measurement or change between two consecutive measurement occasions. As these models involve the calculation of change scores, they inherit well studied limitations of such scores discussed in Section 6.2.

A two stage approach can be used, where trajectories of the TVC are first estimated using a growth model, and then parameters of interest derived from these trajectories (for example, rate of change) are included as covariates in a second model that describes changes in the primary outcome [18]. However, relevant information, such as random effects variances, are not taken into account when transitioning between these models.

Longitudinal mediation models are relatively new and provide an excellent opportunity to test additional important hypotheses. Mediation models are used, in general, to describe how one variable has an effect on another through a third variable. So, for example, how does physical activity relate to BP through BMI? Robittaille and colleagues [19], employed this approach using data from several longitudinal studies of ageing to test the processing speed hypothesis; this states that changes in processing speed mediate age-related changes in memory. They reported significant within-person indirect effects of changes in age predicting changes in the cognitive outcomes through changes in speed, although results were not consistent across studies. That is, increasing age relates to lower speed which, in turn, relates to lower performance on other cognitive outcomes (across repeated measures).

Multilevel structural equation models (MSEMs) used to fit mediation models take advantage of both multilevel models (focus on the differentiation between level 1 and level 2 components) and SEM features (focus on means and covariances) to analyse longitudinal data [20,21]. In the MSEM, regression paths between the variables are included at level 1 and level 2, allowing examination of direct and indirect effects both within and between individuals, each controlling for the other [21,22]. Technical and applied aspects of mediation models are thoroughly discussed in MacKinnon [23].

6.5.2 Modelling change in multiple outcomes

We now consider the scenario where we are interested in modelling change in two outcomes. We regard both variables collected repeatedly as equal, as opposed to the models discussed in the preceding sections, where the emphasis was in understanding change in a single primary outcome. As the ageing process does not occur on a single dimension, understanding change in multiple domains is crucial for gaining a better understanding of ageing and testing long standing hypotheses such as the common cause hypothesis.

Q4. What is the covariation between two processes measured over time? For example, do individuals who have a faster rate of BMI change also have a faster rate of BP change?

Multivariate LGM models, an extension of the univariate LGM model and also known as correlated models of change, permit the evaluation of such questions. Deary and colleagues [24] employed bivariate models to test associations between grip strength and verbal reasoning in older individuals showing that although their levels were correlated, their rates of change were not.

Correlated models of change describe the trajectory of each of the outcomes of interest, allowing the shape parameters of both trajectories (e.g. level and rate of change) to be correlated. These models account for within-person change, between-person changes in initial level, and rate of change; are flexible regarding the curves fitted to each of the processes; and can be fitted to model change in more than two outcomes. The correlations derived from these models do, however, need to be interpreted with care, as they depend on the placement of the intercept. Therefore, only correlations between rate of change, in the case of a model assuming change occurring at a constant rate, are meaningful, as they are independent of the location of the intercept. In models that assume an accelerating or decelerating trajectory (quadratic models), the growth rate is given by a combination of the linear and quadratic terms and depends on the value of the time variable. Therefore, correlations between linear terms of each outcome, or between the intercept of one outcome and the linear term of the other, are meaningless.

6.6 **Relevant considerations when modelling change**

In this section, we discuss two important challenges that need to be addressed when modelling trajectories of change, regardless of which of the models previously presented is employed. These are: (1) age-based vs. process-based models; and (2) choice of parametric shape to best describe the data.

6.6.1 **Age-based vs. process-based models**

It has long been suggested [25] that chronological age does not have any explanatory value in characterizing individuals' functioning, and therefore, modelling change as a function of chronological age may not be optimal. Although the choice of a suboptimal time metric to describe change does not impact the estimation of individual trajectories (changing the time metric represents a simple re-centring of the time index), the estimated mean curve obtained from such models will be biased. This is because data from individuals will be misaligned according to a time metric that does not reflect the process that is driving change.

Sliwinski and colleagues [26], for example, when analysing data from individuals with dementia, showed that models that described change as a function of time to dementia diagnosis fitted the data better than models that described change as a function of chronological age. Similarly, when analysing data from a deceased sample, models describing change as a function of time to death may fit the data better than models that described change as a function of age [26]. The use of time to event metrics may be limited where the event cannot be identified reliably. For example, dementia diagnosis may not reflect the onset of the disease, as individuals usually start experiencing symptoms a long time before being formally diagnosed.

When change is modelled as a function of alternative time metrics, the sole inclusion of baseline age does not separate between-individual from within-individual sources of information adequately (Section 6.4). For instance, when investigating the terminal decline hypothesis and modelling change as a function of distance to death, we are interested in understanding the differences between individuals who join the study closer to death and those who join the study further from death. In this case, Piccinin and colleagues [27] proposed the simultaneous inclusion of baseline age and distance to death at baseline. Further work is needed to identify the best ways to separate such sources when other possible time metrics are considered.

6.6.2 **Choice of parametric shape**

When analysing repeated measures collected on at least three occasions, a range of parametric curves and non-parametric approaches (such as Bayesian adaptive splines [28]) could be used to describe the evolution of the outcome variable. The choice of which curve best describes the evolution of a process is often conducted via comparison of fit indices such as the Bayesian Information Criterion [29] over a series of candidate models. Theoretical considerations are also important as are design features, such as the number of occasions in which measures were collected, that may restrict the spectrum of polynomial curves that can be used to describe change. For example, identifiability of a model describing change following a polynomial curve of order p requires at least p + 2 waves of data [3]. Models that describe an accelerating or decelerating trajectory, exponential, and s-shaped models, parametric functions with cycles, and change point models, are other popular options with interpretable parameters.

Change point models are an example of models that describe non-linear change that have become increasingly popular in the epidemiological literature, as they permit the identification of the onset of a change in velocity. They can be employed to answer relevant life course questions, such as whether early life factors are associated with a later onset of rapid age-related decline. Change point models often describe two phases of a process where individuals decline at different rates in each. In fixed change point models, the change point is fitted as a fixed effect, and therefore assumes that all individuals experience a change in their rate of change at the same point in time [30]. This very strong assumption of a common onset may limit their applicability. More flexible formulations that regard the change point as a random effect, allowing each individual to have a different change point, have also been developed [31,32].

Bivariate versions of change point models [33] that identify the onset of a change in velocity in two outcome variables and estimate the correlation between such onsets, have also been developed. These models permit researchers to test hypotheses related to the temporal ordering of the onset of change in rate of decline and answer longstanding questions such as, 'does it all go together when it goes?'. Most applications of multivariate models have examined the effect of time independent exposures on the outcome trajectory. However, from a theoretical perspective, there are no limitations to including TVCs in each of the sub-models of the correlated model of change.

In some models, parameter interpretation may depend on the location of the intercept. For example, in a quadratic growth curve model, the linear term is usually interpreted as the instantaneous rate of change at time $t = 0$, whilst at other times, the rate of change is a combination of the linear and quadratic terms that depends on time (first derivative of the level 1 equation with respect to t).

Linear transformation of the time metric has been suggested as a way of testing whether covariates have a differential effect at particular stages of a process. For example, this can be achieved by placing the intercept at the end, rather than at the beginning, of the observational period. However, this may result in biased results in studies with missing data. Linear and other transformations of the time metric are discussed in Bollen and Curran [11].

6.7 **Missing data**

Missing data, whether due to design, dropout or death, are unavoidable in longitudinal and life course studies of ageing and can bias estimates if not accounted for properly. Although much research is based on complete case analysis where only individuals with complete data are included in models, methods exist to deal with incomplete data. Amongst *ad hoc* methods, the most commonly used methods are imputation of simple mean, regression mean imputation, and last observation carried forward. These methods do not consider statistical principles and have been shown to result in misleading conclusions [34].

We first introduce some notation. Let R_{ij} be an indicator that takes the value of 1 if person i is observed at time j and 0 if the person was not observed at time j, $\mathbf{R}'_i = (R_{i1}, R_{i2}, \ldots R_{in})$, a vector of missing data indicators and $\mathbf{y}'_i = (y_{i1}, y_{i2}, \ldots y_{in})$, the vector of complete dependent variable. This vector can be partitioned into an observed component $\mathbf{y}_i^O$ and unobserved $\mathbf{y}_i^M$, where $\mathbf{y}_i^O$ is the observed vector of person i and $\mathbf{y}_i^M$ the component of $\mathbf{y}'_i$ that although planned to be observed, was not.

The most basic missing data mechanism is one that assumes that missing observations *are missing completely at random* (MCAR), that is, when the probability of an observation being missing does not depend on either the observed or the unobserved data. A MCAR mechanism implies that the missing data indicators R_{ij} are independent of both $\mathbf{y}_i^O$ and $\mathbf{y}_i^M$, or that $[R \,|\, Y, X] = [R]$.

Missing at random (MAR), instead, allows the missingness to depend on both fully observed model covariates and the observed dependent variable. It assumes that, conditional on these, the missing data are not related to the unobserved dependent variable. In this case, missing observations depend on $\mathbf{y}_i^O$, that is, $[R \,|\, Y, X] = [R \,|\, X]$. Finally, a missing data mechanism is said to be *missing not at random* (MNAR) when the missingness depends on the unobserved dependent variable, that is, when missingness depends on $\mathbf{y}_i^M$, once observed variables such as covariates and observed outcome are considered. In practical terms, it is impossible to test whether the missing data mechanism is MAR or MNAR, as unobserved data are part of both definitions. Related to these definitions is the concept of ignorable missing data. Missing data are said to be ignorable if the missing data are MAR and the parameters of the data model and those of the missing mechanism are distinct [35].

Methods for analysis of longitudinal data discussed in the previous section can be employed with incomplete data under certain assumptions. RE models produce estimates that are robust in the presence of ignorable missing data, whilst GEE make more restrictive assumptions and provide robust estimates under MCAR.

Multiple imputation is one of the most popular methods of dealing with missing data [36], and is particularly recommended when missing observations occur in the covariates. Multiple copies of completed datasets are created and analysed, and estimates obtained from the analysis of each of these completed datasets combined according to Rubin's rules. Guidelines on how and when to perform multiple imputation have been discussed thoroughly [37], and multiple imputation can be conducted in most statistical software packages. Strategies of multiple imputation in longitudinal studies have been discussed by Spratt and colleagues [38].

Models for non-ignorable missing data are of particular interest as this is a missing data mechanism likely to be present in longitudinal studies of ageing. Several methods have been developed in the context of longitudinal models with non-ignorable missing data [39,40].

The shared RE parameters model has been considered in ageing research to account for non-ignorable missing data [41]. It formulates a model composed of two sub-models: one describing change in the outcome variable and the other describing the missing data. Both sub-models are linked via a term that relates the random effects from the longitudinal model with the missing data model. This model permits an assessment of both survival and the evolution of the longitudinal ageing process simultaneously, whilst informing us about the association between both processes. For example, we may be interested in determining the probability of survival and good functioning in 5 years' time. An excellent review of shared parameter models can be found in Tsiatis and Davidian [42].

With the increasing application of shared RE models, user friendly routines for their implementation have been developed in some statistical software packages. Examples include the routine JM in Stata, JoinedR in R; and for a comparison of a Bayesian implementation and the routine considered in SAS, see Guo and Carlin [43].

6.8 **Conclusion**

In this chapter, we described a series of models that can be used to describe change in a single outcome and evaluate the effect of time independent and time dependent covariates, and models that describe change in an outcome in the presence of changes in the TVC and multivariate models. We highlighted some of the challenges related to the modelling of longitudinal data, such as the metric over which to describe change, the separation of between-person from within-person effects, and the choice of the parametric shape that best describes the data. Missing data provide a further particular challenge in life course studies and particularly in longitudinal ageing studies. It is not possible to test whether the missing data mechanism is ignorable or not, and therefore sensitivity analyses are recommended to evaluate the impact of the missing data assumptions on model results.

Throughout the chapter, we alternated the presentation between the traditional random effects model and the SEM framework. While some extensions of the models presented are most naturally conceived within an SEM framework, others are more naturally framed within the traditional hierarchical modelling context.

A variety of software packages are available to users to fit the models discussed in this chapter. Random effects models can be fitted in statistical packages such as MLWin [44], R [45], and Stata [46]. Mplus [47] and Lisrel [48] are two user friendly SEM software packages that can be used to fit most SEM models discussed in this chapter. Stata has recently started to develop add-ons for estimation of SEM models. Available routines are limited although under constant development. Researchers interested in implementing the models discussed here using Bayesian estimation are referred to the different versions of BUGS [49]. Most software packages are under constant development. Therefore, careful consideration of the limitations and capabilities of the different software packages that can be used to fit the models of interest is required before embarking on data analysis.

References

1 Commenges D. Multi-state models in epidemiology. *Lifetime Data Anal* 1999;5:315–27.
2 Bereiter C. Some persisting dilemmas in the measurement of change. In: Harris CW, editor. Problems in Measuring Change. Madison, WI: University of Wisconsin Press; 1963:3–20.
3 Fitzmaurice G. A conundrum in the analysis of change. *Nutrition* 2001;17:360–1.
4 Fitzmaurice G. How to explain an interaction. *Nutrition* 2001;17:170–1.
5 Liang KY, Zeger SL. Longitudinal data analysis using generalized linear models. *Biometrika* 1986;73:13–22.

6 Laird NM, Ware JH. Random-effects models for longitudinal data. *Biometrics* 1982;**38**:963–74.

7 Verbeke G, Molenberghs G. Linear Mixed Models for Longitudinal Data. New York: Springer; 2009.

8 Raudenbush SW, Bryk AS. Hierarchical Linear Models: Applications and Data Analysis Methods. Thousand Oaks: Sage Publications; 2001.

9 Wang L, et al. Investigating ceiling effects in longitudinal data analysis. *Multivariate Behav Res* 2008;**43**: 476–96.

10 Muniz-Terrera G, et al. Analysing cognitive test data: distributions and non-parametric random effects. *Stat Methods Med Res* 2012;**6**:6.

11 Bollen KA, Curran PJ. Latent Curve Models. Hoboken, NJ: Wiley-Interscience; 2006.

12 Muniz-Terrera G, et al. One size fits all? Why we need more sophisticated analytical methods in the explanation of trajectories of cognition in older age and their potential risk factors. *Int Psychogeriatr* 2010;**22**:291–9.

13 Wills A, et al. Population heterogeneity in trajectories of midlife blood pressure. *Epidemiology* 2012;**23**:203–11.

14 Hoffman L, et al. On the confounds among retest gains and age-cohort differences in the estimation of within-person change in longitudinal studies: a simulation study. *Psychol Aging* 2011;**26**:778–91.

15 Lindwall M, et al. Dynamic associations of change in physical activity and change in cognitive function: coordinated analyses of four longitudinal studies. *J Aging Res* 2012;**2012**:493598.

16 Lindsey JK. Models for repeated measurements. Oxford: OUP Catalogue; 2011.

17 Hoffman L, Stawski RS. Persons as contexts: evaluating between-person and within-person effects in longitudinal analysis. *Res Hum Dev* 2009;**6**:97–120.

18 Griffin MA. Interaction between individuals and situations: using HLM procedures to estimate reciprocal relationships. *Journal of Management* 1997;**23**:759–73.

19 Robitaille A, et al. Multivariate longitudinal modeling of cognitive aging: associations among change and variation in processing speed and visuospatial ability. *GeroPsych* 2012;**25**:15.

20 Mehta PD, Neale MC. People are variables too: multilevel structural equations modeling. *Psychol Methods* 2005;**10**:259–84.

21 Preacher KJ, et al. A general multilevel SEM framework for assessing multilevel mediation. *Psychol Methods* 2010;**15**:209–33.

22 Zhang Z, et al. Testing multilevel mediation using hierarchical linear models: problems and solutions. *Organizational Research Methods* 2009;**12**:695–719.

23 MacKinnon DP. Introduction to Statistical Mediation Analysis. New York: Erlbaum Psych Press; 2008.

24 Deary IJ, et al. Losing one's grip: A bivariate growth curve model of grip strength and nonverbal reasoning from age 79 to 87 years in the Lothian Birth Cohort 1921. *J Gerontol B Psychol Sci Soc Sci* 2011;**66**:699–707.

25 Birren JE. Handbook of Aging and the Individual. Chicago, IL: University of Chicago Press; 1959.

26 Sliwinski MJ, et al. Modeling memory decline in older adults: the importance of preclinical dementia, attrition, and chronological age. *Psychol Aging* 2003;**18**:658–71.

27 Piccinin AM, et al. Terminal decline from within- and between-person perspectives, accounting for incident dementia. *J Gerontol B Psychol Sci Soc Sci* 2011;**66**:391–401.

28 DiMatteo I, et al. Bayesian curve-fitting with free-knot splines. *Biometrika* 2001;**88**:1055–71.

29 Raftery AE. Bayesian model selection in social research. *Sociol Methodol* 1995;**25**:111–64.

30 Hall CB, et al. A change point model for estimating the onset of cognitive decline in preclinical Alzheimer's disease. *Stat Med* 2000;**19**:1555–66.

31 Muniz-Terrera G, et al. Random change point models: investigating cognitive decline in the presence of missing data. *J Appl Stat* 2011;**38**:705–16.

32 Muniz-Terrera G, et al. Investigating terminal decline: results from a UK population-based study of aging. *Psychol Aging* 2013;**28**:377–85.

33 **Hall CB, et al.** Estimation of bivariate measurements having different change points, with application to cognitive ageing. *Stat Med* 2001;**20**:3695–714.

34 **Kenward MG, Carpenter J.** Multiple imputation: current perspectives. *Stat Methods Med Res* 2007;**16**: 199–218.

35 **Rubin DB, Little RJA.** Statistical analysis with missing data. Hoboken, NJ: J Wiley & Sons; 2002.

36 **Schafer JL.** Multiple imputation: a primer. *Stat Methods Med Res* 1999;**8**:3–15.

37 **Carpenter J, Kenward M.** Multiple Imputation and its Application. New York: J Wiley & Sons; 2013.

38 **Spratt M, et al.** Strategies for multiple imputation in longitudinal studies. *Am J Epidemiol* 2010;**172**: 478–87.

39 **Wu MC, Carroll RJ.** Estimation and comparison of changes in the presence of informative right censoring by modeling the censoring process. *Biometrics* 1988;**44**:175–88.

40 **De Gruttola V, Tu XM.** Modelling progression of CD4-lymphocyte count and its relationship to survival time. *Biometrics* 1994;**50**:1003–14.

41 **Muniz Terrera G, et al.** Joint modeling of longitudinal change and survival: an investigation of the association between change in memory scores and death. *GeroPsych* 2011;**24**:177.

42 **Tsiatis AA, Davidian M.** Joint modeling of longitudinal and time-to-event data: an overview. *Stat Sin* 2004;**14**:809–34.

43 **Guo X, Carlin BP.** Separate and joint modeling of longitudinal and event time data using standard computer packages. *Am Stat* 2004;**58**:16–24.

44 **Rasbash J, et al.** A User's Guide to MLwiN (version 2.26). University of Bristol: Centre for Multilevel Modelling; 2012.

45 **R Development Core Team.** R: A Language and Environment for Statistical Computing. Vienna, Austria: R Foundation Statistical Computing; 2009.

46 **StataCorp.** Stata 12 help for mlogit. 2011.

47 **Muthén LK, Muthén BO.** Mplus User's Guide. 7th ed. Los Angeles, CA: Muthén & Muthén; 1998–2012.

48 **Jöreskog KG, Sörbom D.** LISREL 7: A Guide to the Program and Applications. Chicago: SPSS Publications; 1989.

49 **Spiegelhalter DJ, et al.** BUGS: Bayesian Inference Using Gibbs Sampling, Version 0.50. Cambridge: MRC Biostatistics Unit; 1995.

Chapter 7

Modelling repeat exposures: some examples from life course epidemiology

Andrew Wills and Kate Tilling

7.1 **Motivation and background**

Repeat measures of an exposure from different life stages provide an opportunity to model the role of developmental trajectories and age-related patterns of exposure on health and function in later life. For example, studies have linked patterns of postnatal and pubertal growth to cardio-metabolic risk [1,2], and cognitive and physical capability in later life [3,4], while the risk of knee osteoarthritis is thought to accumulate through a prolonged exposure to high body weight during adulthood [5]. Such associations may also act in both directions across the life course—for example, studies have shown midlife cognitive performance to be related to later physical performance [6], and physical disability to be related to later cognitive function [7]. Conceptualizing health and disease through a life course framework has become increasingly popular [8], and alongside the increasing availability of longitudinal data, has led researchers to ask more specific questions on the nature of the exposure–outcome relationship. Typical questions include whether risk accumulates uniformly over the life course; whether there are sensitive periods when exposure is particularly detrimental; whether a change in exposure poses a particular risk; and whether aspects of a trajectory such as peak lifetime exposure are important. Where two outcomes are considered (for example physical and cognitive decline with ageing), hypotheses may include a dynamic relationship between them, or a common process underlying both [9]. Addressing such questions can offer an insight into pathways for disease and inform interventions for prevention.

In this chapter, we use the same dataset to illustrate several possible approaches to the analysis. The setting is repeat measures of body mass index (BMI) at different life stages and systolic blood pressure (SBP) at 53 years. Midlife blood pressure is an important outcome as it has been shown to be related to both cognitive (dementia risk [10], cognitive decline [11]) and physical (muscle strength decline [12]) outcomes in older age. Our focus is on the utility and interpretation of each analytical approach, although in contrasting each model we also highlight the key statistical issues which might influence the choice of method(s). We do not discuss confounding or biological aspects of the exposure that might affect interpretation, for example, whether BMI measures have different interpretations at different life stages.

Data are from the MRC National Survey of Health and Development (NSHD). To facilitate the comparison of each method we restrict the sample to males and complete cases (n = 501). SBP (mmHg) was measured at 53 years and BMI (weight/height^2) was calculated from measured height and weight at 2, 4, 6, 7, 11, 15, 36, 43, and 53 years and from self-reported height and weight at 20 and 26 years. Data were collected at relatively fixed ages and for the 4, 6, 7, 11, and 15 year follow-ups, information on age of measurement (in months) was available.

7.2 **Raw approaches: reparameterizations of the general linear model**

We describe the approaches in this section as raw in the sense that they do not estimate a statistical model for the exposure trajectory. They merely consist of a multivariable regression model(s) relating the outcome to the observed exposures or linear functions of them.

One motivation behind the models described in this section is to compare the associations between outcome and exposure (BMI) at different ages. Since a unit difference in exposure can have different meanings at different life stages, and to adjust for small age differences at each follow-up, we normalized and internally standardized the BMI observations by their variance at each age using the LMS method [13], creating a set of BMI z-scores. While beyond the scope of this chapter, it is worth noting that the use of standardized scores to examine trajectories can generate some statistical issues; a useful overview can be found elsewhere [14,15]. We omitted measures at 6, 11, 26, and 43 years from the models in this section to reduce the dimensionality of the dataset but retain intervals of interest: childhood (2–4 and 4–7 years), childhood to adolescence (7–15 years), adolescence to early adulthood (15–20 years), early adulthood (20–36 years) and mid adulthood (36–53 years). Table 7.1 describes the dataset.

7.2.1 **Multivariable models of size and change**

Two models that have been used to study the role of growth are: (1) a model containing each repeat measure [16]—a multivariable model of size; and (2) a model containing the baseline exposure and all subsequent periods of change in exposure [17]—a multivariable model of change. The size model can be written as:

$$E(SBP) = \alpha + \sum_{j=1}^{7} \beta_j \, zBMI_j \tag{1}$$

where $zBMI_j$ is the BMI z-score on occasion $j = 1, 2, \ldots, 7$, corresponding to ages 2, 4, 7, 15, 20, 36, and 53 years respectively. Using similar notation, the change model can be written as:

$$E(SBP) = \alpha + \theta_1 zBMI_1 + \sum_{j=2}^{7} \theta_j \left(zBMI_j - zBMI_{j-1} \right) \tag{2}$$

These models estimate associations of later blood pressure with size at each age (model 1) or change during each interval (model 2) independent of size or changes throughout the rest of life. The results from each are presented in Table 7.2. Model 1 suggests that current BMI and earlier adult BMI (36 years) are positively associated with SBP independent of BMI at other ages across life, and that BMI in infancy, childhood, adolescence, and younger adulthood are not independently associated with later SBP. In contrast, model 2 suggests that BMI at 2 years and changes in BMI throughout the life course are positively associated with later SBP, mutually adjusted for changes in all other intervals. The size of these associations increases with age, up to age 36.

The coefficients in models 1 and 2 have different interpretations. In the size model, the coefficient for BMI at age j represents the mean difference in SBP between two people, one of whom has a BMI one unit higher at age j but with the same BMI at all other ages. In the change model, the corresponding coefficient estimates the mean difference between two people, one of whom has a one unit increase in BMI between age $j - 1$ and age j with no other changes during all future intervals. The change model thus asks a cumulative question: what is the effect of shifting up the BMI distribution by a z-score in a given interval and maintaining

Table 7.1 Correlation matrix and means and SDs for several BMI size and change variables (kg/m^2) from the NSHD dataset

	BMI size							BMI change					
Age (years)	**2**	**4**	**7**	**15**	**20**	**36**	**53**	**2 to 4**	**4 to 7**	**7 to 15**	**15 to 20**	**20 to 36**	**36 to 53**
BMI size													
2	1												
4	0.27	1											
7	0.23	0.38	1										
15	0.16	0.30	0.58	1									
20	0.14	0.25	0.38	0.62	1								
36	0.15	0.20	0.31	0.55	0.64	1							
53	0.08	0.13	0.19	0.45	0.49	0.78	1						
BMI change													
2 to 4	−0.65	0.55	0.10	0.10	0.08	0.03	0.03	1					
4 to 7	−0.04	−0.56	0.55	0.25	0.12	0.09	0.05	−0.40	1				
7 to 15	−0.07	−0.07	−0.40	0.51	0.29	0.30	0.30	0.00	−0.30	1			
15 to 20	−0.03	−0.08	−0.25	−0.48	0.39	0.07	0.02	−0.03	−0.16	−0.28	1		
20 to 36	0.03	−0.04	−0.06	−0.03	−0.35	0.49	0.40	−0.05	−0.02	0.03	−0.36	1	
36 to 53	−0.10	−0.11	−0.19	−0.18	−0.26	−0.38	0.28	0.00	−0.07	0.00	−0.09	−0.16	1
Mean	18.1	16.3	15.8	19.7	22.6	24.9	27.6	−1.8	−0.5	3.8	2.9	2.2	2.7
SD	2.7	1.6	1.3	2.5	2.4	3.3	4.1	2.8	1.6	2.1	2.1	2.6	2.6

Table 7.2 Mutually adjusted regression coefficients from model 1 for BMI size (β), model 2 for BMI change (θ), and the conditional BMI change model (ε) (see models 8 and 9). Coefficients are the mean difference in SBP (mmHg) per z-score increase in each BMI size, change, or conditional change variable

BMI size				BMI change				Conditional BMI change	
Age (years)	β	95% CI	p	Age period	θ	95% CI	p	ε	95% CI
2	−1.30	(−3.02, 0.41)	0.137	2	3	(0.23, 5.77)	0.034	−0.99	−2.61, 0.64
4	0.14	(−1.86, 2.14)	0.893	2 to 4	4.3	(1.62, 6.99)	0.002	0.33	−1.54, 2.19
7	−1.59	(−3.91, 0.73)	0.179	4 to 7	4.17	(1.62, 6.72)	<0.001	−0.64	−2.61, 1.33
15	−0.59	(−3.12, 1.94)	0.648	7 to 15	5.76	(3.34, 8.17)	<0.001	2.76	0.68, 4.85
20	−1.08	(−3.64, 1.47)	0.407	15 to 20	6.35	(3.72, 8.98)	<0.001	2.17	−0.10, 4.44
36	3.64	(0.57, 6.72)	0.021	20 to 36	7.43	(5.08, 9.78)	<0.001	6.50	4.25, 8.75
53	3.79	(1.01, 6.57)	0.008	36 to 53	3.79	(1.01, 6.57)	0.008	3.79	1.01, 6.57
Model SS	19312			Model SS	19312			Model SS	19312

SS = sum of squares.

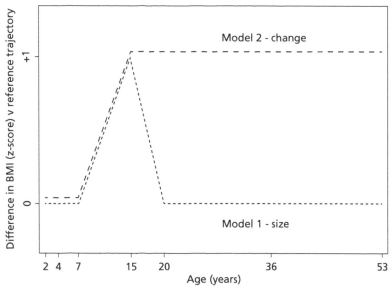

Figure 7.1 Illustration of the trajectory contrast tested by the coefficient for 15 years in model 1 (BMI size) and the coefficient for 7 to 15 years in model 2 (BMI change).

that position across the life course? Figure 7.1 illustrates the contrast from each model in terms of their trajectory. This shows the link between the coefficients in models 1 and 2; for example the coefficient for the interval 7 to 15 years in model 2 (θ_4) is 5.76, which equals the sum of the coefficients at ages 15, 20, 36, and 53 in model 1 (−0.59 − 1.08 + 3.64 + 3.79 = 5.76). More generally, coefficients from model 2 can be written in terms of those from model 1 as:

$$\theta_j = \sum\nolimits_{k=j}^{7} \beta_k \qquad (3)$$

And coefficients from model 1 can be rewritten in terms of model 2:

$$\beta_j = \theta_j - \theta_{j+1} \qquad (4)$$

Thus these models are just reparameterizations of each other; they explain the same amount of variation in the outcome and hence have the same model sum of squares (MSS) (Table 7.2).

7.2.2 **Duality of size and growth and the life course plot**

Nested within models 1 and 2 is an identification issue that complicates the attribution of size and change effects. This has been well discussed in the context of the developmental origins of health and disease (DOHAD) hypothesis [18], where it has been termed the *duality of size and growth* [16], and arises in any setting where there is a third variable of interest that is a linear function of the other two. In the context of DOHAD these three variables are birthweight (BWT), current weight (CWT), and change in weight (ΔWT). Given that ΔWT = CWT − BWT, once the values of two of these variables are known the third can be calculated algebraically. This redundancy means it is impossible to estimate mutually distinct effects for all three. An analogous example exists in attempting to disentangle age, period, and cohort effects because of the logical dependency age = period − cohort.

To illustrate the implications using BMI at ages 2 and 53 years from our dataset, we fitted the following model (using the same notation as described in Section 7.2.1):

$$E(SBP) = \alpha + \beta_1\, zBMI_1 + \beta_7 zBMI_7 \tag{5}$$

which estimates β_1 (standard error) as -1.4 mmHg (0.8), suggesting that, given current BMI, men with a lower BMI in infancy have a higher SBP on average, hence implicating infant size or the period up to and including infancy. However, the same model also implicates post-infant growth because among men of the same current BMI, those with a lower BMI at age 2 also had greater gains from age 2 to 53. A rearrangement of equation 5 illustrates this alternative interpretation of β_1:

$$E(SBP) = \alpha - \beta_1 \big(zBMI_7 - zBMI_1\big) + (\beta_1 + \beta_7)zBMI_7 \tag{6}$$

It can thus be useful to visualize this dual interpretation graphically. This is the basis of the life course plot, which consists of plotting the regression coefficients from model 1 against their respective ages and joining the points [16,19]. Each point on the plot represents the association with size and, as has been shown before [19], the difference between adjacent points is proportional to the regression coefficient for change conditioned on mean weight between the two ages:

$$E(SBP) = \alpha + \frac{(\beta_7 - \beta_1)}{2}\big(zBMI_7 - zBMI_1\big) + (\beta_1 + \beta_7)\frac{(zBMI_1 + zBMI_7)}{2} \tag{7}$$

So the slope of the line provides an indication of the association between the outcome and change in exposure between the two ages.

Figure 7.2 (left) shows the life course plot in our example. It confirms our earlier results with the emphasis on BMI in later life being important but also shows the influence of change in BMI from early life to mid-adulthood. Two issues are evident from this plot. First, the estimated coefficients

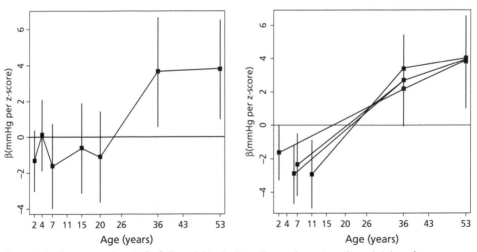

Figure 7.2 Life course plots. Left, full model including all ages (equation 1); and right, after removing those ages that were conditionally uninformative. Several models (represented by the different lines) are presented as a sensitivity analysis. For clarity, the confidence intervals from the adult ages have been removed in the plot on the right, from all models except those for the model containing ages 7,43, and 53 years, but all coefficients had a p-value <0.06.

lack precision. This inflated variance is a statistical problem caused by the strong correlations among the exposures, often referred to as collinearity. Regression textbooks advise against including highly correlated variables for this reason. Second, since the purpose of the life course plot is to visualize the dual interpretation of the coefficients, it is misleading to include ages that are conditionally uninformative, i.e. do not improve model fit conditional on all other variables included in the model, particularly with regard to interpreting the slopes in the plot.

To address these issues, uninformative ages were removed from model 1 and re-entered individually, reassessing model fit. Four different life course plots are presented in Figure 7.2 (right); each model contains BMI at 36 and 53 years and a solitary BMI measure from infancy or childhood. Selecting a single age to represent infancy or childhood dealt sufficiently with multicollinearity to allow us to make inference on these life stages. The confidence intervals for size at ages 36 and 53 are still wide, potentially because BMI measures at these two ages are very highly correlated (Table 7.1).

The life course plot represents the age-specific adjusted association with SBP of being one z-score above the median and is suggestive of growth profiles linked to the highest SBPs in later life. So, those with lower BMIs in infancy or childhood and higher BMIs from mid-adulthood had higher mean SBPs. Alternatively, using the change interpretation, those with larger gains in BMI from childhood to mid-adulthood also had on average higher SBPs. One problem of interpretation with this plot occurs because the model includes size at all ages—and thus size at a later age is conditioned on interpreting the coefficient for size at an earlier age. This practice of adjusting for a later measure of body size when investigating the association between birthweight and a distal health outcome has been the subject of much debate. If birthweight has a positive association with later body size, which is itself positively related to the outcome, then the association between birthweight and outcome can change from positive to negative upon conditioning on the later body size variable (termed the 'Reversal Paradox' [20,21]) .

7.2.3 Conditional change

A common model for repeat exposures in life course research is one that can be referred to as conditional change or conditional size [1,22–25]. The idea is to remove the influence of earlier exposure on the present and assess each exposure from a purely prospective view point, targeted at the question: what is the effect of the present independent of the past?

This approach derives estimates of size at each occasion which are uncorrelated with the other conditional measures of size. The conditional change scores are simply the residuals from the regressions of BMI at each age on all earlier BMI measures, i.e. from the following six models:

$$E(z\,BMI_2) = \alpha_2 + \gamma_{2,1}\,z\,BMI_1$$
$$E(z\,BMI_3) = \alpha_3 + \gamma_{3,1}\,z\,BMI_1 + \gamma_{3,2}\,z\,BMI_2$$
$$\cdots$$
$$\cdots$$
$$E(z\,BMI_7) = \alpha_7 + \sum_{j=1}^{6}\gamma_{7,j}\,z\,BMI_j$$

(8)

By definition, the residuals are completely uncorrelated with the dependent variables and thus by construction, each conditional change variable is entirely uncorrelated with conditional change in all other periods. Effectively, the BMI trajectory is partitioned into a series of discrete independent intervals of change. In our example, the conditional scores can be seen as the change in BMI above or below that expected in our cohort given earlier BMI.

The analysis model is a regression of the outcome on the earliest BMI measure and all the conditional change variables, as follows:

$$E(SBP) = \alpha + \eta_1 zBMI_1 + \sum\nolimits_{j=2}^{7} \eta_j E_j \qquad (9)$$

where η_j are the coefficients for baseline BMI and each conditional change variable (E_j). We would get the same results if we instead used a set of univariable models for each exposure because of the zero correlation structure. We can also estimate each η_j using a sequence of regression models of SBP on $zBMI_j$ and all earlier BMI variables; the coefficient for the most contemporaneous exposure in each model is interpreted and is equivalent to each η_j in equation 9. Similarly, the set of variables in the change model (equation 2) can be applied in the same way to obtain each η_j.

Table 7.2 shows the results from this model. There is some evidence that conditional increases in BMI during all intervals from ages 11 to 53 are positively associated with SBP at 53. Since all exposures are in the same model, we can formally compare the size of the coefficients to test whether there are sensitive periods when BMI increases are particularly detrimental. Wald tests suggest that the period from 20 to 36 years was more strongly associated with SBP compared to the periods from 7 to 15 years (difference in η = +3.7 mmHg; 95% CI: 0.7, 6.8) and 15 to 20 years (difference in η = +4.3 mmHg; 95% CI: 1.1, 7.5).

In this conditional model, the coefficient for BMI at age j represents the mean difference in SBP between two people, with identical BMI up to age $j – 1$, one of whom has a BMI one z-score higher than the other at age j. By removing the association of the past from the present, the coefficients in this model do not suffer from the dual interpretation of size and change as in model 1. However, the conditional change model contains exactly the same information as models 1 and 2 (the MSS is the same) and so is still a reparameterization, meaning nothing new has been gained. The β_j parameters from model 1 can be shown to be related to the parameters in equations 8 and 9 by:

$$\beta_j = \eta_j - \sum\nolimits_{k=j+1}^{7} \gamma_{k,j} \eta_k. \qquad (10)$$

The internal nature of the conditional score calculation means the comparison is between subjects within a population, hence it is not possible to define a growth trajectory that can be referenced externally; this is a limitation. However, the interpretation as the change above or below expectation based on what we know from the past means that it may be a useful method for capturing accelerated or restricted growth.

7.2.4 Path analysis

Path analysis, where the causal relationships between exposures are depicted explicitly in a graph, allow associations to be decomposed into direct effects (those paths linked directly to the outcome), indirect effects (the sum of paths from the exposure to outcome that run through the intermediary variables), and total effects (the sum of direct and indirect effects). The terms direct and indirect effects refer to associations which are 'not mediated' and 'mediated' through other variables in the model respectively, rather than having a causal interpretation. Path analysis has been advocated as a superior method for analysing the relationships between lifetime body size and a distal outcome [26].

Figure 7.3 (left) shows the saturated path model in our example. Each measure of BMI is dependent on all earlier measures and SBP is dependent on all BMI measures. This model contains seven regression equations: six for the BMI measures from ages 4 to 53 (where each BMI is viewed as an intermediate outcome); these equations are the same as those used to estimate the conditional change variables (equation 8), and one equation for the main outcome SBP; similarly this equation is the same as the size model (equation 1). So the saturated path model is a combination of the conditional change model parameterization and the size model parameterization.

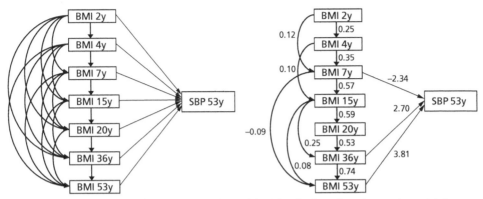

Figure 7.3 Path diagrams. Left: saturated path model. Right: final parsimonious path model (best fitting) and estimated path coefficients. BMI is in z-score units and SBP in mmHg.

The direct and total effects of BMI on SBP from the saturated path model are presented in Table 7.3 (estimated in MPlus using maximum likelihood). In our example, because the same variables are included in all sets of models, the direct effects are equivalent to those reported from the model for size (model 1) (Table 7.2). Likewise, the total effects are equivalent to the coefficients obtained using the conditional change approach (Table 7.2). The minor differences in the confidence intervals are a consequence of the different estimation method.

Many terms were conditionally uninformative in the saturated model. In Table 7.3 and Figure 7.3 (right), the results from a more parsimonious model are shown. This model fits the data as well as the saturated model and has a higher Akaike's Information Criterion than other models containing a direct effect for BMI at 2 or 4 years instead of age 7. Conclusions from this model were similar to the saturated path model in terms of the positive direct associations of BMI at ages 36 and 53 with SBP, and with the positive total effects from age 15. However, BMI at 7 years is now inversely and directly associated with SBP, exactly as shown in the life course plot (Figure 7.2).

By simplifying the path model the regression coefficients are more precise. A path model is not more efficient than the conditional change model as has been suggested [26]; the improvement in precision is because there is less collinearity in the more parsimonious model— the conditional change model and parsimonious path model are now no longer equivalent.

7.2.5 **Further considerations**

We illustrated that these models are all reparameterizations of the same underlying model. In fact there are infinite possible reparamterizations. An alternative to the prospective conditional approach is a retrospective conditional approach. Whereas the prospective viewpoint may be useful for screening (e.g. given what we know about your exposure history, what is your future risk of disease?), a retrospective viewpoint might be useful for questions concerning extant morbid groups (e.g. given your disease, is your past likely to tell us anything more about prognosis?). Interactions may also be considered, although given the potential number of interactions these should be carefully chosen beforehand.

Several statistical issues with these approaches should be mentioned. There is an inherent redundancy to merely using all the raw exposures; we refer to this as multiplicity. The high correlations between exposures cause uncertainty in the regression coefficients. However, tackling multiplicity and collinearity by removing ages means that exposure periods are selected based on statistical rather than biological considerations. More recently, partial least squares regression has been proposed as a way of overcoming multiplicity and collinearity although this method, which

Table 7.3 Estimated direct and total effects from the saturated path model and from a more parsimonious model after removing uninformative terms. The coefficients are the mean change in SBP for a z-score increase in BMI

Saturated (a priori) path model					Final (parsimonious) path model*			
Age (years)	Direct effect	95% CI	Total effect	95% CI	Direct effect	95% CI	Total effect	95% CI
2	-1.30	-3.00, 0.40	-0.99	-2.68, 0.71			-0.07	-0.46, 0.32
4	0.14	-1.84, 2.12	0.33	-1.61, 2.27			0.08	-0.62, 0.77
7	-1.59	-3.89, 0.71	-0.64	-2.69, 1.41	-2.34	-4.23, -0.45	-0.73	-2.57, 1.11
15	-0.59	-3.09, 1.92	2.76	0.61, 4.92			3.40	2.30, 4.50
20	-1.08	-3.62, 1.45	2.17	-0.17, 4.51			2.89	1.85, 3.93
36	3.64	0.59, 6.69	6.50	4.26, 8.74	2.7	-0.04, 5.44	5.51	3.75, 7.26
53	3.79	1.03, 6.55	3.79	1.03, 6.55	3.81	1.06, 6.56	3.81	1.06, 6.56

* χ^2 test for a difference between the a priori (saturated) and final model: χ^2 [14] = 12.52; p = 0.56; Comparative fit index (CFI) = 0.99.

is a data reduction technique similar to a principle components analysis, is still data driven [27]. Measurement error in the exposures will dilute regression coefficients towards the null. Where measurement error is differential across age it may bias comparisons between life stages. Linearity was also assumed in all models although this can be relaxed by including non-linear terms. Lastly, a major limitation is that every subject needs to have the exposure measured at the same age, and at all measurement occasions, although missing data methods such as multiple imputation could be used to 'balance' a dataset under certain assumptions concerning the missingness [28].

7.3 **Growth trajectory modelling**

The two approaches discussed in this section, multilevel models (MLMs) and latent class analysis, involve two steps: first, fitting a model to the repeat exposure data, then using aspects of this model as explanatory variables in an analytical regression model with the outcome. These steps can be carried out separately, or as part of one multivariate or structural equation model. Both examples illustrated in this section used all available waves of data.

7.3.1 **Multilevel models**

Multilevel models (Chapter 6) are an efficient way to estimate an underlying trajectory for each individual, and examples are common in the life course literature [29–32].

There are several ways of specifying the form of the trajectory. We used two fourth order polynomials, splitting the data from 2 to 20 and 20 to 53 years to allow for the complex shape of BMI. Exact age at measurement was used where available. The model contained all possible random effects thereby allowing each individual to have their own quartic polynomial curve for each period. The random coefficients were allowed to be correlated and the occasion level errors were assumed to be independent. From each individual's *fitted* trajectory, we derived a set of summary statistics in an attempt to extract definable features of the trajectory that may vary between individuals; Figure 7.4 illustrates these.

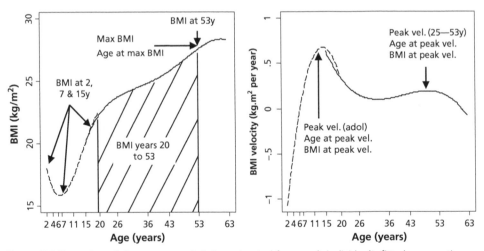

Figure 7.4 Illustration of the summary statistics extracted from each individual's fitted curve estimated from the multilevel model. The line represents the trajectory for the so-called average subject in our cohort. The left panel is the curve for BMI and the right panel is the curve for BMI velocity (vel.). The x-axis shows the age at each follow-up visit. Calculus was used to extract the area under the curve and velocity statistics.

The new features of the trajectory that we have estimated using the MLM were strongly correlated with values taken at cross-sectional ages, for example, BMI velocity in adolescence was strongly correlated with early adulthood BMI (r = 0.69), and cumulative BMI years during adulthood was strongly correlated with current BMI (r = 0.94), BMI at 20 years (r = 0.86), maximum BMI during adulthood (r = 0.94), and BMI at maximum velocity during adulthood (r = 0.59). This makes it difficult in an analytical model to detect whether there is anything special about any of these features or whether they are just markers of the trajectory as a whole. The conditional interpretation of a multivariable analytical model containing these derived variables would also be difficult, as highlighted in the previous section, and therefore the choice of which variables to derive needs to be made *a priori*.

To exploit the novelty of this approach we explored one of the variables that we were unable to estimate using the raw approaches—peak adolescent BMI velocity. One question might be whether there is anything special about this peak or if it is just a marker for adult BMI, which we know to be important. There was evidence for a positive association between peak adolescent BMI velocity and later SBP when taking a prospective viewpoint and estimating the net effect of peak BMI velocity going forward adjusting for the earlier BMI measures in a similar fashion to the conditional change approach (β per 0.5 kg.m^2/year increase in velocity: 8.8 mmHg; 95% CI: 0.1, 17.5). After allowing for current BMI, there was no evidence for an association between peak BMI velocity in adolescence and SBP (β per 0.5 kg.m^2/year increase in velocity: −1.5 mmHg; 95% CI: −7.4, 4.3).

MLMs have several key statistical advantages over raw approaches. First, they are not restricted to data from fixed ages. Second, they use all available data and so easily handle incomplete cases under an assumption that the data are missing at random (MAR) [33]. Third, they account for measurement error by borrowing information from the population average to fit individual trajectories such that each individual's estimated trajectory is shrunk towards the mean; the more shrinkage towards the mean, the more strength is borrowed from the population estimate, and the more correction is made for measurement error. For example, the unadjusted coefficient using the unstandardized BMI value at 53 in our example was 1.31 mmHg, while using the fitted MLM estimate it was 1.46 mmHg.

Alternative techniques for modelling the shape of the trajectory are worth noting. Linear splines [29,31,32,34] are easy to interpret since the model parameters can be constructed to represent size and velocities between knot points. Penalized cubic splines are another semi-parametric method and are useful for modelling complex shapes in a smooth fashion [30,35]. SITAR (SuperImposition by Translation and Rotation) [36] is a parametric method that describes individual variation from the population mean in terms of three random effect parameters (thereby reducing dimensionality): a vertical translation (size shift), a horizontal translation (tempo shift), and a shrinking or stretching of the age scale (velocity shift) [36]. The type of data and number and density of measures may affect the fit of each of these models, so are key factors that might determine the choice of technique. Some approaches may also enable the measurement and analytical model to be fitted in one step using a multivariate multilevel model or a structural equation model; this may reduce bias from shrinkage due to unbalanced measures.

7.3.2 **Latent class models**

Latent class analysis is a popular approach for identifying subgroups of individuals that share an underlying trajectory. There are several examples of their use with BMI [37–39]. Distinctions can be made between different types of latent class models such as latent class growth analysis (LCGA) and growth mixture models (GMM); statistical descriptions of these models can be found elsewhere [40]. However, they all share a common idea—the identification of clusters of people with shared response patterns. Some researchers have thus described their use as a person-centred as opposed to variable-centred approach [41,42].

A latent class model was fitted to our data from ages 2 to 53. Due to the complex patterns of BMI change over life, we did not specify a function for the shape of the BMI trajectory but merely extracted latent classes as if the data were cross-sectional, hence technically we modelled profiles not trajectories. The covariance structure within each class was fixed to zero, meaning that individual trajectories within each class were considered homogenous. This is a similar specification to the LCGA described by Nagin [43]. A sequence of models containing an increasing number of classes up to eight was then estimated using maximum likelihood. We ultimately selected a four-class model based on parsimony, having classes with distinct life course profiles and having a reasonable sample size in each class. The model entropy (a measure of how well the classes separate individuals) was high (0.88), although the Bayesian information criterion (BIC) continued to fall appreciably up to eight classes, indicating improvements in fit. Each individual was assigned their most likely class using the posterior class membership probabilities. The classes were then related to SBP in a separate analysis regression model and were weighted by the posterior probabilities to account for the uncertainty in class assignment.

Figure 7.5 shows the estimated mean trajectory in each of the four classes. The size of each class is shown in Table 7.4, indexed by the level of BMI at age 53 (lowest to highest), along with the model-based mean SBP in each class and differences in SBP between classes. Classes 3 and 4 had the highest mean BMI at age 53 and had a mean SBP more than 10 mmHg higher than the other classes. Compared to class 4, class 3 had a lower BMI in childhood (difference at 7 years: −1.2 kg/m²) and a substantially lower BMI in adulthood (difference at 53 years: −4.4 kg/m²). Despite this difference in BMI trajectories, there was no evidence for a difference in SBP between classes 3 and 4 (mean difference: −0.1 mmHg; 95% CI: 6.3, 6.1). Similarly there was no evidence to suggest a difference between classes 1 and 2 (Table 7.4) despite substantially different mean BMI trajectories in these classes. Compared to class 1, class 2 had a higher mean BMI throughout life (difference at 7 years: +2 kg/m²; difference at 53 years: +2.6 kg/m²). The BMI trajectories in classes 2 and 3 mainly differed in early

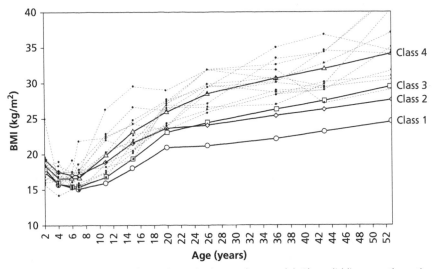

Figure 7.5 Extracted latent BMI classes from the latent class model. The solid lines are the estimated means in each class and the dashed lines are a random subset of individuals from class 4.

Table 7.4 Mean SBP (mmHg) in each latent class and differences in SBP between classes

Class	Class no:	N	Means	Differences	
			Mean SBP (95% CI)	Difference versus class 1 (95% CI)	p
Lowest BMI at 53 years	1	203 (40.5%)	137.8 (135.1, 140.5)	Reference	
	2	97 (19.4%)	139.1 (135.2, 142.9)	1.3 (–3.4, 6.0)	0.5
	3	150 (29.9%)	149.1 (145.9, 152.3)	11.3 (7.2, 15.5)	<0.001
Highest BMI at 53 years	4	51 (10.2%)	149.1 (143.9, 154.5)	11.4 (5.5, 17.4)	<0.001

life—class 3 had a substantially lower BMI up to age 15, and interestingly, class 3 also had a higher mean SBP compared to class 2 (mean difference: +10.1; 95% CI: 5.1, 15.0).

These results suggest that quite different life course trajectories of BMI may lead to the same SBP and support the findings from the raw approaches and MLM based approach. If the classes had contained different trajectories (e.g. all identified classes shared the same mean BMI up to age 36, for example) we may not have been able to make inference on the role of early BMI. By allowing the data to generate the contrast, it is not possible to specify the comparison in an *a priori* analysis strategy, and we rely on the latent class model producing groups that enable us to learn something about the outcome. The comparison is with the entire trajectory so care needs to be taken when attributing an association to particular features of the classes. Hence this approach might be most useful when the question relates to an entire growth trajectory or when hypotheses are unspecific to life stages. There was a degree of subjectivity in choosing a four-class model, although in our example, similar groups were present in higher class models and similar results found.

In terms of statistical advantages, this method deals with multiplicity—each individual's entire trajectory is summarized by a single variable. Latent class models can also explicitly model measurement error, and can allow for missing data under the assumption they are missing at random. However, they do still require data at relatively fixed ages if the exposure changes a lot with age. The model can also be extended to allow subjects to have their own individual trajectory (i.e. allowing within-class variation). It is also possible to model the class structure and link them to the outcome in one step. Combining this with within-class variation allows a further extension of the model to examine between-class and within-class effects. For example, one may hypothesize that effects are not equal across the population distribution. Each of these extensions results in a different model so may give different classes and different conclusions.

7.4 Testing conceptual life course models: structured modelling approach

Mishra and colleagues [44] outlined an approach to assess the statistical support for several conceptual models of how an exposure affects an outcome over the life course; for example, does risk accumulate from prolonged exposure over life? The example given concerned a binary exposure measured at three occasions over life. The idea is to define a trajectory for each individual based on their exposure at each occasion, so for three measurement occasions this gives $2^3 = 8$ possible trajectories, and to compare models corresponding to each life course conceptual hypothesis against a saturated model where each possible trajectory is allowed to influence the outcome. This approach has been used to relate socioeconomic position to BMI [45] and locomotor function [46], and also to suggest that prolonged exposure to high BMI during adulthood is related to knee osteoarthritis in midlife [5]. We present results using our example dataset in the Supplementary web material at www.halcyon.ac.uk.

One advantage of this method is that it forces the researcher to specify each life course model algebraically and hence the research question unambiguously. However, we still cannot separate change effects from size. For example, those that moved into the top tertile of BMI from childhood to adulthood were by definition those that started life in the lower tertiles, so change is conditional on the starting point. With more than two time points and sufficient variation in exposure trajectories, it may be possible to distinguish between change and size [44]. While results should be interpreted qualitatively, it is ultimately p-value driven and sufficient power in each trajectory is required to make fair statistical contrasts across models, particularly given that some of the models involve interaction terms. On the other hand, if we have enough people, the most complex model is also likely to fit the data best. Approaches for choosing the best model which are not based on p-values could be investigated. Lastly the exposures have been dichotomized, thus losing some information, and findings may be sensitive to the choice of cut-off.

7.5 **Summary and conclusions**

In our example, all the methods discussed lead to approximately the same conclusions regarding how life course BMI might be linked to later SBP, namely that those with higher BMI in adulthood tend to have higher SBP, and that a lower BMI in childhood or a greater increase in BMI from childhood to adulthood may be related to later SBP. We have shown that the same underlying regression model can lead to very different coefficients depending upon which variables are conditioned on [47]. Causal diagrams may be useful to help select which variables to condition on [48,49]. For example, much discussion has taken place on whether current weight should be adjusted for when examining the association between birthweight and a later outcome [20,21].

The raw approaches have three major disadvantages in that they require balanced data, may be biased by measurement error, and may suffer from multiplicity/collinearity if exposure was measured on many occasions. The latter point could be dealt with by using expert knowledge to decide *a priori* which time points to include in all models.

The trajectory methods can be used to reduce the dimensionality of the data, model measurement error and to identify pre-specified summary measures of interest (such as maximum velocity, etc.). These methods can deal with unbalanced data under the assumption that the data are missing at random (MAR). Where the trajectories are summarized in one step and then those summaries related to the outcome in a separate model, there may be bias due to shrinkage of residuals towards the mean (if the data are unbalanced), and underestimation of standard errors if the uncertainty in estimating the summaries is not taken into account [50]. Modelling the trajectories and relating them to the outcome in one model overcomes both these problems (Chapter 6).

This is not an exhaustive list of all possible methods available for summarizing time-varying exposures and relating them to later outcomes; other examples include Markov transition models [51], partial least squares [27], and recently there is interest in whether within subject variability in measures such as BP over time might contribute to health over and above mean BP [52,53]. The choice of approach is likely to be guided by the *a priori* hypothesis, and the data structure. For example, if weight and height were measured for everyone at birth and aged 5 and 10 years, then one might not gain much by using the more complex methods. This is because the dataset is balanced and of fairly low dimension. On the other hand, if weight and height were extracted from child health records (thus a very unbalanced dataset), then the dimensionality of the data would need to be reduced, and growth modelling might be a good choice. In practice, several approaches may be followed and used as sensitivity analyses, as has been advocated [54]. For all approaches, care is needed in the interpretation of coefficients, particularly with regard to the variables conditioned on in a given model.

References

1 Eriksson JG, et al. Early growth and coronary heart disease in later life: longitudinal study. *BMJ* 2001;**322**:949–53.

2 Tzoulaki I, et al. Relation of immediate postnatal growth with obesity and related metabolic risk factors in adulthood. *Am J Epidemiol* 2010;**171**:989–98.

3 Kuh D, et al. Developmental origins of midlife physical performance: evidence from a British birth cohort. *Am J Epidemiol* 2006;**164**:110–21.

4 Richards M, et al. Birthweight, postnatal growth and cognitive function in a national UK birth cohort. *Int J Epidemiol* 2002;**31**:342–8.

5 Wills AK, et al. Life course body mass index and risk of knee osteoarthritis at the age of 53 years: evidence from the 1946 British birth cohort study. *Ann Rheum Dis* 2012;**71**:655–60.

6 Kuh D, et al. Lifetime cognitive performance is associated with midlife physical performance in a prospective national birth cohort study. *Psychosom Med* 2009;**71**:38–48.

7 Rajan KB, et al. Disability in basic and instrumental activities of daily living is associated with faster rate of decline in cognitive function of older adults. *J Gerontol A Biol Sci Med Sci* 2013;**68**:624–30.

8 Ben Shlomo Y, Kuh D. A life course approach to chronic disease epidemiology: conceptual models, empirical challenges and interdisciplinary perspectives. *Int J Epidemiol* 2002;**31**:285–93.

9 Clouston SA, et al. The dynamic relationship between physical function and cognition in longitudinal aging cohorts. *Epidemiol Rev.* 2013;**35**:33–50.

10 Launer LJ, et al. Midlife blood pressure and dementia: the Honolulu-Asia aging study. *Neurobiol Aging* 2000;**21**:49–55.

11 Beeri MS, et al. The effects of cardiovascular risk factors on cognitive compromise. *Dialogues Clin Neurosci* 2009;**11**:201–12.

12 Stenholm S, et al. Long-term determinants of muscle strength decline: prospective evidence from the 22-year mini-Finland follow-up survey. *J Am Geriatr Soc* 2012;**60**:77–85.

13 Cole TJ. The LMS method for constructing normalized growth standards. *Eur J Clin Nutr* 1990;**44**:45–60.

14 Plewis I. Statistical methods for understanding cognitive growth: a review, a synthesis and an application. *Br J Math Stat Psychol* 1996;**49**:25–42.

15 Plewis I. Analysing Change: Measurement and Explanation using Longitudinal Data. Chichester: John Wiley & Sons; 1985.

16 Cole TJ. Modeling postnatal exposures and their interactions with birth size. *J Nutr* 2004;**134**:201–4.

17 Skidmore PML, et al. Life course body size and lipid levels at 53 years in a British birth cohort. *J Epidemiol Community Health* 2007;**61**:215–20.

18 Lucas A, et al. Fetal origins of adult disease—the hypothesis revisited. *BMJ* 1999;**319**:245–9.

19 Cole TJ. The life course plot in life course analysis. In: Pickles A, Maughan B, Wadsworth M, editors. Epidemiological Methods in Life Course Research. Oxford: Oxford University Press; 2007: 137–55.

20 Tu YK, et al. Why evidence for the fetal origins of adult disease might be a statistical artifact: the 'Reversal Paradox' for the relation between birth weight and blood pressure in later life. *Am J Epidemiol* 2005;**161**:27–32.

21 Weinberg CR. Invited commentary: Barker meets Simpson. *Am J Epidemiol* 2005;**161**:33–5.

22 Adair LS, et al. Size at birth, weight gain in infancy and childhood, and adult blood pressure in 5 low- and middle-income-country cohorts: when does weight gain matter? *Am J Clin Nutr* 2009;**89**:1383–92.

23 Hardy R, et al. Birthweight, childhood growth, and blood pressure at 43 years in a British birth cohort. *Int J Epidemiol* 2004;**33**:121–9.

24 Keijzer-Veen MG, et al. A regression model with unexplained residuals was preferred in the analysis of the fetal origins of adult diseases hypothesis. *J Clin Epidemiol* 2005;**58**:1320–4.

25 Wills AK, et al. Trajectories of overweight and body mass index in adulthood and blood pressure at age 53: the 1946 British birth cohort study. *J Hypertens* 2010;**28**:679–86.

26 Gamborg M, et al. Life course path analysis of birth weight, childhood growth, and adult systolic blood pressure. *Am J Epidemiol* 2009;**169**:1167–78.

27 Tu YK, et al. Assessing the impact of body size in childhood and adolescence on blood pressure: an application of partial least squares regression. *Epidemiology* 2010;**21**:440–8.

28 White IR, et al. Multiple imputation using chained equations: issues and guidance for practice. *Stat Med* 2011;**30**:377–99.

29 McCarthy A, et al. Birth weight; postnatal, infant, and childhood growth; and obesity in young adulthood: evidence from the Barry Caerphilly Growth Study. *Am J Clin Nutr* 2007;**86**:907–13.

30 Silverwood RJ, et al. BMI peak in infancy as a predictor for later BMI in the Uppsala Family Study. *Int J Obes* 2009;**33**:929–37.

31 dos Santos Silva, et al. Pre-natal factors, childhood growth trajectories and age at menarche: implications for lifecourse epidemiology. *Int J Epidemiol* 2002;**31**:405–12.

32 Tilling K, et al. Is infant weight associated with childhood blood pressure? Analysis of the Promotion of Breastfeeding Intervention Trial (PROBIT) cohort. *Int J Epidemiol* 2011;**40**:1227–37.

33 Little R, Rubin D. Statistical Analysis with Missing Data. Chichester: John Wiley; 1987.

34 Naumova EN, et al. Tutorial in Biostatistics: evaluating the impact of 'critical periods' in longitudinal studies of growth using piecewise mixed effects models. *Int J Epidemiol* 2001;**30**:1332–41.

35 Silverwood R. Issues in Modelling Growth Data Within a Life Course Framework. London: London School of Hygiene and Tropical Medicine; 2008.

36 Cole TJ, et al. SITAR—a useful instrument for growth curve analysis. *Int J Epidemiol* 2010;**39**:1558–66.

37 Li C, et al. Developmental trajectories of overweight during childhood: role of early life factors. *Obesity (Silver Spring)* 2007;**15**:760–71.

38 Ostbye T, et al. Body mass trajectories through adulthood: results from the National Longitudinal Survey of Youth 1979 Cohort (1981–2006). *Int J Epidemiol* 2011;**40**:240–50.

39 Ventura AK, et al. Developmental trajectories of girls' BMI across childhood and adolescence. *Obesity (Silver Spring)* 2009;**17**:2067–74.

40 Bollen KA, Curran P. Latent curve models: a structural equation perspective. New Jersey: John Wiley & Sons; 2006.

41 Jung T, Wickrama KAS. An introduction to latent class growth analysis and growth mixture modeling. *Social and Personality Psychology* 2008;**2/1**:302–17.

42 Muthen B. Latent variable analysis: growth mixture modeling and related techniques for longitudinal data. In: Kaplan D, editor. The SAGE Handbook of Quantitative Methodology for the Social Sciences. London: Sage; 2004: 345–67.

43 Nagin DS. Analyzing developmental trajectories: a semiparametric, group-based approach. *Psychol Methods* 1999;**4**:139–57.

44 Mishra G, et al. A structured approach to modelling the effects of binary exposure variables over the life course. *Int J Epidemiol* 2009;**38**:528–37.

45 Gustafsson PE, et al. Socio-economic disadvantage and body mass over the life course in women and men: results from the Northern Swedish Cohort. *Eur J Public Health* 2012;**22**:322–7.

46 **Birnie K, et al.** Socio-economic disadvantage from childhood to adulthood and locomotor function in old age: a lifecourse analysis of the Boyd Orr and Caerphilly prospective studies. *J Epidemiol Community Health* 2011;**65**:1014–23.

47 **Tu YK, et al.** Simpson's paradox, Lord's paradox, and suppression effects are the same phenomenon—the reversal paradox. *Emerg Themes Epidemiol* 2008;**5**:2.

48 **Greenland S, et al.** Causal diagrams for epidemiologic research. *Epidemiology* 1999;**10**:37–48.

49 **Hernan MA, et al.** Causal knowledge as a prerequisite for confounding evaluation: an application to birth defects epidemiology. *Am J Epidemiol* 2002;**155**:176–84.

50 **Macdonald-Wallis C, et al.** Multivariate multilevel spline models for parallel growth processes: application to weight and mean arterial pressure in pregnancy. *Stat Med* 2012;**31**:3147–64.

51 **Muenz LR, Rubinstein LV.** Markov models for covariate dependence of binary sequences. *Biometrics* 1985;**41**:91–101.

52 **Rothwell PM.** Limitations of the usual blood-pressure hypothesis and importance of variability, instability, and episodic hypertension. *Lancet* 2010;**375**:938–48.

53 **Elliott MR, et al.** Associations between variability of risk factors and health outcomes in longitudinal studies. *Stat Med* 2012;**31**:2745–56.

54 **De Stavola BL, et al.** Statistical issues in life course epidemiology. *Am J Epidemiol* 2006;**163**:84–96.

Chapter 8

Propensity score matching and longitudinal research designs: counterfactual analysis using longitudinal data

Sean AP Clouston

8.1 Introduction to counterfactual analysis

Causation is the backbone of science, yet scientific analysis is replete with examples of studies that make conclusions based on two variables being statistically associated. A simple association does little to help us determine why an association exists. Instead, researchers must rely on critical analysis, clear mechanisms, known causal linkages, and prior research to consider the relevance of an association. This limitation, some methodologists argue, arises due to the counterfactual problem: we cannot simultaneously test two conditions (treatment and control) in the same respondent at the same time [1]. This chapter provides an overview of one type of causal analysis, using propensity scores, and illustrates how the approach can be applied in longitudinal studies. Other approaches for addressing causality are briefly discussed in Chapter 5, Section 5.5.1.

The fact that we cannot observe both factual and counterfactual outcomes (those that did not happen) has been solved in a number of ways. For example, some researchers use genetically similar test subjects (such as cloned mice, or observation of twins). Randomized controlled trials (RCTs) have a long history as the gold standard of scientific evidence within observational studies where genetically similar subjects are unavailable or where generalizability is necessary. In an RCT, respondents are randomly assigned to treatment groups. The benefit of using an RCT framework is that doing so solves a number of methodological problems. First, the likelihood of treatment is equivalent for everyone who participates in the study, effectively eradicating selection bias. Second, randomization theoretically creates comparable groups with respect to both measured and unmeasured confounders, thus eliminating (on average over a number of trials) the problem of confounding.

RCTs cannot address many life course questions of substantial interest, for ethical or practical reasons. This has led to alternative ways to deal with the original counterfactual problem. Observational researchers have begun by making the assumption that 'observational studies (are) . . . experimental designs controlled by someone other than the researcher—quite often, the subjects of the research' [1]. Using that ingenious observation, it becomes theoretically defensible to estimate fact and counter-fact for two hypothetical individuals who sit at the mean of two observed groups – one that has been exposed to a 'treatment' and another that has not – thereby replicating the circumstances of an RCT using observational data. To do so, counterfactual analysis focuses on two qualities of an RCT: randomization evenly distributes selection bias between treatment and control groups, and also ensures that individuals in treatment and control groups are compara-ble. Counterfactual analysis can be accomplished in a number of ways. It is possible, for example, to observe a random set of individuals who are accidentally treated [2]. A *post hoc* statistical option also exists using the probability of treatment, called the propensity score, by using it to approximate a situation where selection bias is evenly distributed throughout treatment and control groups (or subgroups therein). The challenges and practicalities of using such estimates is discussed in Section 8.2 before we return to counterfactual analysis and its application to longitudinal data.

8.2 **The propensity score**

Formally speaking, propensity scores (P_T) are the estimated probability of treatment (sometimes called the population average or marginal probability) predicted using observed covariates: $P_T = \Pr(T = 1 \mid X = x)$, where x are the observed values for covariates X, and T is a dichotomous treatment indicator ($T = 1$ if treated and $T = 0$ if untreated).

Propensity scores are gaining in popularity, and have been used in topics from examining the impact of environmental regulation [3] or labour market policies [4], to understanding the health implications of precarious unemployment [5], or the developmental implications of concentrated disadvantage [6]. They are also relevant for testing life course hypotheses in rela-tion to health and ageing, as will be demonstrated in this chapter. Caliendo and Kopeinig pro-vide a good practical guide to this rapidly growing literature [7]. Nevertheless, broad usage of counterfactual methods has been slow [8], in part because of critiques that show the similarity of propensity score model results with results from more standard models. For instance, Shah and colleagues carried out a systematic review of publications where both regression models and propensity scores were used in studies of the impact of medical interventions on mortality [9]. They found that propensity score matching (PSM) generally provided results that were in similar directions to those from regression models, but with estimates that were smaller in size. They further suggested that because few people know when and how to use propensity scores, their use is limited. On the other hand, it has been suggested that wildly different results may occur because of differences in how the propensity score is specified [10]. The issue of speci-fication raises an important point: like any statistical estimation, the selection equation can be mis-specified, and thus the selection equation should be transparently reported. Nevertheless, a recent meta-analysis comparing results from RCTs to those from propensity score analyses found that they generally provide similar results [11], suggesting that PSM can provide robust results.

Balance is a statistical term describing when two groups are not statistically different in terms of observed characteristics. In observational data, balance is often ensured by classifying the sample into subgroups (blocks), within which treated and untreated respondents are similar in terms of the propensity score and are not known to differ depending on covariates. There are a number of ways to generate balanced blocks. Achy-Brou and colleagues suggest using quintiles of the pro-pensity score, while excluding outlying observations to ensure balance [12]. Becker and Ichino suggest starting with five groups whose propensity scores have a defined range of 0.20, testing balance by using t-tests to assess whether each covariate differs by treatment group ($\alpha = 0.05$), and then consecutively cutting blocks at the halfway point until balance is attained, being sure to exclude any groups containing only treated or only control cases [13].

To get an unbiased estimate of treatment effect using balanced data, Rosenbaum and Rubin suggest incorporating the propensity score into statistical models in one of three ways: covariate adjustment on the propensity score, matching pairs of individuals on their propensity score, or subclassification using the balanced blocks described above [14]. Covariate adjustment includes the propensity score put directly into regression analyses as a control variable. Matching can be done at the individual level, where individual i is matched to individual(s) j, who differ only on the treatment. However, other options for matching exist; Becker and Ichino provide a very good explanation of a variety of matching methods including, for example, nearest neighbour matching and kernel matching algorithms [13]. Finally, subclassification, though often discussed separately from matching methods, effectively matches a group of treated individuals with a group of control individuals. Because 'covariates are balanced and the assignment to treatment can be considered random' thus treatments and controls within these blocks are not different because of observed selection bias [13: p. 364].

Like most forms of statistical analysis, counterfactual analysis relies on estimating an average treatment effect (ATE) and therefore the Stable Unit Treatment Value Assumption (SUTVA) must be made [1]. SUTVA acknowledges the implicit assumption that in order to take an average, the treatment must in theory have a stable effect across the distribution of possible outcomes, regardless of who is being treated. Thus, if it is believed that treatment only benefits a subset of the sample, then estimating an average treatment effect is meaningless. Here we consider the case where there is only one treatment, though such an assumption is not necessary. With multiple treatments, counterfactual analysis can appropriately compare groups but analysts must be careful to discuss how those groups should be compared, and estimate the propensity scores accordingly, either by rank-ordering from least to most effective treatment, or by creating different propensity scores for each treatment that might account for mutually exclusive treatments. For ease of interpretation, our analysis will focus on the dichotomous situation where one treatment is compared to one control.

8.3 **Propensity scores in longitudinal models**

When using causal modelling in a longitudinal context, we are faced with trying to match individuals based on selective criteria. In some longitudinal models, treatment will have occurred prior to observation and matching need only occur once. However, in cases where treatment occurs at multiple observations, longitudinal propensity scores in relation to treatment may change over time. Temporal change in the propensity score can follow at least three patterns: monotonic, random [12], and timed [15], each with different substantive and methodological implications (Figure 8.1).

8.3.1 **Monotonic rates**

In most ageing research, the likelihood of experiencing many forms of potential treatment begin at a particular level and then change at a rate (r_p) that can be described as an injective function of age: put simply, if we know a value of age we can calculate a unique likelihood, and if we know the likelihood we can always calculate a unique value for age. In this instance either $r_p > 0$, meaning that the likelihood of treatment is increasing linearly with age, $r_p < 0$, meaning that the rate is decreasing with age, or $r_p = 0$, suggesting that the likelihood of treatment is independent of age under observation. If the propensity score changes predictably with age, we can make the reasonable assumption that matching at baseline will lead to the same match protocol as those done later in observation, and thus methods of accounting for cross-sectional matches can be interpreted directly into longitudinal models either using subclassification, weighting, or adjustment at baseline.

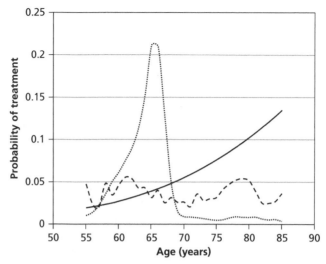

Figure 8.1 Hypothetical changes in propensity scores that change over time. Solid line: monotonic increasing propensity scores; dotted line: timed propensity scores; dashed line: random propensity scores.

8.3.2 **Random rates**

This type of propensity score, discussed by Achy-Brou and colleagues [12], is relevant when propensity scores can change randomly as a function of a temporal outcome (e.g. side effects) during observation. In this instance, the propensity for getting treatment is known, but the propensity for a particular treatment may change rapidly within individuals. To account for this, the authors suggest calculating time-specific propensity scores and using them to weight the stratified expected values when calculating the overall average treatment effect. To account for shifting treatments during observation, they use weights to adjust estimates of change from one regimen to another during observation.

8.3.3 **Timed propensity scores**

If rates can increase and later decrease with time (if the relationship between treatment and time is not injective), then propensity scores calculated at baseline are misleading; a person could reliably have the same propensity for treatment at more than one time in their lives. However, the propensity for treatment could be rising in one instance, and declining in the other. This may be problematic if the average treatment effect (ATE) depends not only on values of x, but also on timing of treatment: $ATE = f(x, t_T)$. A language for timed treatments has been developed when considering technological adoption that distinguishes 'early adopters', when the propensity for adoption may be low because no one is sure what the is value of a new technology, as compared to 'late adopters', where the likelihood of adopting a new technology is low because few people remain without the adoptive devices. If individuals can select treatment timing, it is possible that ill-timed treatments are less beneficial than well-timed ones. Should this be true, then SUTVA does not hold, and individuals with similar propensity scores should not necessarily be matched. Instead, it may be more useful to compare treatments of early adopters to non-adopters *and* to that of optimal or late adopters, suggesting that analysts calculate a cumulative distribution propensity function for use in matching, rather than using the more traditional probability density function.

8.4 **Longitudinal counterfactual analysis**

Using counterfactual analysis on cross-sectional data cannot guarantee causal results if unobserved variation (measures not included in the model or the dataset) defines the propensity score. This may be solved by using life course data, which may include variables measured prior to treatment, or by being careful to measure all variables of interest prior to treatment. However, counterfactual methods cannot differentiate between causation and selection on the dependent variable (called 'direct selection', to differentiate it from selection on other health relevant factors such as education, race, or lifestyle [16]). Such differentiation can be important; for example, Clouston and Quesnel-Vallée used longitudinal data to find that health differences relating to marital partnerships can result because of indirect and direct health selection, coupled with partnership benefits in a way that depends on social policy [17]. If direct selection is plausible, then longitudinal analysis is necessary to understand the role of both selection and causation. Furthermore, reliance on cross-sectional methods can be particularly detrimental when studying development, ageing, health, and mortality, which are known to depend on cohort, age, and historical era [18].

Studies have recently begun incorporating counterfactual methods into a longitudinal context. For instance, Colman and colleagues developed propensity scores from life course data from the MRC National Survey of Health and Development (1946 British birth cohort study) to show that antidepressants and anxiolytics had long term benefits to mental health [19]. Clouston and colleagues used propensity scores to find that a university education has a substantial impact on levels of adult fluid cognition in three life course studies, after adjusting for early life selective factors including adolescent cognition, gender, and parental social class [20]. Blundell and colleagues used propensity scores to show that higher education provides substantial returns both in log-hourly wages and in the likelihood of employment, in the National Child Development Study (1958 British birth cohort study) [21]. Robins proposed an approach called Marginal Structural Models (MSMs) when analysing longitudinal models of change [22]. MSMs use the inverse probability of treatment weights to overweight individuals whose probability of observed treatment outcome is low, and to reduce the influence of individuals whose treatments were predictable. Sampson, Sharkey and Raudenbush put such models to practice in a longitudinal context [6] and convincingly showed that structural disadvantage accumulates over time, limiting children's cognitive development. One problem not often discussed is the extent to which overweighting is appropriate; for example, should weights for some individuals be 50 times larger than others? [6] The use of stabilized weights which limit the potential influence of extreme weights have been proposed to address this [23].

Achy-Brou and colleagues (also Segal and colleagues [24]) further argue that weighting models is not an efficient way to adjust for selection bias and instead used propensity score adjustment to analyse the effectiveness of two different diabetes treatment regimens over 6 months with measurement every third month [12]. They used time-varying propensity scores and regression in a Bayesian framework. In their analysis, they used treatment regimens that did not differ over time (either TTT or CCC, but not TCT where T=treatment and C=control). To ensure balance, Achy-Brou and colleagues removed individuals outside the overlapping region (only 5% of the sample). They calculated propensity scores and transition probabilities at each time point, though we should note that Arpino and Mealli have shown the feasibility of using multilevel logistic regression to specify time-varying propensity scores [25].

Using robust longitudinal methodology, Retelsdorf and colleagues used propensity score matching in a 3-year study of development in children's reading capabilities among students who were tracked in academic and non-academic educational institutions [26]. To model longitudinal change they used latent growth curve modelling on a balanced subsample without further adjustment for the propensity score, and found that individuals in academic tracking programmes gained faster in terms of decoding speed but not in terms of reading ability. Leite and colleagues provide an excellent test of longitudinal propensity scores in latent growth curve models [27]; however, in doing so they compare four models that specify fundamentally different assumptions about treatment and selection. While longitudinal research using propensity scores has begun, no studies have yet provided a detailed discussion of the substantive implications of longitudinal treatments and outcomes. This lack of detail may be problematic if researchers assume that different models have similar implications.

8.4.1 **Longitudinal treatments**

In longitudinal observational research, treatment can occur in two different ways: (1) observation after treatment, and (2) treatment during observation. In the first case, treatment occurs prior to measurement of outcomes and propensity scores are time-invariant (a special case of monotonic propensity scores). For instance, treatment (T) occurs at some point (call it τ) and outcomes (O_t) are measured repeatedly (at times (t) = $\tau +1, \tau + 2 \ldots$) afterward. This yields a conceptual framework whereby changes in outcomes result from either treatment or the factors that lead to treatment. Treatment occurs prior to observation and may have already had an effect on the outcome, and thus it has the potential to cause differences at baseline (intercept) between $O_{T,1}$ and $O_{C,1}$ (C=control), and also differences in rates of change over time (slope). Differences in intercepts may result from a number of factors. If the data are properly balanced, remaining effects must be selection on the dependent variable, selection on unobserved covariates, or observed treatment effects.

Causal analysis becomes more difficult when we examine treatments that change longitudinally during observation. In such a case, the decision to match treatments and controls requires adjustment not only for between-person differences but also for within-person measurement time. When treatment occurs during observation, cases have one explicit and one implicit control: those individuals who were not treated can be explicitly matched, while within-individual observations occurring prior to treatment are implicitly useful in examining change, in that they provide us with an individual average prior to beneficial change. Modelling tactics remain similar to those used when treatment occurs prior to observation, except that a further piecewise treatment variable needs to be incorporated into the model that allows either linear or stepwise differential effects following the change in the observed treatment outcome. Examples of this type of model are increasingly popular when examining the role of life course transitions (e.g. marriage, children) on happiness or self-rated health [16,28,29].

8.5 **Example**

An example is now described, highlighting the use of propensity scores in longitudinal analysis, and how we apply these methods to life course data from the Wisconsin Longitudinal Study (WLS), addressing the impact of educational attainment on change in cognition. We estimate selection into education using gender, parental socioeconomic position, adolescent cognition, and adolescent non-cognitive (soft) skills. We use subclassification to estimate the role of treatment before observation (educational attainment) on level and change in adult fluid cognition.

8.5.1 **Methods**

First, we focus on creating two comparable groups: treated (T) and control (C). Second, we explicitly estimate the propensity score using covariates that include early life factors (x): $P_T = \Pr(T = 1|X = x)$, where x contains an n by $k+1$ matrix of covariates used to predict the probability of treatment. Insofar as our propensity score is well specified, this provides an estimate of an individual's likelihood of experiencing treatment, which we use to create balanced blocks. Finally, we incorporate these balanced blocks as a level in the multilevel mixed effects models (MLMs) (Chapter 6).

Incorporating the propensity score into MLMs, counterfactual analysis provides two pieces of information. First, balanced blocks define groups within which individuals have comparable propensities for treatment. Blocks represent sampling groups with propensity scores that define different rates of selection into treatment *between* but not *within* groups. Theoretically speaking, each block therefore makes up a small RCT where the selection bias is equivalent, but each small RCT in the sample is subject to different selection biases. As such, each group has a random intercept, but the benefits of treatment are believed to be generalizable under SUTVA.

To specify a propensity score in a MLM, we suggest using subclassification. This assumes that treatment effects are equivalent for all who are treated, though allowing differences in pre-treatment levels (intercepts). This leads us to model selection as a random between-group process, thereby incorporating a third level into the generalized MLM equation for longitudinal analysis:

$$Y_{kit} = \beta_{0ik} + \beta_{1i}T_{it} + \varepsilon_{itk} \tag{1}$$

Hence equation 1 describes the change in outcome Y for individual i over time t within treatment block k as predicted by some parametrization of time T subject to some error ε. Individual level parameters for intercept (β_{0ik}) and slope (β_{1i}) are modelled (equation 2) according to individual level covariates (X) and we assume that the random effects (v) are normally distributed with mean zero. Here β_{11} is the mean slope and β_{00k} is the mean within block intercept when all covariates are zero.

$$\begin{cases} \beta_{0ik} = \beta_{00k} + \gamma_0 X_0 + v_{0ik} \\ \beta_{1i} = \beta_{11} + \gamma_1 X_1 + v_{1i} \end{cases} \tag{2}$$

Finally, we model block-level differences in intercepts where β_{00} is the mean intercept when all covariates are zero (equation 3). We estimate the block-level intercept (β_{00k}) using factors (δ) implicated at the group-level (G_0) and further assume that the group-level error (η_{00k}) is normally distributed, with mean zero.

$$\beta_{00k} = \beta_{000} + \delta_0 G_0 + \eta_{00k} \tag{3}$$

Further details and results from the analysis using data from the WLS are presented in Supplementary web material at www.halcyon.ac.uk.

8.5.2 **Limitations**

Life course data are extremely helpful because they provide information on variation that is often unobserved in cross-sectional or late life ageing studies alone. Although SUTVA is necessary when providing an average treatment effect [1], treatment effects can be modified, and much of the most interesting analyses interrogate this problem. For example, the quality of a treatment (e.g. marital partnerships, educational investments) may play a role in the benefits received from such treatments. In this case, measuring and modifying the treatment may be integral to providing a true estimate of the effect, and any treatment effect calculated prior would underestimate any potential benefits. Finally, sample mortality can bias models if not accounted for because mortality is itself subject to many forces that impact on other health outcomes [30], and may further lead to overestimates of the impact of social treatments on health outcomes because of the influence of terminal decline [31,32]. Further incorporating estimates and measures of mortality would help researchers to provide less biased results.

8.6 Conclusion

This chapter has shown how propensity scores can be used in longitudinal analyses, highlighting the multiple options available and the decisions that have to be made in the analysis process. A longitudinal mixed effects model has been defined that uses subclassification based on balanced subgroups to provide a longitudinal estimate of the causal impact of treatment. An example of such a model using life course data from the Wisconsin Longitudinal Study, examining change in adult fluid cognition between ages 53 and 70, was presented. In this example, support was found for the view that education is highly selective on adolescent cognitive and non-cognitive factors, including gender and parental social class and further, that education causes beneficial increases in adult fluid cognition but does little to impact the rate of decline in that cognition.

References

1 **Morgan SL, Winship** C. Counterfactuals and Causal Inference: Methods and Principles for Social Research. Cambridge: Cambridge University Press; 2007.

2 **Glymour MM, et al.** Does childhood schooling affect old age memory or mental status? Using state schooling laws as natural experiments. *J Epidemiol Community Health* 2008;**62**:532–7.

3 **List JA, et al.** Effects of environmental regulations on manufacturing plant births: evidence from a propensity score matching estimator. *Rev Econ Stat* 2003;**85**:944–52.

4 **Lechner M.** Program heterogeneity and propensity score matching: an application to the evaluation of active labor market policies. *Rev Econ Stat* 2002;**84**:205–20.

5 **Kim MH, et al.** Is precarious employment damaging to self-rated health? Results of propensity score matching methods, using longitudinal data in South Korea. *Soc Sci Med* 2008;**67**:1982–94.

6 **Sampson RJ, et al.** Durable effects of concentrated disadvantage on verbal ability among African-American children. *Proc Nat Academy Sci* 2008;**105**:845.

7 **Caliendo M, Kopeinig S.** Some practical guidance for the implementation of propensity score matching. *J Econ Surveys* 2008;**22**:31–72.

8 **Rubin DB.** Estimating causal effects from large data sets using propensity scores. *Annals Int Med* 1997; **127**:757–63.

9 **Shah BR, et al.** Propensity score methods gave similar results to traditional regression modeling in observational studies: a systematic review. *J Clin Epidemiol* 2005;**58**:550–9.

10 **Baser O.** Too much ado about propensity score models? Comparing methods of propensity score matching. *Value Health* 2006;**9**:377–85.

11 **Dahabreh IJ, et al.** Do observational studies using propensity score methods agree with randomized trials? A systematic comparison of studies on acute coronary syndromes. *Eur Heart J* 2012;**33**:1893–901.

12 **Achy-Brou AC, et al.** Estimating treatment effects of longitudinal designs using regression models on propensity scores. *Biometrics* 2010;**66**:824–33.

13 **Becker SO, Ichino A.** Estimation of average treatment effects based on propensity scores. *The Stata Journal* 2002;**2**:358–77.

14 **Rosenbaum PR, Rubin DB.** The central role of the propensity score in observational studies for causal effects. *Biometrika* 1983;**70**:41.

15 **Atalay K, Barrett G.** The impact of age pension eligibility age on retirement and program dependence: evidence from an Australian experiment. Social and Economic Dimensions of Aging Population Research Paper Series 295: McMaster University, Canada; 2012.

16 **Goldman N.** Marriage selection and mortality patterns: inferences and fallacies. *Demography* 1993;**30**: 189–208.

17 **Clouston S, Quesnel-Vallée A.** The role of defamilialization in the relationship between partnership and self-rated health: a cross-national comparison of Canada and the United States. *Soc Sci Med* 2012;**75**:1342–50.

18 **Hofer SM, et al.** Evaluating the interdependence of aging-related changes in visual and auditory acuity, balance, and cognitive functioning. *Psychol Aging* 2003;**18**:285–305.

19 **Colman I, et al.** Psychiatric outcomes 10 years after treatment with antidepressants or anxiolytics. *Brit J Psychiatr* 2008;**193**:327–31.

20 **Clouston SAP, et al.** Benefits of educational attainment on adult fluid cognition: international evidence from three birth cohorts. *Int J Epidemiol* 2012:**41**:1729–36.

21 **Blundell R, et al.** The returns to higher education in britain: evidence from a British cohort. *Econ J* 2000;**110**:82–99.

22 **Robins JM.** Association, causation, and marginal structural models. *Synthese* 1999;**121**:151–79.

23 **Robins JM, et al.** Marginal structural models and causal inference in epidemiology. *Epidemiol* 2000;**11**: 550–60

24 **Segal JB, et al.** Using propensity scores subclassification to estimate effects of longitudinal treatments: an example using a new diabetes medication. *Med Care* 2007;**45**:S149.

25 **Arpino B, Mealli F.** The specification of the propensity score in multilevel observational studies. *Comp Stat Data Analysis* 2011;**55**:1770–80.

26 **Retelsdorf J, et al.** Reading development in a tracked school system: a longitudinal study over 3 years using propensity score matching. *Br J Educ Psychol* 2012:**82**:647–71.

27 **Leite WL, et al.** An evaluation of latent growth models for propensity score matched groups. *Structural Equation Modeling: A Multidisciplinary Journal* 2012;**19**:437–56.

28 **Zimmermann AC, Easterlin RA.** Happily ever after? Cohabitation, marriage, divorce, and happiness in Germany. *Pop Develop Rev* 2006;**32**:511–28.

29 **Myrskylä M, Margolis R.** Happiness: before and after the kids. Rostock, Germany: Max Planck Institute for Demographic Research Working Paper; 2012.

30 **Harel O, et al.** Population inference with mortality and attrition in longitudinal studies on aging: a two-stage multiple imputation method. *Exp Aging Res* 2007;**33**:187–203.

31 **Piccinin AM, et al.** Terminal decline from within-and between-person perspectives, accounting for incident dementia. *J Gerontol B: Psychol Sci Soc Sci* 2011;**66**:391–401.

32 **Thorvaldsson V, et al.** Onset of terminal decline in cognitive abilities in individuals without dementia. *Neurology* 2008;**71**:882–7.

Chapter 9

Understanding healthy ageing using a qualitative approach: the value of narratives and individual biographies

JD Carpentieri and Jane Elliott

9.1 Introduction to understanding healthy ageing using a qualitative approach

How can narrative methods be used in life course research on healthy ageing, and in what ways can they provide insights not available through quantitative data? How can qualitative and quantitative approaches to studies of the life course be combined in order to shed additional light on healthy ageing? These questions form the focus of this chapter, which draws on material from qualitative biographical interviews with members of the MRC National Survey of Health and Development (NSHD) and the Hertfordshire Cohort Study (HCS), to provide narrative case histories. This chapter highlights the methodological value of such narratives when seeking to understand older people's own experiences of health and ageing. It does so by first introducing key themes and concepts in narrative research, and then discussing those themes in relation to three individual case studies, each of which has been anonymized (Section 9.4).

9.2 What is a narrative?

The most concise definition of narrative is a story with a beginning, a middle, and an end—this description has been traced back to Aristotle in his *Poetics* [1–3]. However, a successful narrative is more than just a sequence or chronicle of events. Indeed, Labov and Waletzky [4: p. 12] suggested that although a sequence of actions is sufficient for a minimal narrative, such a narrative is 'abnormal: it may be considered as empty or pointless'. They argued that a defining feature of a typical narrative is that the teller does not just list events or actions; he or she interprets them. The narrator makes sense of those experiences both for him or herself and for the audience.

Given the specific interest for many qualitative researchers in understanding the *meanings* of events and experiences from an individual's perspective, it is clear why narrative can be seen as a powerful and useful tool for understanding healthy ageing from a life course perspective. Narratives do not just tell us what has happened; they tell us what those events or happenings mean to the narrator. They can therefore provide valuable information about older people's diverse experiences of health and ageing.

9.2.1 Big stories and small stories

Within the field of narrative analysis, distinctions can be made between 'big stories' and 'small stories' [5–7]. Big stories are the grand, biographical narratives of lives; they tend to focus on major events, experiences and turning points. These events and experiences are connected to form a life story [7]. In contrast, small stories tend to focus on mundane events and everyday occurrences. Whereas big stories tend to be elicited by interviewers, small stories occur more naturally—these are the type of anecdotes that might occur in everyday conversation. Such anecdotes also occur in open and semi-structured interviews, but are unlikely to appear in the carefully structured interviews most often used to collect quantitative data.

In the context of the research discussed here, which involved qualitative biographical interviews with members of established cohort studies, researchers might expect congruence between the big story, told by the interviewee, and the information that could be derived from the prospective longitudinal data in constructing a case study of a particular individual. For example, one of the case studies in this chapter centres on Patricia, a 72 year-old woman. In her qualitative interview, Patricia's life story includes the following key events: getting married in her early forties to a man who was considerably older than her and who already had three children; never having children of her own; enjoying a successful working life; and retiring in her early sixties when her husband suffered a stroke. These key structuring elements of the life story are all likely to have been recorded in the cohort study's quantitative longitudinal data (although the meaning for the individual is more likely to be shared in a qualitative interview). In contrast, the *small stories* are those which provide insights into experiences of daily life and the significance of those experiences. These are very unlikely to be captured in the more structured quantitative longitudinal data. The case studies below provide more examples of these small stories and exemplify how they might shed light on the lived experiences of healthy ageing or, conversely, the impact of poor health and capability on an individual's quality of life and wellbeing.

A major advantage of conducting qualitative interviews with individuals who are already part of a large scale quantitative study is that it is possible to place these individual cases and narratives in context. Each individual's big story and small stories can be understood against the backdrop of the detailed quantitative data collected from the larger sample. Therefore, for each of the case studies we provide some brief information from their quantitative record.

9.3 **Narratives of health, ageing and illness**

9.3.1 **Healthy ageing**

Much of the now considerable literature on healthy ageing draws on qualitative research evidence [8–13], and some of this takes an explicitly narrative approach [8,14]. Indeed, much of this is discussed elsewhere (Chapters 1 and 4).

Narrative has featured in the literature on health behaviour and health education [15,16]. Within the field of the sociology of health, there has been a focus on lay perspectives of disease and patients' own experiences of ill health. In particular, for those suffering from chronic disease, the idea of an 'illness career' has been a useful analytic tool and can be readily expressed in the form of a narrative.

In Chapter 1, healthy ageing is defined as encompassing 'healthy biological ageing and high levels of psychological and social wellbeing'. When looking at the key themes that older people themselves focus on as central to healthy ageing, qualitative researchers have found an emphasis on being engaged in meaningful activities, having the ability and resources to engage in activities and having a positive attitude (Chapter 4). For example Bryant et al. [9] found that some older people conceptualized healthy ageing as 'going and doing something meaningful'; this in turn required a balance between 'abilities and challenges'. This has clear resonances with Laslett's original work conceptualizing the third age, which stresses the importance of self-actualization [17].

9.3.2 **Narrative identity**

An interest in narrative in qualitative research has clear resonances with theoretical work on the concept of narrative identity [18–22]. The term 'identity' can be understood in two ways. On the one hand there is the notion of identity as *exactly* the same, equivalent or identical (the Latin *idem*). Alternatively, identity can be used to refer to continuity or something that can be traced through time. The Latin *ipse* or 'self same' (*soi-même* in French) suggests this sense of identity as *permanence* without *sameness* through time [23]. Narrative fits with this conceptualization of individual identity as 'self-same', in that it provides the practical means by which a person can understand themselves as living through time, a human subject with a past, present and future, made whole by the coherence of the narrative plot with a *beginning, a middle, and an end* [20]. The narrative constitution of the self suggests that subjectivity is neither an incoherent stream of events, nor is it immutable and incapable of evolution [21].

9.3.3 Narrative gerontology

Narrative gerontology and an emphasis on healthy or active ageing might be thought of by some as the 'new' gerontology [24], but its origins can be traced back to at least the mid-1990s [25]. It is based on the concept, or metaphor, of life as story and therefore has similarities with narrative psychology. Much of the work that is influenced by narrative gerontology is linked to qualitative or theoretical work on what it *means* to be old, and on how to work with, and care for, older adults. There is therefore an emphasis on using narrative gerontology in practice and with practitioners. Narrative gerontology puts an emphasis on the wisdom of the old and the advantages in old age of having greater life experience and more disposable time in which to reflect on and make sense of that life experience [26]. It also encourages an awareness of the stereotypical discourses of decline and ageing that inform much of societal thinking about what it means to be old [27]. Narrative gerontology suggests that individuals need to have 'narrative capital', or 'a good strong story', in order to enable them to maintain levels of wellbeing. A central tenet of narrative gerontology is that identity development is a lifelong process; the self is seen as a story that is continually developing [28–30]. A key goal of active or healthy ageing is to avoid 'narrative foreclosure', or the sense that life is becoming hopeless and worthless [30–34]. Narrative foreclosure is the 'premature conviction that one's life story has effectively ended' [35]. The individual's biographical development has stalled; the big stories have effectively ended, and only small stories remain. The narrator has moved into 'epilogue time' [36: p. 193].

Another way of looking at this process is in terms of biographical disruption. Several researchers have investigated the impact of chronic ill health on individuals' sense of identity [37–42]. In particular, Bury [43] showed unexpected chronic illness as biographically disruptive: the sufferer's narrative thread linking past, present, and expected future is broken by poor health. However, ill health does not necessarily have the same impact on all sufferers' identities. Bury's original work was with younger adults suffering from arthritis—an unexpected condition for that age group. For older adults, serious health problems may be perceived as biographically reinforcing or continuous. Pound and colleagues [44] found that elderly men and women in a working-class section of London experienced stroke as a 'normal crisis', one that, while unwanted, was not necessarily unexpected. Likewise, Sinding and Wiernikowski [45] found that many older people did not experience cancer as disruptive to the 'story of their life': the disease was seen as a normal, biographically continuous part of the ageing process.

9.4 Collecting individual biographies and narrative through cohort studies

Cohort studies have some clear narrative properties [46,47,57]. They enable us to follow individuals' lives through time and allow for the estimation of models that focus on how earlier life experiences and environments may impact on later outcomes. However, the quantitative data collected as part of a cohort study could be thought of as being closer to a chronicle than a narrative. Events, experiences and dates are recorded, but the individual respondents are not typically asked to make meaning out of this information, or to provide their own narrative account of their life. Rather, narratives may be constructed by researchers, who aim to make sense of the detailed data from a large sample within the framework of their own research questions. A major advantage of these qualitative interviews over other collections of narrative biographical data, is that it is possible to locate individuals within the context of a large representative sample and to understand to what extent their experiences may be shared by others with similar characteristics. By carrying out qualitative interviews with cohort members, it was intended to give the individuals themselves an opportunity to provide an account of their life that would complement the quantitative data that had been collected from and about them ever since they were born. Qualitative biographical interviews were carried out with small subsamples of the HCS (30 interviews in total), the MRC NSHD (30 interviews), and the National Child Development Study (the 1958 British birth cohort) (220 interviews, not used in this chapter). For further details of the sample selection and interview process see Elliott et al. [48,49]

9.5 **How were the narrative case studies chosen for this chapter?**

As the focus of this book is on healthy ageing, the aim was to select cases from the interviewed subsample that could shed light on healthy ageing and barriers to it. Three variables were used to identify cases, with two focusing on physical health and one on wellbeing. First was self-rated health (SRH), a single variable with five response categories ranging from excellent to poor. SRH is a simple but reliable tool for assessing general health and predicting future health issues, including mortality [50]. The second physical indicator was self-reported physical capability: a score was derived from a series of six questions about capability in daily life, ranging from being able to bathe and dress oneself to being able to run for a bus.

Among the 60 interviewees in the NSHD and HCS, seven rated their health as excellent, 26 as 'very good', 21 as 'good', and six as 'fair'. None of those interviewed rated their health as poor. In total there were five individuals with excellent self-rated health and good physical capability (one from the HCS and four from the NSHD) and four with 'fair' self-rated health and poor physical capability (two from the HCS and two from the NSHD).

Third, to take account of psychological and social factors, cohort members' Warwick-Edinburgh mental wellbeing scores—possible range 14 (lowest) to 70 (highest)—were also considered [51]. There was considerable heterogeneity in wellbeing among these small groups of individuals, with wellbeing scores ranging from 38 to 70. However, individuals with excellent self-rated health and good physical capability had wellbeing scores ranging from 52 to 70, and those with only 'fair' health and poor physical capability ranged from 38 to 46. There was no overlap between the two groups.

Based on this initial analysis of the quantitative data, three cases were selected for detailed narrative analysis in this chapter: two females from the HCS and one male from the NSHD. Doreen is a 76 year-old woman with only fair self-rated health, poor physical capability and a wellbeing score of just 41. Patricia is a 72 year-old woman with excellent self-rated health and good physical capability and a wellbeing score of 52. Alan is a 64 year-old man with excellent self-rated health, high physical capability and a wellbeing score of 70. These cases are discussed in turn in Sections 9.5 to 9.7. Each case has been anonymized to avoid the possibility of identifying the individuals concerned. Names have been changed, and a few biographical details have been altered to obscure individual identities. Written consent was provided by each individual for their interview to be recorded, and for extracted quotations to be reproduced in publications, reports, web pages, and other research outputs.

These three case studies provide examples of different narratives of health and ageing. One interviewee tells a tale of unhealthy ageing. The second interviewee's narrative is of a good level of physical health but lower than expected psychological and social wellbeing. The third narrative is of very healthy and active ageing.

9.6 Doreen: 'This unfortunate 76 year-old': a narrative of decline

Doreen is 76 and lives with her husband. Doreen and her husband have been living in the same house in a small town in Hertfordshire for nearly 40 years. They have three grown children who live fairly nearby and three grandchildren. Doreen left education at age 15, but enjoyed her subsequent career as a shorthand typist. She was forced by ill health to retire at age 61.

In the quantitative interview, Doreen rated her own health as fair, and indicated that it had declined greatly over the last year. Indeed, she was the only individual of the 30 interviewed from the HCS whose health had declined greatly, with 20 of 30 individuals stating that their health was about the same. Doreen has a body mass index (BMI) of 35 kg/m^2, i.e. Grade 2 obesity (BMI $\geq$ 35), which is associated with higher all-cause mortality than Grade 1 obesity (BMI of 30 – < 35) [52]. Doreen's Warwick-Edinburgh wellbeing score is 41; this is more than one standard deviation (SD) lower than the sample mean for the whole cohort (51.7, SD 8.02) [53], but is average for those in the sample with fair health and poor physical capability. The health problems that Doreen cites include obesity, breast cancer, diabetes, 'gouty' arthritis, an ovarian cyst, swollen hands and feet, and a recent knee replacement. When asked how she would describe her health, Doreen quotes her doctor: '[He] says I'm a very unfortunate 76 year-old, 'cause I've had so much go wrong with me . . . a lot of complications'.

Doreen's physical problems means she struggles with many routine activities of daily living, such as getting up and down stairs and bathing herself. Her husband, in turn, suffers from Alzheimer's disease. She is physically reliant on him; he is mentally reliant on her. As she observes, they are mutually dependent: '*I'm his brain most of the time and he helps me to do the things that I can't do*'.

Doreen's poor health is the central theme of her interview: almost every narrative becomes an illness narrative. This is true no matter what the topic or time period. For example, when asked if she had a sweet tooth as a child, Doreen quickly brings the question back to her current health problems: '*No more than average, I would say—no, not more than average. I've got Type 2 diabetes, since I've been in my sixties*'. Health problems provide a form of global coherence to her interview [54], exerting a seemingly inexorable gravitational pull on her narratives.

This is perhaps unsurprising, given the vicious downward spiral she finds herself in: her health problems reduce her capability, and her reduced capability, in turn, makes it very difficult to engage in behaviours that would lessen her health problems. Her lack of health makes it nearly impossible to live healthily. For example, Doreen understands that she should be more active and do more exercise, but her weight, and problems with her swollen feet and ankles, make this extremely challenging. As she explains: '*I wish I was more mobile, that's for sure. Everybody keeps telling me I should walk and do this and all that, but when it hurts, it's very difficult*'. These problems are exacerbated by her susceptibility to falling, which Doreen partly attributes to the antidepressants she is taking. Her health, capability and psychological wellbeing all negatively influence each other.

This troublesome spiral has had a strongly negative effect on her sense of self. In particular, she no longer views herself as a 'coper'. While Doreen has suffered health problems for decades, she had always viewed herself as someone who coped well with them. In Doreen's narrative, there is a sense that there was a 'past self' that was psychologically capable of triumphing over health problems: '*I took—, having cancer very well. You know, I mean it was serious, and it frightens you, but I think I took it very well*'. However, since her knee replacement a year ago, she feels she has gone downhill rapidly, and is now much more easily overwhelmed. Instead of being incorporated into her sense of self, ill-health is now overwhelming it.

In Doreen's 'big story' there is a major rupture between past and present. A key theme throughout Doreen's narrative is the contrast between her former self and her current self, the difference between then and now. In discussing her younger days, Doreen emphasizes her active engagement with the world, whether through work—she starts the life story section of the interview by saying, '*I loved work, I loved my job*'—or through play. She tells a number of small stories emphasizing activity: as a child, playing outside, building tree houses, tobogganing and throwing snowballs; as an adult, going dancing and shopping. These stories are contrasted with her lack of capability and her immobility in her old age. She repeatedly begins small stories with the phrase, '*I used to*', emphasizing what she can no longer accomplish. '*I wish we had done a bit more really*', she laments. Her big story seems to have come to an unexpectedly early end, replaced by a series of small stories about the challenges of day-to-day life.

The stark contrast between Doreen's past self and her current one fits with the once prevailing view of ageing as a decline into decrepitude and incapability (as discussed by Laslett [17] and Gullette [55]), or narrative foreclosure.

9.7 **Patricia: 'I know what to watch for': a narrative of control**

Patricia is age 72 and lives with her husband Donald, who is fifteen years older. In the quantitative interview, Patricia described her health as excellent, just as it was a year ago. She has a high level of physical capability and a BMI of 26 kg/m², i.e. just slightly above the recommended range. Her Warwick-Edinburgh wellbeing score is 52, which is very close to the mean score for this cohort of 51.7 (SD: 8.02) [53]. However, it is the lowest of anyone with excellent self-rated health and good physical capability.

Patricia describes an active childhood in which she enjoyed playing, and swam regularly and with some skill. As an adult, she had an interesting career as an administrator, a job she loved. She had no children of her own, but has stepchildren through her husband. Like Doreen, Patricia retired earlier than planned—not because of her own health problems but because of her husband's. Since retirement, she has continued to lead an active life, playing bridge and bowls every week. She also enjoys gardening and exercises regularly. As she says:

> '*I do that (stretching exercises) pretty regular actually. I've got all the videos and all the discs. I've done Pilates, I've done yoga . . . I've done it all; I do anything to keep my weight down*'.

Patricia's qualitative interview provides indications why her wellbeing is lower than expected, given her good physical health and active life. Her husband had a stroke over 10 years ago and is now in a wheelchair; his incapacity means that Patricia has major caring responsibilities. These responsibilities constrain her life in a number of ways. For example, the couple have recently moved to a house with a smaller garden. While the new house is better suited to their capabilities, the move has left Patricia feeling socially isolated. As she says:

> '*I've been so busy getting this thing sorted out and I keep thinking, I must phone Barbara, I must phone Jean, I must get in contact with them, and they've sort of left me alone I think, really*'.

In contrast to Doreen, health does not dominate Patricia's narratives. However, it does play an important role—particularly her husband's health problems and their impact on her own life. In particular, Patricia tells a number of small stories that provide insights into the negative impacts of her husband's health on her own wellbeing. In the following extract, for example, Patricia explains somewhat ruefully that driving holidays used to be a major part of the couple's life together, but no longer are:

> 'I don't know whether we'll go anymore, I don't particularly—, he likes to go weekends away to hotels in England, but it's all drive, drive, drive for me. I have to pack his scooter, his wheelchair, his toilet seat riser, his backrest; all that has to go, for about 3 or 4 days; drive along the M25, down the M3 if you're going south or up that way, and you've got—, it's a hassle and I just don't really want to do it anymore, you know. Getting old [laughs]'.

A second key theme of Patricia's narratives is her proactive approach to her own health as she ages. Patricia is very candid about the fact that she would not expect her stepchildren to take care of her in later life. She is therefore already planning to move into sheltered accommodation when she is older:

> 'Probably when I get to about 80-odd I might move into one of these complexes for the elderly, because I haven't got any children, you see; I've got stepchildren but it's not the same as your own children, and I feel that I'd be looked after that way. If I didn't get up in the morning someone would wonder why, wouldn't they?'

It is striking that Patricia uses the age of 'about 80-odd' as a benchmark for when she will need to move. In this way she underlines her rationality, realism and ability to plan, but also distances herself from being 'elderly' or in the fourth age, the age of decrepitude and decline [17,56]. There is also, of course, an implicit optimism here in expecting that she will live to be at least '80-odd', in comparison with her parents, who died in their mid-seventies.

This plan highlights another powerful contrast between the life course narratives of Doreen and Patricia. Doreen's 'disrupted biography' is evident in her reluctance to look ahead. When asked a question about the future, she sidesteps the question. In contrast, Patricia's narratives focus not just on the past and present, but on her plans for the future. Implicit in this planning is Patricia's desire to exert as much control as possible over her health, in order to minimize decline. This control is manifested through planning, exercise and medical care. In her narratives, Patricia's independence, capability and rationality is often constructed in contrast to other lives that have been dominated by ill health and incapacity. For example, after briefly discussing her father's sudden death, she provides a detailed narrative of her mother's chronic ill health, which persisted from her forties until she died in her mid-seventies. Likewise, Patricia tells the interviewer that, like her husband, she suffers from eye problems, but implies that she has learned from his experiences:

> 'I know what to watch for so that if there is a problem I know, just go straight and get it seen to'.

9.8 Alan: 'I usually get up and walk . . . about 3 miles': striding on—a narrative of healthy ageing

Alan is 64 and lives with his wife. They have a son and daughter and several grandchildren, who all live in Canada. Despite this distance, they are a close family, speaking regularly on the phone and through Skype, and visiting each other every year. Alan has recently retired after a successful career as a teacher and then Head of Year. He enjoys a very active life including chess club, helping to run a youth group at church, singing in a choir, and regularly walking for pleasure.

In the quantitative interview, Alan described his general health as excellent and as about the same as a year ago. He also was scored as having high capability. His Warwick-Edinburgh wellbeing score was the maximum possible score of 70, an unusually high score for this cohort (who have a mean of 51.9 and SD of 7.85). He has a BMI of 23 kg/m^2, i.e. within the normal range.

Alan's overarching narrative is one of enviable good health and high levels of physical activity. His body is 'dys-appearing' somewhat—i.e. making itself more apparent through aches, pains and other assorted other indicators of ageing [57]—but he has no serious health concerns and is highly active. '*In the morning,*' he says, '*I usually get up and walk . . . for an hour or so . . . about 3 miles.*' He regularly goes on longer walks, as well—for example, a 5-day hike in Northern England. He and his wife, who is also in good health, are very socially engaged: '*We go out quite a lot visiting,*' he notes, adding, '*We've a lot of friends in the area*'.

While his excellent health and high levels of activity could in theory be attributed to his relatively young age compared to Doreen and Patricia, it is worth noting that Alan is several years older than Doreen was when she was forced to retire due to ill health. He appears to be on a markedly different health trajectory than she was at his age.

In contrast to Doreen and Patricia, health and illness have barely any presence in Alan's narratives. This is particularly noteworthy given the central place of physical activity in these narratives. In contrast to Patricia, this activity is presented not as a strategy for keeping his weight down and maintaining good health, but as enjoyable for its own sake. For example, when asked what he gets out of walking, Alan highlights aesthetic, psychological and physical pleasures, but does not overtly point to health gains: '*It's just beautiful, nature; all the animals and birds that you see, and it makes you feel good*'. Throughout his interview, health—and its corollary, illness—are in the distant background, if they have a presence at all.

However, in one small story about his chess club, Alan does highlight his awareness of the long-term benefits of staying active and engaged:

> '*I suppose it's good for your mind, but that's not the reason [I play]. When you get older, you think, well, I'll just continue with that. There's a guy who's now 90 who plays in the league; you wouldn't think he was 90 . . . He still plays a very high standard of chess. He says without the chess, he would have been like these other ones* [laughs]'.

Since retirement, Alan has, if anything, grown more active and engaged. As he observes, his good health allows him to live a more dynamic, rewarding life, one that is biographically continuous with his younger self: '*[Good health means] you can enjoy retirement more; to retire and to not be healthy would be a bit of a shame. I don't want to stop doing the things that I'm doing*'.

In part, his good physical and psychological health is due to maintaining his lifelong interest in walking. However, Alan has also taken advantage of the extra time available to him in retirement to take up new activities, e.g. leading a local music group. Instead of facing narrative foreclosure, like Doreen, he is able to add a new chapter to his life. '*I really loved teaching [and] thought I would miss it, but I don't*', he says, somewhat surprised. '*Now I'm retired, [I'm] finding other things to do*'. This fits closely with Ricoeur's [21] concept of individual identity developing through time, maintaining *permanence* without *sameness*.

In some ways, Alan's health has actually improved with age. In one of the few health-focused stories he tells, Alan mentions that he has had asthma since he was an adolescent, and that it used to '*be a problem occasionally*'. Because of a new generation of medication, this is no longer the case. Now, he says, '*it doesn't stop me doing anything*'. This is a useful reminder that individual biographies unfold within a broader historical context; medical advances play a central role in influencing healthy ageing.

9.9 **Discussion**

The 'big stories' exemplified in these three case studies contain a number of other narratives, and a number of key themes. Doreen's story is a narrative of decline—reinforcing, perhaps, the traditional view of old age as a period of physical decrepitude and disappearance from social engagement and public life. Patricia's narrative is one of control. She seeks to manage her health and slow any decline. She seeks to prepare for a predicted future when she will be unable to care for herself. She cannot stop the ageing process, but she can manage it to a certain degree. Alan's narrative is one of very active ageing: the modern ideal.

It is striking that in none of these case studies is there a clear message, or narrative, about the early life experiences that might have influenced health in later life. None of these three individuals reflect on how past experiences or behaviours may have impacted on their current health and wellbeing. Rather, in Doreen's case the ageing process is conceptualized as having transformed her from an individual who copes well with ill health to someone who is severely limited by health problems and lack of mobility. In contrast, both Patricia and Alan are currently still actively working to maintain health and capability. Indeed, one way of characterizing the three narratives is the different way that each individual makes a link between past, present and future. Doreen's poor health means that she focuses on looking back at her past life—her narrative focuses on the past and has the recurrent theme of, '*I used to*'. The fact that Patricia's husband is significantly older and in poor health encourages her to look forward, so that her narrative focuses around the future and the statement, '*I will*'; whereas Alan's excellent health allows him to live in the present, continuing to do what he always has, while adding new activities—his narrative is much more present focused and keeps returning to the statement, '*I do*'.

There are perhaps two main ways in which this more narrative approach to data collection and analysis can be seen to complement the quantitative longitudinal approaches exemplified by other chapters.

First, in contrast to structured quantitative data collection, semi-structured and in-depth interviews provide evidence about the everyday lives and experiences of older people. Doreen's case study, in particular, provides a good exemplar of how we can gain an insight into the difficulties of daily life through 'small stories' told in the context of a biographical interview. Many of these stories are habitual or exemplar narratives which help the interviewer to understand the challenges faced by the respondent. In turn, this can lead to an understanding of some of the mechanisms by which poor health and reduced capability can have an impact on wellbeing and quality of life.

Second, by examining individual cases holistically and allowing cohort members to provide the 'big story' of their biography from their own perspective, researchers can be alerted to important factors that influence individuals' lives—factors that may not have been adequately captured in the structured quantitative interviews. As discussed in Sections 9.5 and 9.6, for both Doreen and Patricia, a spouse's health is an important factor contributing to individual wellbeing.

One of the key messages of these case studies is that healthy ageing cannot be looked at only at the individual level. Health must be looked at from a life course, or lifelong, perspective, but also from a 'life wide' perspective. The health of one's partner can significantly affect the quality of one's ageing. Patricia has aged healthily as an individual, but despite her robust health and high level of physical capability, Patricia's wellbeing is relatively low for someone with good physical health. As her narrative indicates, this is influenced by the limitations placed on her life by her partner's poor health. For example, she is no longer able to enjoy valued pastimes such as travelling, and she has grown somewhat isolated from her friends. Observing her older partner's health problems appears to encourage Patricia's natural inclination to be competent and in control, and to make plans to reduce the negative impacts of her own ageing on herself and others. Doreen, in contrast, is co-dependent on her husband. Individually, neither could cope, but together, they have sufficient capability for most aspects of daily life. Narratively, their life stories have fused. Both the HCS and the NSHD include brief questions about spouses' health status, but these case studies suggest that as individuals get older, and restricted capability and health problems grow more common, it is important to ask more detailed questions about spouses' health and caring responsibilities in order to understand more about factors influencing wellbeing and quality of life.

These three narratives are consistent with the conceptualization of healthy ageing provided by Bryant and colleagues [9], namely that healthy ageing centres on the ability to 'go and do something meaningful'. Both Patricia and Alan describe several groups and activities with which they are regularly involved—chess, bridge, bowls, and walking provide social contact and a chance to exercise both body and mind. Even though Patricia is somewhat constrained by her disabled older husband she still has excellent self-rated health and good physical capability. The aim in this chapter has been to demonstrate the value of narrative data collection and narrative analysis for developing an understanding of older people's experiences of ageing. Although there are just three case studies presented here, the quantitative studies from which they have been drawn provide the context within which they can be understood. It is clear that Alan and Doreen are situated near the extreme ends of the dimension spanning healthy and unhealthy ageing. They therefore provide helpful 'ideal types' or benchmarks which can be used to help exemplify and understand the contrasting experiences of older adults in Britain today.

References

1 **Chatman S.** Story and Discourse: Narrative Structure in Fiction and Film. Ithaca: Cornell University Press; 1978.

2 **Leitch TM.** What Stories Are: Narrative Theory and Interpretation. University Park, Pennsylvania: The Pennsylvania State University Press; 1986.

3 **Martin W.** Recent Theories of Narrative. Ithaca, NY: Cornell University Press; 1986.

4 **Labov W, Waletzky J.** Narrative analysis: oral versions of personal experience. In: Helm J, editor. Essays on the Verbal and Visual Arts. Seattle, WA: University of Washington Press; 1967:12–44.

5 **Bamberg M.** Stories: big or small: why do we care? *Narrative Inquiry* 2006;**16**:139–47.

6 **Freeman M.** Life 'on holiday'? In defence of big stories. *Narrative Inquiry* 2006;**16**:131–8.

7 **Phoenix C, Sparkes AC.** Being Fred: big stories, small stories and the accomplishment of a positive ageing identity. *Qualitative Research* 2009;**9**:219–36.

8 **Katz S.** Busy bodies: activity, aging, and the management of everyday life. *J Aging Stud* 2000;**14**:135–52.

9 **Bryant LL, et al.** In their own words: a model of healthy aging. *Soc Sci Med* 2001;**53**:927–41.

10 **Reichstadt J, et al.** Older adults perspectives on successful aging: qualitative interviews. *Am J Geriatr Psychiatry* 2010;**18**:567–75.

11 **Prieto-Flores M, et al.** Identifying connections between the subjective experience of health and quality of life in old age. *Qualitative Health Research* 2010;**20**:1491–9.

12 **Duay DL, Bryan VC.** Senior adults' perceptions of successful aging. *Educational Gerontology* 2006;**32**: 423–45.

13 **Rossen EK, et al.** Older women's perceptions of successful aging. *Activities, Adaptation & Aging* 2008;**32**: 73–88.

14 **Faircloth CA, et al.** Energizing the ordinary: biographical work and the future in stroke recovery narratives. *J Aging Stud* 2004;**18**:399–413.

15 **Moffat BM, Johnson JL.** Through the haze of cigarettes: teenage girls' stories about cigarette addiction. *Qualitative Health Research* 2001;**11**:668–81.

16 **Workman TA.** Finding the meanings of college drinking: an analysis of fraternity drinking stories. *Health Commun* 2001;**13**:427–47.

17 **Laslett P.** A Fresh Map of Life: The Emergence of the Third Age. Cambridge, MA: Harvard University Press; 1991.

18 **Ezzy D.** Subjectivity and the labour process: conceptualising 'good work'. *Sociology* 1997;**31**:427–44.

19 **Giddens A.** Modernity and Self Identity: Self and Society in the Late Modern Age. Cambridge: Polity; 1991.

20 **Gubrium JF, Holstein JA.** Grounding the postmodern self. *Sociol Q* 1994;**34**:685–703.

21 **Ricoeur P.** Life in quest of narrative. In: Wood D, editor. On Paul Ricoeur: Narrative and Interpretation. London and New York: Routledge; 1991.

22 **Somers MR.** The narrative construction of identity: a relational and network approach. *Theory Soc* 1994;**22**:605–49.

23 **Ricoeur P.** Time and Narrative. vol. 3. Chicago: University of Chicago Press; 1988.

24 **Holstein MB, Minkler M.** Self, society, and the 'new gerontology'. *Gerontologist* 2003;**43**:787–96.

25 **Gilleard C, Higgs P.** Ageing and the limiting conditions of the body. *Sociological Research Online* 1998;**3**:U56–U70.

26 **Freeman M.** Narrative foreclosure in later life. In: Kenyon G, Bohlmeijer ET, Randall WR, editors. Storying Later Life; Issues, Investigations, and Interventions in Narrative Gerontology. New York: Oxford University Press; 2011:3–19.

27 **Holstein MB, Minkler M.** Critical gerontology: reflections for the 21st century. In: Bernard M, Schwartz T, editors. Critical Perspectives on Ageing Societies. Bristol: The Policy Press; 2007:13–26.

28 **Bohlmeijer ET, et al.** Narrative foreclosure in later life: preliminary considerations for a new sensitizing concept. *J Aging Stud* 2011;**25**:364–70.

29 **Kenyon G, et al.** Narrative Gerontology, Theory, Research and Practice. New York: Springer; 2001.

30 **Polkinghorne D.** Narrative Knowing and the Human Sciences. New York: State University of New York Press; 1988.

31 **Randall WL.** Narrative intelligence and the novelty of our lives. *J Aging Stud* 1999;**13**:11–28.

32 **Polkinghorne DE.** Narrative knowing and the study of lives. In Birren JE, Kenyon GM, Ruth JE, Schroots JJF, Svensson T, editors. Aging and Biography: Explorations in Adult Development. New York: Springer; 1996:77–99.

33 **Gubrium JF, Holstein JA.** Narrative practice and the coherence of personal stories. *Sociol Q* 1998;**39**: 163–87.

34 **Singer JA.** Narrative identity and meaning making across the adult lifespan: an introduction. *J Pers* 2004;**72**:437–60.

35 **Freeman M.** When the story's over: narrative foreclosure and the possibility of self-renewal. In: Andrews M, Slater S, Squire C, Treacher A, editors. Lines of Narrative: Psychosocial Perspectives. Toronto: Captus University Publications; 2000:245–50.

36 **Morson G.** Narrative and Freedom: The Shadow of Time. New Haven: Yale University Press; 1994.

37 **Kleinman A.** The Illness Narratives: Suffering, Healing, and the Human Condition. New York: Basic Books; 1988.

38 **Charmaz K.** Good Days Bad Days: the Self in Chronic Illness and Time. New Brunswick, NJ: Rutgers University Press; 1991.

39 **Kelly MP, Dickinson H.** The narrative self in autobiographical accounts of illness. *Sociological Review* 1997;**45**:254–78.

40 **Williams G.** The genesis of chronic illness: narrative reconstruction. In: Hinchman LP, Hinchman SK, editors. Memory, Identity, Community: The Idea of Narrative in the Human Sciences. Albany, NY: State University of New York Press; 1997:185–212.

41 **Sanders C, et al.** The significance and consequences of having painful and disabled joints in older age: co-existing accounts of normal and disrupted biographies. *Sociol Health Illn* 2002;**24**:227–53.

42 **Sparkes AC, Smith B.** Sport, spinal cord injury, embodied masculinities, and the dilemmas of narrative identity. *Men Masc* 2002;**4**:258–85.

43 **Bury M.** Chronic illness as biographical disruption. *Sociol Health Illn* 1982;**4**:167–82.

44 **Pound P, et al.** Illness in the context of older age: the case of stroke. *Sociol Health Illn* 1998;**20**:489–506.

45 **Sinding C, Wiernikowski J.** Disruption foreclosed: older women's cancer narratives. *Health* 2008;**12**: 389–411.

46 **Elliott J.** The narrative potential of the British Birth Cohort Studies. *Qualitative Research* 2008;**8**:411–21.

47 **Elliott J.** Using Narrative in Social Research: Qualitative and Quantitative Approaches. London: Sage; 2005.

48 **Elliott J, et al.** The design and content of the 'Social participation' study: a qualitative sub-study conducted as part of the age 50 (2008) sweep of the National Child Development Study. CLS Working Paper Series 2010/3. London: Centre for Longitudinal Studies; 2010.

49 **Elliott J, et al.** The design and content of the HALCyon qualitative study: a qualitative sub-study of the National Study of Health and Development and the Hertfordshire Cohort Study. CLS Working Paper 2011/5. London: Centre for Longitudinal Studies; 2011.

50 **Idler EL, Benyamini Y.** Self-rated health and mortality: a review of twenty-seven community studies. *J Health Soc Behav* 1997;**38**:21–37.

51 **Tennant R, et al.** The Warwick-Edinburgh Mental Well-being Scale (WEMWBS): development and UK validation. *Health Qual Life Outcomes* 2007;**5**:63.

52 **Flegal KM, et al.** Association of all-cause mortality with overweight and obesity using standard body mass index categories. A systematic review and meta-analysis. *JAMA* 2013;**309**:71–82.

53 **Gale CR, et al.** Neighbourhood environment and positive mental health in older people: the Hertfordshire Cohort Study. *Health Place* 2011;**17**:867–74.

54 **Linde C.** Life Stories: the Creation of Coherence. Oxford: Oxford University Press; 1993.

55 **Gullette M.** Aged by Culture. Chicago: University of Chicago Press; 2004. <http://www.press.uchicago.edu/ucp/books/book/chicago/A/bo3625122.html>

56 **Baltes PB, Smith J.** New frontiers in the future of aging: From successful aging of the young old to the dilemmas of the fourth age. *Gerontology* 2003;**49**:123–35.

57 **Crossley N.** In the gym: motives, meaning and moral careers. *Body & Society* 2006;**12**:23–50.

Part III

Healthy ageing in body systems, organs, and cells

Chapter 10

A life course approach to neuroendocrine systems: the example of the HPA axis

Yoav Ben-Shlomo, Michael Gardner, and Stafford Lightman

10.1 Endocrine overview

Ageing is associated with a progressive decline in both cognitive and musculoskeletal performance. The fundamental mechanisms underlying this decline are unclear but neuroendocrine mechanisms are excellent candidates for mediating some of the phenotypic changes, though other pathways clearly contribute as well. There are a variety of different endocrine systems that could be included and which are briefly considered. The growth hormone/insulin-like growth factor-I (GH/IGF-I) and gonadal steroid systems have been studied in most detail as they are clearly important factors for muscle protein synthesis. GH pulse amplitude falls by about 14% every 10 years from the age of 30 [1,2], and IGF-I falls in proportion. Indeed, IGF-I levels fall below the accepted lower limit of normal for young adults in about 30% of older adults [3]. The fall of testosterone in males shows a very similar pattern, with levels falling below 11.2 nmol/L in 20% of men above 60, to over 50% in men aged above 80 [4].

The impact of ageing on the insulin and thyroid axes is less clear. There is certainly an age-related reduction in glucose tolerance [5,6], and glucose stimulated insulin secretion [7] (Chapter 11), and older individuals with global and central adiposity are at risk of glucose intolerance unrelated to low muscle mass [8]. With respect to the hypothalamic–pituitary–thyroid axis, there are data not only from cross-sectional studies but also from larger longitudinal studies suggesting that even in the absence of thyroid disease, ageing is associated with increased thyroid-stimulating hormone (TSH) concentrations but no change in thyroxine (T4) [9].

The hypothalamic–pituitary–adrenal (HPA) axis is an endocrine system that can have powerful effects not only on musculoskeletal function but also on cognitive abilities. Dysregulation of adrenal glucocorticoid secretion can cause sarcopenia, glucose intolerance, osteoporosis, cardiovascular disease, cognitive decline and mood disturbance, features that are all seen in older populations. There is now a moderate literature suggesting that chronic stress, through activation of the HPA axis, can increase the 'wear and tear' or allostatic load and mediate many of the effects of chronic stress on the medical disorders associated with ageing [10]. Chronic stress increases the risk of metabolic disorder [11], and may increase insulin resistance [12] and cellular ageing [13].

The HPA axis is normally tightly regulated by a peripheral hourly pituitary adrenal oscillatory mechanism [14] and a central circadian oscillator located in the brain (suprachiasmatic nucleus of the hypothalamus). Functional weakening of the central oscillator with ageing is well recognized in rodents [15] and primates [16], while reduced amplitude of rhythms has been reported during ageing in man [17]. Decline in clock function not only contributes to sleep disturbance [18], but also sleep independent cognitive decline. With respect to the HPA axis, older individuals have a reduced circadian gradient of cortisol [19]. Given the widespread effects of the HPA axis on age-related traits, we have chosen to use this system as an exemplar for examining endocrine influences on ageing. This in no way implies that the other endocrine systems are any less important. and it is reasonable to suppose that there may be additive or synergistic effects across the different endocrine systems; so that considering any one in isolation, as is generally the case, is overly simplistic. For example both Maggio and colleagues [20] and Friedrich and colleagues [21] found an additive effect of being in the lowest quartiles for IGF-I and testosterone (Maggio also included dehydroepiandrosterone-sulfate; DHEA-S) on increased risk of all-cause mortality.

10.2 **How can we measure the HPA axis?**

It is the very dynamics of the HPA axis that create challenges for investigators. Levels of cortisol are markedly different at different times of the day (high in the morning and low at night), so that knowledge about the timing of samples is critical. Furthermore, in addition to the well-known circadian rhythmicity, there is a powerful approximately hourly ultradian rhythm that results in considerable variation over short periods of time and between the same time on different days [22]. Ideally one should collect samples at multiple time points across multiple days [23] as a measure of 'usual' exposure, as well as the reactivity of the system to an acute stressor, be it psychological (e.g. Trier Social Stress Test) or physical (carbon dioxide (CO_2) breath test). However, pragmatism and financial constraints often dictate the final sampling design.

Ninety five percent of cortisol is bound to cortisol binding globulin (CBG) and albumin—so only 5% of circulating cortisol is in the active free form. Since CBG is an acute phase protein that can increase during acute stress and fall during chronic illness [24], care needs to be taken when interpreting total cortisol levels in anyone other than healthy volunteers. The question that arises is how best to measure basal levels of cortisol and cortisol reactivity—both of which may be critical for health. For epidemiological studies, it is clearly best to perform non-invasive studies that can easily be repeated on several occasions. Fortunately free cortisol in the blood is also measurable within the salivary fluid. Since salivary glands have high levels of beta hydroxysteroid dehydrogenase, a major proportion of salivary cortisol is converted to cortisone [25] but, despite this, there is a good correlation between salivary cortisol and total blood cortisol.

There has been much discussion as to the best protocols for measuring salivary cortisol. These can vary from detailed dynamic tests with very regular venous sampling that require admission to a day ward to large scale population sampling using salivary samples (see review paper by Adam and Kumari for more details [26]). Studies tend to go down one of two avenues; either a challenge test paradigm or measure of daily diurnal variability, and a few studies try to incorporate both approaches. Most studies that measure diurnal variability will obtain anywhere between two to six samples measured over 1 to 3 days. More recent studies have tried to link detailed diary measures of stressful events with repeated measures. Whilst there are a multitude of different parameters that can be generated from such data, most studies focus on two dynamic measures: (1) the size of the diurnal drop calculated from the difference between peak levels in the morning and nadir levels at night; and (2) the cortisol awakening response (CAR; the difference between the level on wakening and the level 30 minutes later). What this represents is uncertain, but some infer that it is a measure of 'the response to the stress of waking up' and have suggested that CAR is larger in healthy individuals [27] and may reflect an adaptive boost response enabling the body to deal with the stresses of the upcoming day [28]. The validity of CAR can be particularly problematic, as it is dependent on good compliance with specific instructions regarding the timing of samples; this issue has been shown in younger people [29], so that a blunted CAR may be observed when it is merely an artefact due to failure to capture the correct timing of samples. It is likely that this issue is also present in older populations, especially if there is mild cognitive impairment, though perhaps to a lesser degree due to better compliance with instructions.

10.3 **How does one interpret measures of HPA function?**

The large body of empirical research linking chronic stress and HPA function is often contradictory, with some studies reporting increased activation and others reporting a reduction in activity. Some of this variability reflects different methodologies, random noise, under-powered small studies and publication bias (i.e. the tendency for small positive findings to be more likely to appear in the scientific literature). A meta-analysis of this literature [30] concluded that much of the variability is attributable to stressor and person features. As the authors state, 'timing is an especially critical element, as hormonal activity is elevated at stressor onset but reduces as time passes. Stressors that threaten physical integrity, involve trauma, and are uncontrollable elicit a high, flat diurnal profile of cortisol secretion' [30: p.25]. We share their viewpoint and would further extend this idea by postulating that there is a 'natural history' of cortisol responsiveness (Figure 10.1).

Considering Figure 10.1, let us assume that there is a 'normative' diurnal profile, as shown by line (a), for all individuals, though the absolute magnitude of this will differ between subjects. In the early stages of exposure there is an appropriate heightened CAR but with preserved diurnal variability, as shown by line (b). If the exposure is removed, the individual will revert to their normative profile. With more chronic exposure, there is a subsequent reduction in diurnal variability, such that night time levels are now elevated compared to the normative pattern: line (c). Finally, there may be a stage of reduced variability with both a diminished CAR and reduced diurnal variability, leading to greater 24-hour cortisol exposure and a larger area under the curve, shown by line (d), as the reduction in diurnal variability is more important than the reduction in CAR. Therefore, when comparing different populations, it is important to consider how these different patterns of response may be represented in the population sample and whether this could explain discrepant results between studies.

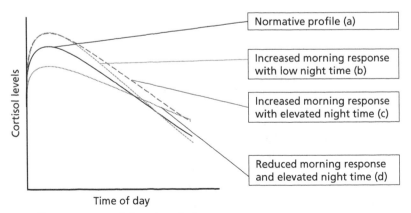

Figure 10.1 Different patterns of diurnal cortisol response.

10.4 **Associations with age, gender and socioeconomic position**

We have already highlighted how age alters the rhythmicity of the HPA axis [31]. A large study of 2802 healthy participants from the Whitehall II cohort (mean age 61 years) used latent variable mixture models to identify 'latent' classes or patterns of cortisol secretion from six measures over 1 day. A two-class solution was the most parsimonious, with a 'normative group' and a 'raised group' who showed elevated CAR but also elevated night time levels and hence a reduced diurnal slope. Participants with an elevated pattern tended to be older, male, smokers, had shorter sleep duration, reported more stressful events, woke up earlier, and walked slower [32]. Male hyper-responsiveness also seems to be a feature in studies of acute stress responsiveness, in direct contrast to the animal literature [33]. Thus, men in general seem to show a greater cortisol response to psychological stressors in laboratory settings, which can be seen even on task anticipation. However, there may be developmental differences, so girls around puberty have been shown to have a bigger cortisol response to corticotrophin releasing hormone than their male counterparts [34]. Kudielka and Kirschbaum argue that sex differences in cortisol production may reflect sexual dimorphism in the limbic brain regions, cognitive processing, circulating sex hormones, and differences in corticosteroid-binding globulin [33].

The relationship between socioeconomic position (SEP) and the HPA axis has been of much interest due to the role of chronic stress and allostatic load [10] in explaining health disparities. A recent review of the literature [35] concluded that there was no consistent relationship, though lower SEP was more consistently associated with a reduction in diurnal variability. Allostatic load showed a stronger relationship with metabolic and cardiovascular markers than the neuroendocrine measures, even though the HPA axis is supposedly an upstream driver of metabolic and cardiovascular mediators.

10.5 **Life course determinants of HPA function**

A life course approach to HPA regulation has been considered both in terms of critical/sensitive period exposures as well as accumulation of risk models (Chapter 1) such as type 2 chronic allostatic overload, as exemplified by lower SEP across life. Most of the research testing early life exposures has either examined physical stressors such as suboptimal development, or psychological stressors during childhood, both in the prenatal period [36] as well as postnatally and in childhood.

10.5.1 **Physical stressors**

Most work in this area has focused on early growth and development. Barker and colleagues had previously highlighted the association between size at birth and cardiovascular disease, diabetes and a range of cardiometabolic risk factors [37]. It was therefore logical that the same group examined whether these associations could be mediated by dysregulation of the HPA axis. Phillips and colleagues [38] demonstrated that lower birthweight was associated with higher fasting cortisol in three populations aged 20, 46 to 54 and 60 to 71 years. In addition, higher cortisol was associated with higher blood pressure, but there was effect modification by obesity, so that the associations were strongest in subjects with a body mass index (BMI) >30 kg/m^2. However, this literature is far from consistent. Kajantie [36] has hypothesized that the birthweight–cortisol relationship can be explained by an interaction between birthweight and gestational age; babies with small size at birth but born before 40 weeks have high adult fasting cortisol, whilst those born at or after 40 weeks have low adult cortisol levels. This could be related to the role of corticotrophin-releasing hormone, which is produced by the placenta and may induce premature delivery. This hypothesis is clearly speculative and requires replication. This association, if valid, may not necessarily reflect the effects of undernutrition, as it is recognized that genetic factors may be involved both in the regulation of fetal growth as well as later life obesity and metabolic factors [39]. It is therefore important that follow-up of the Dutch famine survivors, an extreme 'natural experiment', failed to demonstrate a differential cortisol response to a stress task amongst five groups of exposed participants (born before the famine, exposed in late, mid or early gestation of famine, conceived after famine), or a birthweight association [40]. However, this study did not examine diurnal variability. We know relatively little about the effects of childhood growth and development and pubertal timing on HPA function.

Another stressor of interest, given a body of animal research, is the role of infection load, which can produce both short-term effects (febrile illness) as well as long-term adverse effects on growth and development. In a follow-up study of 25 year-olds (Barry Caerphilly Growth Study) who were seen repeatedly between birth and 5 years, more respiratory infections in early life were associated with lower night time cortisol and a reduced total hormone output, as measured by the area under the curve [41]. In this case, counter to the birthweight example, greater infection load appears to have down-regulated HPA responsiveness. This association was specific to respiratory infection and was not seen with gastrointestinal infection, suggesting that the former was not merely a proxy measure of adverse socioeconomic conditions in childhood.

A systematic review of early life adversity also identified six studies that all found an association between prenatal substance exposure (alcohol, tobacco, cocaine) and childhood cortisol reactivity [42]. However, in some cases associations were positive, i.e. adverse exposure was associated with higher cortisol levels, but in one study this was actually in the opposite direction—thus both over- and under-activity have been observed.

10.5.2 Psychosocial stressors

Not surprisingly, a larger body of literature has examined psychosocial stressors, particularly amongst children. For example, in a study of 357 children (aged between 9 and 15 years), Essex and colleagues [43] found a complex pattern of cortisol responsiveness conditional on exposure to maternal depression and/or family expressed anger in the early and pre-school period. Children exposed to high levels of maternal depression and who also expressed anger showed heightened morning levels and slightly flatter diurnal slopes at around 9 years of age; for 15 year-olds the morning levels were comparable to normal exposure, but their diurnal slopes were much flatter (this is somewhat consistent with our proposed natural history in Figure 10.1). The age-related findings are cross-sectional rather than truly longitudinal, so it remains to be shown that this transition in cortisol profiles truly occurs within individuals. The systematic review by Hunter and colleagues [42] found 13 studies showing that maternal factors such as anxiety and depression during pregnancy, life time history of depression, and poor mother–child attachment were associated with a heightened cortisol response in the offspring, whilst three studies found a decreased response and two found no effect. Three intervention studies were identified. Dozier and colleagues randomized 46 children (just under 2 years of age) from foster homes to either receive a behavioural intervention around attachment or no treatment, and had an additional population of non-foster children [44]. They observed a reduction in baseline cortisol when the children were allocated to a 'strange situation' paradigm designed to elicit stress and attachment behaviour. They found that the first cortisol level was higher in the control foster children and the levels for the intervention children were similar to the non-foster children, suggesting that the intervention had reduced the cortisol response to the strange situation. A poverty alleviation quasi-experimental trial from Mexico found that families that were allocated poverty alleviation had children (aged between 2 and 6 years) with lower baseline cortisol levels, and this was particularly marked for children whose mothers scored high on depressive symptoms (p<0.05 for interaction in fully adjusted model) [45]. A final randomized controlled trial recruited 92 pre-school siblings of adjudicated youths identified from court records. An intensive prevention programme was implemented involving 22 weekly group meetings and 10 bi-weekly home visits and up to six additional home visits [46]. This study uniquely measured both diurnal patterns and pre–post challenge responsiveness. The challenge was similar to the Dozier study in that it involved free play with an unfamiliar group of peers. There was no evidence of any differences at baseline, but after the intervention (time two) there was a significant interaction (p = 0.02) between the anticipatory pre-challenge cortisol level, so that the intervention group showed higher levels than controls. No effects were seen for diurnal variability and post-challenge levels. This pattern is opposite to what the other two trials demonstrated and is open to two conflicting interpretations. Either this anticipatory stress response is a negative marker and hence the intervention has actually worsened the HPA responsiveness, or the lack of response seen in the control group after the intervention is actually what is abnormal, hence the intervention has reinstated a normal anticipatory response.

There are few studies that have attempted to look at the cumulative life course effects of psychosocial stressors. The Midlife in the US (MIDUS) and National Study of Daily Experiences (NSDE) subsample have examined longitudinal data on adult social strain with family and friends over a 10-year period across two data collection waves [47]. They found that at the second data collection point, greater strain was associated with a lower peak level and flatter diurnal variation cross-sectionally. However, when they disaggregated this by persistence of social strain, there was an apparent lag effect, so that subjects just reporting social strain at wave two did not show an effect, whereas those with strain at wave one or persistent strain at both time points had a more pathological pattern of response. Another study, this time using a retrospective design so therefore prone to recall bias, examined associations of self-reported life events across life with diurnal variability in just over 1000 subjects in the Longitudinal Aging Study Amsterdam (LASA) [48]. Once again there was evidence of a differential effect dependent on the timing of exposure. Early adverse life events were associated with a flatter diurnal curve whilst later life events only showed higher morning cortisol, consistent with Figure 10.1.

10.6 **HPA and physical capability**

If dysregulation of the HPA axis is associated with accelerated ageing, one would expect to see associations with worse physical capability, as this is a sensitive biomarker of increased mortality, morbidity, and reduced quality of life (Chapter 2). However, the association between functioning of the HPA axis and physical capability in the normal population is poorly understood and there is a paucity of good epidemiological studies. The best human model of HPA axis over-activity is seen in Cushing's syndrome, where there is overproduction of cortisol (hypercortisolism). Proximal muscle weakness has been detected in 56–90% of such patients [49]. Three population-based studies reporting associations between cortisol levels and physical capability are LASA [50,51], the Whitehall II study (WHII) [32] and the Caerphilly Prospective Study (CaPS) [52]. In WHII and CaPS, participants with less diurnal decline had slower walking speed. In LASA, gender differences were observed, so that men with higher cortisol levels had slower chair rise and walking speeds, whilst women had poorer standing balance [51]. In LASA, higher cortisol was also found to be associated with a loss of grip strength over 4 years [50].

We have recently reported, as part of the HALCyon collaboration <http://www.halcyon.ac.uk>, the largest synthesis of data in this area using an individual participant data meta-analysis [53]. We have been able to include data from the above named studies and add new unpublished data from three additional cohorts: Boyd Orr study, Hertfordshire Cohort Study (HCS), and the MRC National Survey of Health and Development (NSHD). We were able to examine various cortisol measures (morning, night time, diurnal drop, and CAR) with a number of different tests of physical performance and strength (walking speed, chair rises, poor standing balance, and grip strength) and with good statistical power (sample size for analyses ranged from 1224 to 8448) with participants ranging in age from 50 to 92 years. In simple age- and sex-adjusted models we found that slower walking speed was associated with lower morning cortisol, higher night time cortisol, smaller diurnal drop, and a smaller CAR. Slower chair rise speed was also associated with a lower morning cortisol, higher night time cortisol, and smaller diurnal drop. Poor balance was only predicted by higher night-time levels, and grip strength was not associated with any of the cortisol measures. In a fully-adjusted model, conditioning on age, sex, smoking status, and body mass index, the strongest and most consistent predictor was diurnal variability, so that smaller drop was associated with worse walking speed (Figure 10.2) and chair rise time. The appropriateness of adjustment for body mass index is debatable, as this may be a confounder or an intermediary between any observed association, and hence the adjusted estimates may actually be over-adjusted. The lack of an association with grip strength is interesting, as grip strength is a simpler task than walking and chair rises (Chapter 2), which require neuromuscular speed and control using proximal rather than

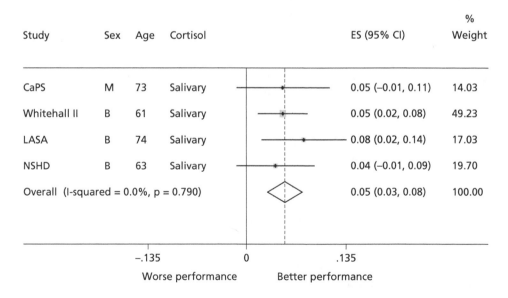

Difference in standardized walk speed per SD increase in diurnal drop adjusted for age and sex

Figure 10.2 Meta-analysis of the association between diurnal drop and walking speed adjusted for age and gender.

distal muscles and upper body strength [54]. In contrast, the ability to balance requires not just proximal muscle strength but also a more complex interplay between sensory inputs and motor outputs controlled by the brain. This greater complexity may explain the weaker associations of balance with the HPA axis.

The associations between cortisol and physical performance in these meta-analyses were cross-sectional and hence reverse causation could not be ruled out. However, in CaPS we were able to examine the relationship between repeat cortisol measures over 20 years and physical performance in later life [52]. This study found that higher fasting clinic morning cortisol at phase one was associated with faster walking speed at phase five (20 years later). Interestingly at phase one, age was inversely associated with morning cortisol whilst at phase five, where cortisol was measured at home under non-stressed conditions, it was positively associated with cortisol. We had, *a priori*, assumed that higher morning cortisol would suggest a less healthy HPA axis, but in this case the ability to mount a good stress-induced response may actually be a marker of a more reactive and healthier system.

10.7 **HPA axis and cognition**

Chronic stress can accelerate cognitive decline [55]. In the case of patients with Cushing's syndrome, chronic exposure to elevated levels of cortisol is associated with deficits in several areas of cognitive performance, including visual and spatial information and non-verbal memory [56]. We recently undertook a systematic review of the literature for studies which examined the association between measures of diurnal cortisol patterns and cognitive performance (Ben-Shlomo et al., in preparation). Eligible study populations were community-dwelling older adults, with a minimum of 100 participants. We identified 16 studies to be included in the review. Whilst there was some evidence that higher morning cortisol was associated with worse cognitive performance [57,58], other studies showed little evidence of an association between morning cortisol and cognitive performance [59]. Furthermore, whilst participants with less diurnal decline had poorer cognitive performance [60,61], most studies did not measure diurnal decline. The outcome measures of cognitive performance across the 16 studies were heterogeneous, including verbal memory, verbal fluency, object recognition and executive function.

We went on to undertake an individual participant data meta-analysis to overcome some of the methodological issues with interpreting the heterogeneous published literature. The meta-analysis included three cohorts from the original HALCyon research programme: CaPS; the National Child Development Study (NCDS 1958 British birth cohort); and NSHD; and in addition, two large scale cohorts identified through the HALCyon collaboration: LASA and WHII. The cortisol measures used were the same as those in tests of the associations between the HPA axis and physical capability (Section 10.6), i.e. morning cortisol (serum or salivary), night-time cortisol (salivary), diurnal decline, and CAR. We classified cognitive performance into two measures: crystallized capability and fluid capability. Crystallized capability is stable in maturity and represents acquired knowledge over life (Chapter 3). In CaPS and NSHD, the crystallized capability measure was the National Adult Reading Test [62]; in WHII it was the Mill Hill Vocabulary Test [63], and in LASA the Groninger Intelligentie Test [64]. Fluid capability requires performance-based skills, typically involving on the spot problem solving requiring focused attention, mental manipulation and other challenging cognitive processes (Chapter 3). For each cohort, three fluid cognition measures were included in the study and these were subsequently used to derive one fluid capability measure per study. In CaPS and WHII, the Alice Heim test was used to measure verbal and mathematical reasoning [65]. In LASA, the Raven's Coloured Progressive Matrices [63] assessed the ability to deal with new information, and in NCDS and NSHD the verbal memory task was letter cancellation [66].

A greater diurnal decline was associated with better fluid capability (standardized coefficient per SD increase 0.037, 95% CI: 0.008, 0.065, p = 0.01; age and gender adjusted). Furthermore, higher night-time cortisol was associated with worse fluid capability (standardized coefficient per SD increase −0.063, 95% CI −0.124, −0.002, p = 0.04; age and gender adjusted). Both these associations were attenuated after further adjustment for BMI, smoking status and socioeconomic position. No associations were found between morning cortisol, night-time cortisol or diurnal decline and crystallized capability (Ben-Shlomo et al., in preparation). A bigger CAR was weakly associated with better fluid and crystallized capability.

These associations were again cross-sectional in nature and hence reverse causation could not be ruled out. Indeed, worse cognitive ability at age 16 in the NCDS [67] and at age 20 in The Vietnam Era Twin Study of Aging [68] predicted elevated midlife cortisol levels and flatter diurnal variability. Hence the direction of effect may be complex, with neurodevelopment influencing the HPA axis and vice versa.

10.8 **Future research directions and conclusions**

There is much we still do not understand about the regulation of the HPA, its life course determinants and, most importantly, the longer term sequelae of dysregulation of the HPA both on physical, cognitive, and psychological morbidity. We have not covered the large literature on cortisol and depression, for example, as this is not specifically related to ageing *per se*, but two studies have presented evidence that maternal anxiety and depression in pregnancy were associated with less diurnal variability [69] and a blunted response to a CO_2 challenge [70]. In the former study, this appeared to mediate the association with offspring anxiety in adolescent teenage girls [69]. Several researchers have advocated that the HPA axis is an obvious candidate pathway for explaining socioeconomic gradients in health outcomes and 'how experience gets under the skin' [71], and its pleiotropic effects make it very suitable when considering age-related changes in morbidity and function [31,72]. There is clearly evidence that different life course experiences, both physical and psychosocial, can influence the HPA axis so that it may over- and under-respond to stressors and have an altered diurnal pattern. In this respect, the plasticity of the HPA axis makes it ideally suited for any theoretical model of allostasis. However, there are still serious gaps in our empirical evidence base over the implications of these observations. Firstly, most studies, including those with prospective follow-up, usually have cortisol measured at one or maybe two time points. Therefore, it is unclear as to how robust some of these findings are over time, and what would be the true natural history of cortisol responsiveness to a prolonged adverse exposure compared to a transient one. We clearly need longitudinal studies that have better characterization of both acute response as well as diurnal patterns. This very plasticity also means that current studies have a large degree of measurement error in the cortisol measures, so that true associations should be larger. This may or may not explain the very modestly sized associations seen between cortisol and physical capability and cognition, which may have only limited clinical significance. In contrast, the few studies that have examined cortisol with mortality, or cardiovascular disease, have shown larger effects [73,74] though further studies are required. Looking at cortisol alone may be less informative than in combination with other biomarkers such as in the MacArthur studies of Aging [75] or as cortisol to testosterone ratio [76]. Given that the endocrine system has evolved to maintain biological homeostasis it is unsurprising that dysregulation in one system may, to some degree, be counterbalanced by adaption in other systems. Future studies must consider the interplay across various endocrine systems and model the effects of dysregulation across more than one, which may have a far greater than additive effect, eventually leading to a tipping point and accelerated decline.

Technological developments will enable future research to address the HPA hypothesis using at least two different approaches. One will be the enhanced ability to repeatedly sample micro-aliquots of blood using a device that can be worn under normal conditions at work or home. This will enable repeated sampling across the day as well as in conjunction with the recording of naturalistic stressors (e.g. argument with the wife, work-related stress, etc.) which have far greater salience than laboratory-based tasks. The challenge here will be to synthesize and analyse such a wealth of data into simpler exposure measures. The second approach will use our rapidly advancing knowledge of genetics, epigenetics and metabolomics to overcome some of the current difficulties in characterizing the HPA axis. For example, could one demonstrate whether adverse environmental exposures over the life course result in different methylation patterns, thereby silencing or activating different genes, and these in turn are associated with HPA dysregulation? [77] Similarly, to what degree do individuals with HPA dysregulation show different metabolomic profiles compared to a normative group?

In public health terms, it currently remains unclear how best to use cortisol measures. They could be one of a potential bank of prognostic markers and used for risk stratification, so that high-risk subjects could be identified for targeting interventions. Rather than using them to predict future ill-health and frailty, they may be more useful as markers of how well individuals with existing disease or ill-health could cope with a future stressor such as surgery or chemotherapy. At this moment in time, the added value of knowing an individual's cortisol profile has yet to be proven. Finally, there is a real need to undertake more intervention studies to see whether one can modify existing HPA response patterns and whether these are potential mediators for health outcomes.

References

1 **Zadik Z, et al.** The influence of age on the 24-hour integrated concentration of growth hormone in normal individuals. *J Clin Endocrinol Metab* 1985;**60**:513–6.

2 **Veldhuis JD, et al.** Differential impact of age, sex steroid hormones, and obesity on basal versus pulsatile growth hormone secretion in men as assessed in an ultrasensitive chemiluminescence assay. *J Clin Endocrinol Metab* 1995;**80**:3209–22.

3 **Leifke E, et al.** Age-related changes of serum sex hormones, insulin-like growth factor-1 and sex-hormone binding globulin levels in men: cross-sectional data from a healthy male cohort. *Clin Endocrinol (Oxf)* 2000;**53**:689–95.

4 **Harman SM, et al.** Longitudinal effects of aging on serum total and free testosterone levels in healthy men. Baltimore Longitudinal Study of Aging. *J Clin Endocrinol Metab* 2001;**86**:724–31.

5 **Andres R.** Aging and diabetes. *Med Clin North Am* 1971;**55**:835–46.

6 **Basu R, et al.** Mechanisms of the age-associated deterioration in glucose tolerance: contribution of alterations in insulin secretion, action, and clearance. *Diabetes* 2003;**52**:1738–48.

7 **Ihm SH, et al.** Effect of donor age on function of isolated human islets. *Diabetes* 2006;**55**:1361–8.

8 **Ramachandran R, et al.** Selective contribution of regional adiposity, skeletal muscle, and adipokines to glucose disposal in older adults. *J Am Geriatr Soc* 2012;**60**:707–12.

9 **Bremner AP, et al.** Age-related changes in thyroid function: a longitudinal study of a community-based cohort. *J Clin Endocrinol Metab* 2012;**97**:1554–62.

10 **McEwen BS, Wingfield JC.** The concept of allostasis in biology and biomedicine. *Horm Behav* 2003;**43**:2–15.

11 **Chandola T, et al.** Chronic stress at work and the metabolic syndrome: prospective study. *BMJ* 2006; **332**:521–5.

12 **Rosmond R.** Role of stress in the pathogenesis of the metabolic syndrome. *Psychoneuroendocrinology* 2005;**30**:1–10.

13 **Epel ES, et al.** Accelerated telomere shortening in response to life stress. *Proc Natl Acad Sci USA* 2004; **101**:17312–5.

14 **Walker JJ, et al.** The origin of glucocorticoid hormone oscillations. *PLoS Biol* 2012;**10**:e1001341.

15 **Froy O.** Circadian rhythms, aging, and life span in mammals. *Physiology (Bethesda)* 2011;**26**:225–35.

16 **Zhdanova IV, et al.** Aging of intrinsic circadian rhythms and sleep in a diurnal nonhuman primate, Macaca mulatta. *J Biol Rhythms* 2011;**26**:149–59.

17 **Hofman MA, Swaab DF.** Living by the clock: the circadian pacemaker in older people. *Ageing Res Rev* 2006;**5**:33–51.

18 **Reddy AB, O'Neill JS.** Healthy clocks, healthy body, healthy mind. *Trends Cell Biol* 2010;**20**:36–44.

19 **Kumari M, et al.** Identifying patterns in cortisol secretion in an older population. Findings from the Whitehall II study. *Psychoneuroendocrinology* 2010;**35**:1091–9.

20 **Maggio M, et al.** The hormonal pathway to frailty in older men. *J Endocrinol Invest* 2005;**28**(11: Suppl Proceedings):15–19.

21 **Friedrich N, et al.** Improved prediction of all-cause mortality by a combination of serum total testosterone and insulin-like growth factor I in adult men. *Steroids* 2012;**77**:52–8.

22 **Young EA, et al.** Cortisol pulsatility and its role in stress regulation and health. *Front Neuroendocrinol* 2004;**25**:69–76.

23 **Hellhammer J, et al.** Several daily measurements are necessary to reliably assess the cortisol rise after awakening: state- and trait components. *Psychoneuroendocrinology* 2007;**32**:80–6.

24 **Cameron A, et al.** Temperature-responsive release of cortisol from its binding globulin: a protein thermocouple. *J Clin Endocrinol Metab* 2010;**95**:4689–95.

25 **Perogamvros I, et al.** Salivary cortisone is a potential biomarker for serum free cortisol. *J Clin Endocrinol Metab* 2010;**95**:4951–8.

26 **Adam EK, Kumari M.** Assessing salivary cortisol in large-scale, epidemiological research. *Psychoneuroendocrinology* 2009;**34**:1423–36.

27 **Kudielka BM, Kirschbaum C.** Awakening cortisol responses are influenced by health status and awakening time but not by menstrual cycle phase. *Psychoneuroendocrinology* 2003;**28**:35–47.

28 **Adam EK, et al.** Day-to-day dynamics of experience-cortisol associations in a population-based sample of older adults. *Proc Natl Acad Sci USA* 2006;**103**:17058–63.

29 **Halpern CT, et al.** Challenges of measuring diurnal cortisol concentrations in a large population-based field study. *Psychoneuroendocrinology* 2012;**37**:499–508.

30 **Miller GE, et al.** If it goes up, must it come down? Chronic stress and the hypothalamic–pituitary–adrenocortical axis in humans. *Psychol Bull* 2007;**133**:25–45.

31 **Seeman TE, Robbins RJ.** Aging and hypothalamic–pituitary–adrenal response to challenge in humans. *Endocr Rev* 1994;**15**:233–60.

32 **Kumari M, et al.** Identifying patterns in cortisol secretion in an older population. Findings from the Whitehall II study. *Psychoneuroendocrinology* 2010;**35**:1091–9.

33 **Kudielka BM, Kirschbaum C.** Sex differences in HPA axis responses to stress: a review. *Biol Psychol* 2005;**69**:113–32.

34 **Stroud LR, et al.** Sex differences in cortisol response to corticotropin releasing hormone challenge over puberty: Pittsburgh Pediatric Neurobehavioral Studies. *Psychoneuroendocrinology* 2011;**36**:1226–38.

35 **Dowd JB, et al.** Socio-economic status, cortisol and allostatic load: a review of the literature. *Int J Epidemiol* 2009;**38**:1297–309.

36 **Kajantie E.** Fetal origins of stress-related adult disease. *Ann N Y Acad Sci* 2006;**1083**:11–27.

37 **Barker DJP.** Mothers, Babies and Health in Later Life. 2nd ed. London: Churchill Livingstone; 1998.

38 **Phillips DI, et al.** Low birth weight predicts elevated plasma cortisol concentrations in adults from 3 populations. *Hypertension* 2000;**35**:1301–6.

39 **Sovio U, et al.** Association between common variation at the FTO locus and changes in body mass index from infancy to late childhood: the complex nature of genetic association through growth and development. *PLoS Genet* 2011;**7**:e1001307.

40 **de Rooij SR, et al.** Cortisol responses to psychological stress in adults after prenatal exposure to the Dutch famine. *Psychoneuroendocrinology* 2006;**31**:1257–65.

41 **Vedhara K, et al.** Relationship of early childhood illness with adult cortisol in the Barry Caerphilly Growth (BCG) cohort. *Psychoneuroendocrinology* 2007;**32**:865–73.

42 **Hunter AL, et al.** Altered stress responses in children exposed to early adversity: a systematic review of salivary cortisol studies. *Stress* 2011;**14**:614–26.

43 **Essex MJ, et al.** Influence of early life stress on later hypothalamic-pituitary-adrenal axis functioning and its covariation with mental health symptoms: a study of the allostatic process from childhood into adolescence. *Dev Psychopathol* 2011;**23**:1039–58.

44 **Dozier M, et al.** Effects of an attachment-based intervention on the cortisol production of infants and toddlers in foster care. *Dev Psychopathol* 2008;**20**:845–59.

45 **Fernald LC, Gunnar MR.** Poverty-alleviation program participation and salivary cortisol in very low-income children. *Soc Sci Med* 2009;**68**:2180–9.

46 **Brotman LM, et al.** Effects of a psychosocial family-based preventive intervention on cortisol response to a social challenge in preschoolers at high risk for antisocial behavior. *Arch Gen Psychiatry* 2007;**64**:1172–9.

47 **Friedman EM, et al.** Social strain and cortisol regulation in midlife in the US. *Soc Sci Med* 2012;**74**:607–15.

48 **Gerritsen L, et al.** Early and late life events and salivary cortisol in older persons. *Psychol Med* 2010;**40**:1569–78.

49 **Fernandez-Rodriguez E, et al.** The pituitary-adrenal axis and body composition. *Pituitary* 2009;**12**:105–15.

50 **Peeters GM, et al.** The relationship between cortisol, muscle mass and muscle strength in older persons and the role of genetic variations in the glucocorticoid receptor. *Clin Endocrinol (Oxf)* 2008;**69**:673–82.

51 **Peeters GMEE, et al.** Relationship between cortisol and physical performance in older persons. *Clin Endocrinol (Oxf)* 2007;**67**:398–406.

52 **Gardner MP, et al.** Diurnal cortisol patterns are associated with physical performance in the Caerphilly Prospective Study. *Int J Epidemiol* 2011;**40**:1693–702.

53 **Gardner M, et al.** Dysregulation of the hypothalamic pituitary adrenal (HPA) axis and physical performance at older ages: an individual participant meta-analysis. *Psychoneuroendocrinology* 2013;**38**:40–9.

54 **Kuh D, et al.** Grip strength, postural control, and functional leg power in a representative cohort of British men and women: associations with physical activity, health status, and socioeconomic conditions. *J Gerontol A Biol Sci Med Sci* 2005;**60**:224–31.

55 **Peavy GM, et al.** Effects of chronic stress on memory decline in cognitively normal and mildly impaired older adults. *Am J Psychiatry* 2009;**166**:1384–91.

56 **Forget H, et al.** Cognitive decline in patients with Cushing's syndrome. *J Int Neuropsychol Soc* 2000;**6**:20–9.

57 **Comijs HC, et al.** The association between serum cortisol and cognitive decline in older persons. *Am J Geriatr Psychiatry* 2010;**18**:42–50.

58 **Kuningas M, et al.** Mental performance in old age dependent on cortisol and genetic variance in the mineralocorticoid and glucocorticoid receptors. *Neuropsychopharmacology* 2007;**32**:1295–301.

59 **Fonda SJ, et al.** Age, hormones, and cognitive functioning among middle-aged and elderly men: cross-sectional evidence from the Massachusetts Male Aging Study. *J Gerontol A Biol Sci Med Sci* 2005;**60**:385–90.

60 **Beluche I, et al.** A prospective study of diurnal cortisol and cognitive function in community-dwelling elderly people. *Psychol Med* 2010;**40**:1039–49.

61 **O'Hara R, et al.** Serotonin transporter polymorphism, memory and hippocampal volume in the elderly: association and interaction with cortisol. *Mol Psychiatry* 2007;**12**:544–55.

62 **Bright P, et al.** The National Adult Reading Test as a measure of premorbid intelligence: a comparison with estimates derived from demographic variables. *J Int Neuropsychol Soc* 2002;**8**:847–54.

63 **Raven J.** The Raven's Progressive Matrices: change and stability over culture and time. *Cogn Psychol* 2000;**41**:1–48.

64 **Comijs HC, et al.** The association between depressive symptoms and cognitive decline in community-dwelling elderly persons. *Int J Geriat Psychiatry* 2001;**16**:361–7.

65 **Elovainio M, et al.** Organisational justice and cognitive function in middle-aged employees: the Whitehall II study. *J Epidemiol Community Health* 2012;**66**:552–6.

66 **Richards M, et al.** Lifetime cognitive function and timing of the natural menopause. *Neurology* 1999;**53**: 308–14.

67 **Power C, et al.** Cognitive development and cortisol patterns in mid-life: findings from a British birth cohort. *Psychoneuroendocrinology* 2008;**33**:530–9.

68 **Franz CE, et al.** Cross-sectional and 35-year longitudinal assessment of salivary cortisol and cognitive functioning: the Vietnam Era Twin Study of Aging. *Psychoneuroendocrinology* 2011;**36**:1040–52.

69 **Van den Bergh BR, et al.** Antenatal maternal anxiety is related to HPA-axis dysregulation and self-reported depressive symptoms in adolescence: a prospective study on the fetal origins of depressed mood. *Neuropsychopharmacology* 2008;**33**:536–45.

70 **Vedhara K, et al.** Maternal mood and neuroendocrine programming: effects of time of exposure and sex. *J Neuroendocrinol* 2012;**24**:999–1011.

71 **Hertzman C, Boyce T.** How experience gets under the skin to create gradients in developmental health. *Annu Rev Public Health* 2010;**31**:329–47.

72 **Aguilera G.** HPA axis responsiveness to stress: implications for healthy aging. *Exp Gerontol* 2011;**46**: 90–5.

73 **Schoorlemmer RM, et al.** Relationships between cortisol level, mortality and chronic diseases in older persons. *Clin Endocrinol (Oxf)* 2009;**71**:779–86.

74 **Kumari M, et al.** Association of diurnal patterns in salivary cortisol with all-cause and cardiovascular mortality: findings from the Whitehall II study. *J Clin Endocrinol Metab* 2011;**96**:1478–85.

75 **Seeman TE, et al.** Price of adaptation-allostatic load and its health consequences. MacArthur studies of successful aging. *Arch Intern Med* 1997;**157**:2259–68.

76 **Davey Smith G, et al.** Cortisol, testosterone, and coronary heart disease: prospective evidence from the Caerphilly study. *Circulation* 2005;**112**:332–40.

77 **Ng JW, et al.** The role of longitudinal cohort studies in epigenetic epidemiology: challenges and opportunities. *Genome Biol* 2012;**13**:246.

Chapter 11

Vascular and metabolic function across the life course

Debbie A Lawlor and Rebecca Hardy

11.1 Introduction

Cardio-metabolic diseases, including coronary heart disease (CHD), stroke and type 2 diabetes, account for the majority of deaths in high income countries and are an increasing cause of morbidity and mortality in low and middle income countries (LMIC). CHD and stroke are rare until middle age and more than half of the deaths due to these causes occur over the age of 70 [1]. Although type 2 diabetes, previously known as adult onset diabetes, has in recent decades been diagnosed in obese children [2], it still remains rare until midlife or older age [3]. Not only do these conditions largely become apparent for the first time in older age, they are major contributors to morbidity and reduced quality of life in older age [1].

In this respect cardio-metabolic ill-health might be considered a disease of old age. However, it has been known for decades that the pathophysiological process of atherosclerosis, which ultimately leads to CHD and ischaemic strokes, begins in childhood and young adulthood [4–6]. Consequently, a growing body of research has highlighted the potential role of pre-adult influences that may operate through various different life course models on cardio-metabolic disease risk (summarized in previous life course book chapters [7–10]). In general this research has focused on the association of pre-adult risk factors with markers of cardio-metabolic health or disease outcomes at one time point in adulthood, with little attention to how markers of cardio-metabolic health and function change as people age from birth through to adulthood.

Understanding how markers of cardio-metabolic function change across life and the characteristics associated with deviation from what might be considered underlying 'normal' age-related change is key to fully understanding the life course epidemiology of these conditions and for identifying means of preventing future disease.

In this chapter our aims are to: (1) describe human life course trajectories in blood pressure (BP), lipids, glucose, insulin and non-invasive assessments of vascular structure and function; (2) explore whether these age-related trajectories differ between males and females and different ethnic groups; (3) review evidence regarding the associations of pre-adult risk factors with these trajectories; (4) explore whether there are key periods of the life course (specifically puberty, pregnancy, and the perimenopause) when these trajectories show distinct changes; and (5) describe how changes with age in these indicators of cardio-metabolic function are related to future cardiovascular disease. Due to space restrictions the summary of evidence for all of these aims in relation to glucose, insulin, and vascular structure and function are available in Supplementary web material at www.halcyon.ac.uk., though summarized in the conclusion here.

Link to supplementary web material

11.2 Life course changes in blood pressure in industrialized countries; gender and ethnic differences

The most detailed study of age-related change in BP within children is Project HeartBeat! [11]. In that study BP was assessed repeatedly—every 4 months for 4 years—in approximately 700 children who were aged 8, 11, or 14 years at recruitment in the early 1990s. Systolic blood pressure (SBP) and two measurements of diastolic blood pressure (DBP)—one based on the 4th (phase four DBP) and one on the 5th (phase five DBP) Korotkoff sound, both of which have been used to measure DBP in infants and children—were assessed. Multilevel models with polynomial terms to account for non-linear change were used to analyse the data. For SBP, levels increased steeply between ages 8 and 16 years and then levelled off, with the rate of increase being greater in males compared with females, but with no notable ethnic differences (Figure 11.1). Increases in both phase four and five DBP were monotonic, but for phase four there was a curvilinear quadratic association, with the rate of increase reducing somewhat after age approximately 13 years, whereas the rate of age-related increase for phase five was more constant over time. Rates of change were similar in males and females and in blacks and non-blacks for both, but levels of phase four DBP were higher in males at all ages, and both phase four and phase five DBP were higher in black children at all ages (Supplementary web material Figure 11.S1) [11].

Several cross-sectional [12–14] and prospective [15–20] studies have modelled repeatedly assessed BP in adults and concluded that SBP increases monotonically across most of adult life, whereas DBP increases to the fifth decade, and thereafter plateaus or declines. These studies also suggest that over midlife the rate of increase in SBP and DBP is greater in women compared to men, so that by the fifth or sixth decade mean levels have become higher in women. Cross-sectional studies cannot take account of secular or birth cohort influences and many of the prospective studies have used regression methods that do not account for correlation between values at different ages in the same people. Furthermore, the different age ranges covered by these different studies, and the fact that most started measurements in the third or fourth decade, make it difficult to make reliable conclusions regarding change across the whole of adult life.

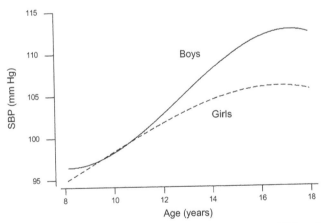

Figure 11.1 Longitudinal age-related change in systolic blood pressure in childhood from one US prospective study (Project HeartBeat!) [11].

Reprinted from *American Journal of Preventive Medicine*, Volume **37**, Issue 1, Labarthe DR, et al. Systolic and fourth- and fifth-phase diastolic blood pressure from ages 8 to 18 years: Project HeartBeat!, pp. S86–96, Copyright © 2009, with permission from Elsevier.

In the Baltimore Longitudinal Study of Aging, SBP and DBP changes from age 17 to 97 years were modelled using appropriate methods in over 2000 participants, with BP assessed at 2-yearly intervals between 1958 and 1991 [21]. SBP was relatively stable in both women and men until the fourth decade, increased in both genders by a similar amount until the seventh decade, and then stabilized in women but continued to increase in men. At all ages mean SBP was lower in women compared to men [21]. DBP changed relatively little in either gender with increasing age, showing a weak increase across the whole of adulthood in men, and a similar weak increase in women to the fifth decade, after which it plateaued and then declined slightly [21]. This greater age-related increase in SBP compared with DBP would inevitably result in age-related increases in pulse pressure and may reflect arterial wall thickening.

By contrast, a recent study that reported change in SBP between age 30 and 64 years from 52 countries, found SBP increased with increasing age in both men and women in all of the countries, but with markedly greater rates of increase in women and a slowing of the increase, or even a decline, beyond approximately age 60 [22]. Similarly, in a recent study that combined data from seven UK prospective cohort studies (30,372 participants, 102,583 SBP observations), each with at least two measurements of BP and each covering different periods of the life course (7 to 80+ years), there was an increase in SBP with increasing age in midlife that was steeper in women than men (Figure 11.2) [23]. Four life course phases were observed: a rapid increase in SBP coinciding with peak adolescent growth, a more gentle increase in early adulthood, a midlife acceleration beginning in the fourth decade, and a period of deceleration in late adulthood where increases in SBP slowed and at very old age appeared to decline [23]. The mean gender difference in SBP from age 7–80 years (Figure 11.3) confirms the more prominent increase in SBP in boys compared with girls in childhood (Figure 11.1) [11], and the greater midlife increase in women compared with men. By the mid-twenties, SBP was markedly higher in men compared with women, but by the late fifties/early sixties mean SBP was higher in women [22,23].

The extent to which the slowing of the increase, or even decrease, in SBP from the seventh or eighth decade, seen in most prospective studies (Figure 11.2) [21–24], is driven by selection bias (those who survive to older age having lower BP across their life course), more effective treatment regimes, or a greater impact of treatments that have been taken for a longer duration, as opposed

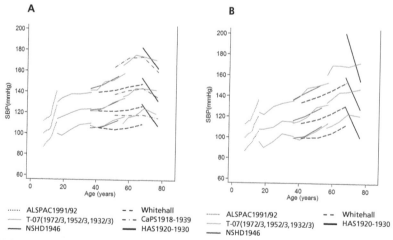

Figure 11.2 Longitudinal age-related change in systolic blood pressure using data from seven UK cohorts coverage age 7–80+ years [23]. Plot A, men; plot B, women.

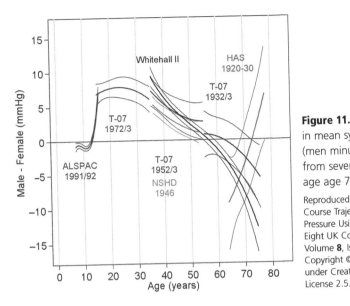

Figure 11.3 Gender difference in mean systolic blood pressure (men minus women) using data from seven UK cohorts cover-age age 7–80 + years [23].

Reproduced from Wills AK, et al., Life Course Trajectories of Systolic Blood Pressure Using Longitudinal Data from Eight UK Cohorts, *PLoS Medicine*, Volume **8**, Issue 6, e1000440, Copyright © 2011 Wills et al, licensed under Creative Commons Attribution License 2.5.

to true age-related physiological changes, is unclear. Sensitivity analyses in the study of seven UK cohorts suggested that survivor bias was unlikely to explain much of the decline [23]. Removal of participants who had ever taken antihypertensive treatment in that study resulted in the decline being less marked [23], and in the Baltimore Longitudinal Study of Aging, in which participants on any treatments that would affect BP or with any cardiovascular, metabolic or renal diseases or evidence of high risk were excluded, SBP leveled off at older age in women but did not decline in either gender [21]. These results suggest that BP treatment and/or co-morbidity may explain some of the decline seen in general population studies. Possible age-related pathophysiological factors explaining the deceleration at very old age include age-related weight loss, arterial stiffening and changes in the autonomic control of blood pressure related to cognitive decline [25].

There is, however, considerable variation around these average trends, and examining mean BP may conceal population subgroups with different underlying trajectories. In a recent latent class analysis of midlife adults, subgroups of BP change between 36 and 53 years were identified [26]. In both men and women and, for both SBP and DBP there was a large 'normal' group, that included over 90% of participants and was characterized by steady annual increases [26]. There was also a smaller group (accounting for 3–6%; 'increaser' group) in whom the rate of increase was three to four times greater than the large 'normal' group. In women only there was an additional subgroup in whom SBP and DBP remained consistently high (accounting for 1–3%) [26].

11.3 Average life course BP trajectories in different populations

The consistent demonstration of generally increasing BP with increasing age in studies of industrialized populations has been interpreted as age-related increases in BP being a 'natural' physiological process. However, studies of non-industrialized subsistence farming populations have shown little age-related increases in adult BP [27,28]. Most of these studies have been cross-sectional and have been criticized as potentially biased because of their small size, selection bias and concerns with how accurately BP and age were assessed [28,29]. A recent large (N = 2248) study of lowland forager horticulturalists from Bolivia that used reliable and accurate methods to assess BP and age, measured BP up to nine times over an 8-year period in adults ranging from

20 to 90 years [29], and found that BP increased with age, in particular for women, but that the rate of increase was less than in a comparison general US population. A further comparison in which BP change in adults from 52 western populations and four non-industrialized populations confirmed little or no age-related changes in the non-industrialized populations was in marked contrast to the increases seen in western populations (Supplementary web material Figure 11.S2) [29]. In a separate study of populations from 52 countries, the magnitude of this increase in SBP with age in midlife varied considerably between countries, from 1.7 to 11.6 mmHg per 10 years in men and from 0.8 to 22.4 mmHg per 10 years in women [22]. None of the populations was an isolated subsistence farming community, and there was no clear linear association between country level income and rate of change, with LMIC tending to fall at the two extremes [22]. Taken together, these findings suggest that there is no clear evidence that marked midlife increases in BP are physiological and that some aspects of western lifestyles likely cause this increase.

11.4 Early life characteristics associated with age-related change in BP

A systematic review of studies examining the association of socioeconomic position (SEP) and BP concluded that there was consistent evidence for an inverse association between adult SEP and BP measured in later adulthood, such that those from the most adverse SEP had the highest mean BP and a greater risk of hypertension [30]. Most cross-sectional and prospective studies have found no association between childhood SEP (i.e. parental SEP) and BP measured in childhood, adolescence or early adulthood [30,31]. By contrast, a number of cohort studies have found that childhood SEP is associated with adult BP, such that those from more adverse childhood SEPs have higher BP in adulthood, independent of adult SEP [32–34]. Few studies have examined childhood SEP in relation to change in BP over life. In the MRC National Survey of Health and Development (NSHD), with repeat measurements of adult BP, there was evidence of amplification of the effect of childhood SEP on adult BP, with the difference in BP between manual and non-manual childhood social class increasing by 1.0 mmHg per 10 years greater age [34]. Amplification of the effect with age could explain why little or no association is found between childhood SEP and BP measured in childhood and early adulthood in many studies, but an association between childhood SEP and adult BP has been found.

It has similarly been suggested that the negative association between birthweight and SBP, although initiated *in utero*, is amplified with age [35]. Though it should be noted that the existence of an inverse association of birthweight with BP has been challenged, with suggestions that it is explained by bias (including publication bias), confounding or postnatal (rather than *in utero*) effects [36,37]. Furthermore, the evidence that this association amplifies with age comes from comparisons of multiple studies with BP measured at different ages [35,38], and so the apparent amplification of the association might actually be a result of stronger associations in historical, compared to more contemporary, birth cohorts. Studies with repeated measures of BP within the same sample in adulthood suggest that the association is constant, i.e. that the magnitude of the association of birthweight with BP is the same at all adult ages [34,39], and two studies have found no amplification of effect between childhood and early adulthood [40,41], though one study suggested an increase in effect between adolescence and early adulthood [42].

Adult height, in particular leg length, can be considered as a biomarker of early life environmental factors, and taller height—driven by longer leg length—is associated with lower adult BP [43,44]. Leg length reflects pre-pubertal growth, and has been related more strongly than trunk length to breastfeeding and higher energy diets in early childhood, and more advantaged early life socioeconomic environment [45,46]. In the MRC NSHD, greater adult height and leg length, but not trunk length, were related to faster age-related increases in BP and pulse pressure during midlife, suggesting that detrimental early life influences on vascular structure and function may increase vulnerability to the effects of ageing on the arterial tree [43].

Greater adiposity at any time of life, including childhood, is associated with higher BP. Greater childhood adiposity is associated with greater adult BP, and in studies with repeat measurements of weight or other indicators of adiposity, those who lose weight have BP levels on average similar to those who started with a healthier weight [33,47–49]. Since BP tracks from childhood to adulthood, it is hard to disentangle length of overweight from any impact of current size [49]. To our knowledge no studies have examined associations between childhood adiposity and BP change later in life.

Infancy may be a sensitive period with respect to the effect of dietary sodium intake on later BP levels, and there is also evidence of associations of greater childhood physical activity and fitness with lower BP [33]. However, these exposures have not been explored in relation to age-related change of BP. Randomized controlled trials and cross-cohort comparisons suggest that the observed association of breastfeeding with reduced BP in later life is not causal [50,51].

11.5 Periods of the life course with specific blood pressure changes

In the Avon Longitudinal Study of Parents and Children (ALSPAC) cohort (South of England birth cohort born in the 1990s) there is some evidence of an increase in the rate of increase of SBP during adolescence (Figure 11.2), but this is not apparent in Project Heartbeat! (US cohort born late 1970s–early 1980s), in which the rate of increase in both SBP and DBP actually flattened at around age 15–16 years (Figures 11.1 and 11.S1). However, population level trends with age may be too crude to identify an effect of puberty, which will occur at different ages in different individuals. Furthermore, these studies may have had insufficient repeat data around the time of puberty to detect a specific effect. In studies with very detailed repeat measurement, a marked increase in SBP, which is more pronounced in males compared to females, has been found that coincides with the pubertal growth spurt in height (a valid proxy for puberty) [52,53]. The close synchrony between pubertal growth spurt, peak weight increase, and peak SBP increase in those studies makes it difficult to determine whether this represents common mechanisms that regulate growth and BP during puberty, or whether the puberty-related increase in weight and height cause the increase in BP [53]. It is also unclear whether any changes in the BP trajectory that might occur in relation to puberty have a subsequent impact on trajectories of adult BP. An earlier age at menarche has been related to cardiovascular disease in girls [54,55], and to higher DBP at 31 years in one study [56], but not to SBP or DBP in midlife in another [57]. In both studies, men who had a late puberty had lower mean BP in midlife than those who had gone through puberty earlier, which was not completely explained by their lower body mass index (BMI) [56,57].

There are a large number of studies that have examined change in BP in normal gestation (usually defined as women who have not experienced pre-eclampsia) using repeat measurements [58]. The majority of studies are small, with most containing fewer than 100 participants, and just three (the Omega Study from the US [59], Generation-R from the Netherlands [60] and ALSPAC [61]) including more than 1000 [58]. Despite different methods used for assessing BP and modelling change with gestational age, studies tend to show very similar patterns for DPB, with a gradual decline in early pregnancy to a nadir at about 18 to 20 weeks and then steady increases to late pregnancy and delivery [58]. Results are less consistent for SBP, with some studies showing continuous increases in SBP across the whole of pregnancy, some an initial decrease in early pregnancy similar to that seen with DBP, and some no change to approximately 18 to 20 weeks, and increases with gestational age thereafter. The vast majority of the studies using repeatedly assessed ambulatory BP assessment suggest a gradual decline to18 to 20 weeks [58], consistent with ALSPAC that included over 12,000 women with a median of 14 BP measurements per woman [61]. The Generation-R study of 8000 women reported a monotonic increase in SBP across pregnancy, but had just three measurements of BP per woman, and so was limited in the extent to which it could model non-linear change [60].

Using the extensive data in ALSPAC it has also been shown that women with existing hypertension, those who develop gestational hypertension and who develop pre-eclampsia begin pregnancy with notably higher BP than other women, with those who develop pre-eclampsia also having a much more marked increase in BP in later pregnancy (Figure 11.4) [61]. Despite these different

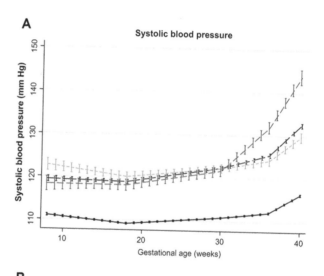

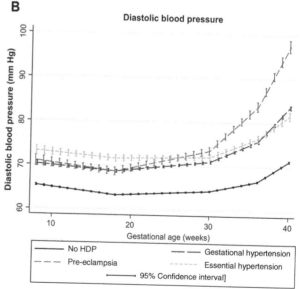

Figure 11.4 Blood pressure change in pregnancy by category of hypertensive disorder, using data from a UK prospective pregnancy cohort study (Avon Longitudinal Study of Parents and Children) [61].

Reproduced from Macdonald-Wallis et al., Blood pressure change in normotensive, gestational hypertensive, preeclamptic, and essential hypertensive pregnancies. *Hypertension*, Volume Number **59**, Issue Number 6, pp. 1241–8, Copyright © 2012 by American Heart Association, Inc., with permission from Wolters Kluwer Health.

trajectories, established pre-eclampsia risk factors, including maternal age, parity, BMI, smoking and pregnancy size, are associated with early pregnancy BP and subsequent rates of change in similar ways to their association with pre-eclampsia [62,63].

Women diagnosed with pre-eclampsia and gestational hypertension (defined as hypertension on at least two occasions after 20 weeks gestation) are at increased risk of future hypertension, other adverse cardio-metabolic risk factors and cardiovascular disease [64,65]. However, the extent to which this is due to normal vascular changes of pregnancy unmasking an existing underlying genetic or environmental risk of hypertension, or to a direct effect of the pregnancy, is unclear [66].

Both SBP and DBP increase more in midlife in women than they do in men (Figures 11.2 and 11.3) and in cross-sectional studies BP is higher in post-menopausal compared with pre-menopausal women after adjustment for age differences [67]. However, the magnitude of the post- versus pre-menopausal difference is small and prospective studies that have modelled repeatedly-assessed SBP and DBP as women go through the menopause suggest little or no specific effect of the menopause *per se*, over and above that due to ageing [67,68]. Furthermore, in the one study with available data, changes in sex hormones related to the menopause were not related to BP change over this period [68]. Thus, available evidence does not support an important impact of the menopause *per se* (and its associated hormonal change) on BP trajectories.

11.6 **Relationship of different life course trajectories of blood pressure with future cardiovascular risk**

Higher BP in late adolescence and early adulthood (ages 18 to 30 years) is associated with later CHD and stroke risk with magnitudes that are similar to those seen with associations of BP measured at older ages [69]. In the Cardiovascular Risk in Young Finns study, SBP assessed between 12 and 18 years was positively associated with carotid intima media thickness (CIMT) assessed at 33 to 39 years, with a magnitude (0.013 mm greater CIMT per 1SD greater childhood SBP; 95% CI: 0.007, 0.019) similar to that of the association with SBP in adulthood (assessed at the same time as CIMT) (0.010 mm per 1SD greater SBP; 95% CI: 0.006, 0.014); neither childhood nor adult DBP was associated with CIMT [70]. These findings suggest that determinants of BP change during infancy and childhood, through their influences on BP level in adolescence and early adulthood, are important for identifying those at risk of future cardiovascular disease. However, we are unaware of any studies which investigate this.

In terms of changes in BP across adult life, the Lifetime Risk Pooling Project found that participants who were consistently hypertensive over at least 10 years and those whose BP increased to the level of hypertension had particularly high cumulative lifetime risk of CHD, while those whose BP decreased to normal levels had an estimated risk similar to those with BP which had always been in the normal range [71]. In one UK study, adults belonging to a subgroup with more marked increases in midlife SBP and DBP were more likely to have undiagnosed angina than other participants [26]. In the same study, greater midlife increases in SBP were associated with poorer cardiac structure and function, including left ventricular function at age 60–64 years [72]. Greater increase between 43 and 53 years was shown to be a stronger risk factor of higher left ventricular mass index than more recent BP increases between 53 and 60–64 years [72]. Whether this finding represents a detrimental impact of rate of increase during a particular sensitive period of adult life, or whether there is a lag effect which is independent of age, remains to be seen. Further, the possibility of reverse causality cannot be ruled out, as the study does not have earlier life cardiac measures.

11.7 **Life course changes in lipids; gender and ethnic differences**

One cross-sectional [73], and one prospective [74] (with repeat measurements in the same children) study, suggest similar patterns of change in lipids across childhood. Levels of total cholesterol (Figure 11.5) and low density lipoprotein cholesterol (LDLc) (Supplementary web material Figure 11.S3) declined with age from 8 to 16 years, with this decline being more rapid in boys than in girls in the prospective study [74]. By contrast, triglyceride levels increased with increasing age, and did so more markedly in boys than girls; in boys there was a monotonic increase with age whereas in girls the increase flattened from age 12 onwards (Supplementary web material Figure 11.S4). Patterns of change in high density lipoprotein cholesterol (HDLc) also differed markedly between girls and boys, with a sinusoidal pattern in boys that produced a peak mean level around age 11 and a trough around age 15, and little change in levels in girls until age 15, after which levels increased (Supplementary web material Figure 11.S5). Thus, by age 15–16, boys had lower total and LDLc, but higher triglycerides and lower HDLc compared with girls [74]. No ethnic differences in mean levels or change in total cholesterol were found [74]. At all ages mean levels of LDLc, HDLc and triglycerides were more adverse (higher LDLc (Figure 11.S3) and triglycerides (Figure 11.S4) and lower HDLc (Figure 11.S5)) in non-black compared with black children, but the patterns of change with age were the same for both ethnic groups [74]. It is important to note that this was the only study that we were able to find that modelled change in lipids measured repeatedly in the same children, and we cannot assume that these results (based on data from US children born in the late 70s/early 80s) would necessarily generalize to other populations.

Studies of age-related changes in lipids in adults have largely been cross-sectional in design and suggest that in western industrialized countries total cholesterol, LDLc and triglycerides increase from the late twenties or early thirties to at least the sixth decade of life and HDLc declines over this period [22,75,76]. Total cholesterol, LDLc and triglyceride levels are greater in men in early adulthood, but the slope of increase from the early thirties to later life is greater in women than in men, and similarly HDLc is lower in men in early adulthood but the decline over adulthood is greater in women [22,75,76]. In a recent study that compared age associations between national

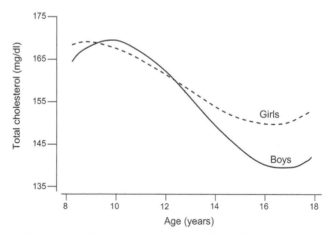

Figure 11.5 Longitudinal changes in total cholesterol in childhood from one US prospective study (Project HeartBeat!) [74].

Reprinted from *American Journal of Preventive Medicine*, Volume **37**, Issue 1, Dai S, et al., Blood lipids in children: age-related patterns and association with body-fat indices: Project HeartBeat!, pp. S56–S64, Copyright © 2009, with permission from Elsevier.

cross-sectional surveys across the globe, it was found that mean total cholesterol levels in early adulthood (age 30 years) and the rate of increase with age (to mid-fifties) were lower in LMIC than in high income countries, though there was some age-related increase in all countries [22]. In high income countries where surveys had been conducted more recently, the magnitude of the increase with age was lower, possibly as a result of increased use of statins or improvements in lifestyle risk factors [22].

11.8 Early life characteristics associated with age-related change in lipids

Lower childhood SEP is associated with more adverse lipid profiles in adulthood [8,77,78], but a recent study of children found that only apolipoprotein B showed socioeconomic differences when lipid-related outcomes were measured in childhood, and this association was largely explained by socioeconomic differences in adiposity [79]. Birthweight is weakly inversely associated with adverse lipid profiles in childhood and adulthood [8]. Greater adiposity at any age is associated with more adverse lipids and, as with BP, there is evidence that weight loss, including in childhood, results in improvements in lipid profiles [48]. Breastfeeding is associated with better lipid profiles in observational studies [8], but to our knowledge studies with better causal designs (e.g. RCTs) have not been conducted and, given that these have shown breastfeeding is not causally related to BP (see Section 11.4), this may also be the case with lipids. Notably, we were unable to find any studies of the association of early life characteristics with age-related change in lipids over life.

11.9 Periods of the life course with specific lipid changes

There is some evidence of an adolescent nadir in total and HDLc in both genders around the age of 14 to 16 years (Figure 11.S5). By contrast LDLc levels may improve at this age, with Project Heartbeat! finding a levelling off of the decline from early childhood at around 16 years in females, though no obvious change in rate of decrease at this time in males (Figure 11.S3). In females, childhood triglyceride levels are static until age 12 years, and thereafter show a continuous decline to age 18; the change at age 12 may represent a very early adolescent/puberty effect, but this is favourable rather than adverse (Figure 11.S4). Hence, there is little evidence of a specific pubertal effect on lipids but, as for BP, these studies may not have sufficient repeated measures to be able to detect such an effect. Existing evidence does not support an important long-term effect of puberty on lipid levels. Where associations between early menarche and a poorer lipid profile in adulthood have been observed, these have generally been small, and may be mediated through BMI, since early menarche is associated with higher adult BMI [80–83]. A Finnish study showed associations between younger age at puberty in men and adverse lipids in adulthood, with that for HDLc remaining after adjustment for childhood and fetal growth [56], but a British study showed no such associations [83].

In response to gestational hormones—progesterone, 17β-estradiol and placental lactogen—in normal pregnancy, blood lipids increase, particularly in the second and third trimesters, to reach peak levels at 31 to 36 weeks gestation [84–89]. Triglycerides increase markedly, commonly doubling, with total cholesterol and LDLc increasing by about 50%, and there is some evidence of a modest decline in HDLc [84–89]. One study suggested that adverse pregnancy-related changes in total cholesterol and LDLc reversed quickly in the postnatal period, but that declines in HDLc following pregnancy persisted for at least 10 years [90]. However, it is unclear whether pregnancy-related lipid changes have any lasting effect on future cardio-metabolic health.

More adverse lipid levels are seen in women who are postmenopausal compared with those who are premenopausal in cross-sectional studies that adjust for age. Consistent with these findings several relatively small prospective studies, with between two and five repeat measures, suggest that lipid profiles change specifically in relation to the menopause, over and above age-related changes [68,91–93]. In one study (of approximately 1000 women), perimenopausal changes in endogenous estrogen and gonadotrophins were shown to be associated with adverse lipid changes over this period, suggesting that there are specific lipid changes in relation to the perimenopause [68,93]. The extent to which these changes persist long-term and go on to affect cardiovascular disease risk is unclear.

11.10 **Associations of life course lipids with future disease**

Adverse lipid profiles in childhood, adolescence and young adulthood are associated with extent of atherosclerosis (arterial fatty streaks or raised lesions) in postmortem studies [94–96], and in the Cardiovascular Risk in Young Finns study, LDLc assessed between ages 12 and 18 years was positively associated with CIMT assessed at age 33 to 39 years, with the magnitude of association (0.010 mm greater CIMT per 1SD greater childhood LDLc; 95% CI: 0.004, 0.016) being greater than that for the association of LDLc in adulthood (assessed at the same time as the CIMT) with this outcome (0.004 mm per 1SD greater LDLc; 95% CI: 0.000, 0.009) [70]. In a subsequent multi-cohort study (including the Young Finns study) higher total cholesterol from the age of 12 years was associated with higher young adult CIMT, with associations at younger ages (3, 6, and 9 years) being weak or null [97]. There is also evidence that higher triglycerides and lower HDLc in childhood (particularly from age 9 years onwards) are associated with adult risk of greater CIMT, CVD events, components of the metabolic syndrome, and type 2 diabetes, though some of these studies had limited statistical power and for metabolic syndrome components and type 2 diabetes the associations were largely driven by greater childhood BMI [97–99]. To our knowledge, there are no studies to date that have examined associations of change in lipid levels across childhood and early adulthood with cardiovascular disease in later life.

11.11 **Conclusions**

For life course epidemiology, a basic understanding of how human systems and function change on average over the whole of life is key to being able to explore plausible times in life when interventions to improve or maintain function are likely to have the greatest impact on healthy ageing and disease prevention. Furthermore, higher BP, LDLc, and fasting glucose in adolescence and early adulthood are associated with adverse cardio-metabolic events in older age, independent of these risk factors in adulthood, and therefore understanding early life influences on trajectories in these risk factors to this age would be valuable. And yet, one of the most striking conclusions of this chapter is the relative paucity of studies that use prospective data from cohort studies to correctly model change in cardio-metabolic function with age in order to understand the ageing process on this system. Whilst we would not expect any currently existing study to have a range of repeatedly assessed cardio-metabolic outcomes from birth/infancy through to late adulthood, we did anticipate greater amounts of research for BP, at least, than we were able to find.

Studies often have repeat measurements of BP, and sometimes other cardio-metabolic markers, across infancy, childhood, and into early adulthood, but they rarely explore factors associated with differences in age-related change of these, or of age-related changes in these with later outcomes, preferring instead to examine associations of exposures and outcomes each assessed at just one age. Where an attempt to explore change is undertaken, the statistical methods used are often less than optimal (Chapter 6).

From available data there is little evidence to suggest a clear pattern of increasing function in early life to a high point of 'peak' cardio-metabolic function around adolescence or early adulthood, followed by a period of relatively static function and then decline at older age. For cardio-metabolic function, this assumed general life course pattern of physiology does not appear to hold true.

In general, BP increases across life from mid-childhood into adulthood, but the rates of this increase vary at different ages. LDLc and HDLc show some evidence of change towards more healthy levels with increasing age across childhood, but triglycerides tend to increase over childhood and little is known about age-related changes in glucose and insulin in early life. In adulthood, the age-related increase in SBP, adverse lipid levels and fasting glucose levels are not found in all populations, and may reflect age-related changes in adverse lifestyles, or an accumulation of the adverse effects of long-term high energy intake and sedentary behaviour over life, in modern industrialized populations. That said, there is some evidence for an insulin-resistant, independent, age-related decline in pancreatic β cell function with increasing adult age (see Supplementary web material). Age-related changes of vascular structure and function are at a very early stage of research, but increasing use of these technologies should make it possible to gain an understanding of how early growth and development impacts this system, and how it then ages across adulthood (see Supplementary web material).

Puberty, pregnancy and the perimenopause may perturb the 'normal' age-related trajectories of cardio-metabolic markers seen in most industrialized countries, but whether such influences are temporary, and whether they largely highlight an underlying vulnerability that would have become apparent at an older age anyhow, is unclear. Importantly, the paucity of research in this area means that, as yet, it is unclear whether individual variation from the mean age-related change in cardio-metabolic markers within populations influences later disease risk.

In summary, despite prospective cohort studies in children and adults often repeatedly measuring cardio-metabolic markers, particularly those that are relatively easy and cheap to assess, such as BP and blood lipids, few have appropriately modelled change with age and explored risk factors for different patterns of age-related change, or of these different patterns with future disease risk. Greater attention to this would help our understanding of how cardio-metabolic function ages across the life course, and how to prevent adverse or accelerated ageing in this system.

References

1 **Frayn K, Stanner S.** The aetiology and epidemiology of cardiovascular disease. In: Stanner S, editor. Cardiovascular Disease: Diet, Nutrition and Emerging Risk Factors. Oxford: Blackwell Publishing; 2005: 1–21.

2 **D'Adamo E, Caprio S.** Type 2 diabetes in youth: epidemiology and pathophysiology. *Diabetes Care* 2001;**34**:S161–5.

3 **US Centre for Disease Control.** CDC facts on diabetes. *CDC Facts* 2012; http://www.cdc.gov/features/diabetesfactsheet/(last accessed September 2012).

4 **Enos MW, et al.** Coronary disease among United States soldiers killed in action in Korea. *JAMA* 1953;**152**:1090–3.

5 **McNamara JJ, et al.** Coronary artery disease in combat casualties in Vietnam. *JAMA* 1971;**216**:1185–7.

6 **Strong JP, et al.** Prevalence and extent of atherosclerosis in adolescents and young adults. Implications for prevention from the pathobiological determinants of Atherosclerosis in Youth Study. *JAMA* 1999;**281**:727–35.

7 **Lawlor DA, et al.** A lifecourse approach to coronary heart disease and stroke. In: Kuh D, Hardy R, editors. A Life Course Approach to Women's Health. Oxford: Oxford University Press; 2002:86–120.

8 **Lawlor DA, et al.** Pre-adult influences on cardiovascular disease. In: Kuh D, Ben-Shlomo Y, editors. A Life Course Approach to Chronic Disease Epidemiology. Oxford: Oxford University Press; 2004:46–70.

9 **Forouhi N, et al.** A life course approach to diabetes. In: Kuh D, Ben-Shlomo Y, editors. A Life Course Approach to Chronic Disease Epidemiology. Oxford: Oxford University Press; 2004:165–88.

10 **Whincup PH, et al.** A life course approach to blood pressure. In: Kuh D, Ben-Shlomo Y, editors. *A Life Course Approach to Chronic Disease Epidemiology*. Oxford: Oxford University Press; 2004:218–39.

11 **Labarthe DR, et al.** Systolic and fourth- and fifth-phase diastolic blood pressure from ages 8 to 18 years: Project HeartBeat! *Am J Prev Med* 2009;**37**:S86–96.

12 **Burt VL, et al.** Prevalence of hypertension in the US adult population. *Hypertension* 1995;**25**:305–13.

13 **Burt VL, et al.** Trends in the prevalence, awareness, treatment, and control of hypertension in the adult US population. *Hypertension* 1995;**26**:60–9.

14 **Bazzano LA, et al.** Blood pressure in westernized and isolated populations. In: Lip GYH, Hall JE, editors. Comprehensive Hypertension. Philadelphia: Mosby, Elsevier; 2007: 21–30.

15 **Harlan WR, et al.** A longitudinal study of blood pressure. *Circulation* 1962;**26**:530–43.

16 **Miall WE, Chinn S.** Blood pressure and ageing; results of a 15–17 year follow-up study in South Wales. *Clin Sci Mol Med Suppl* 1973;**45**:23s–33s.

17 **Svardsudd K, Tibblin G.** A longitudinal blood pressure study. Change of blood pressure during 10 yr in relation to initial values. The study of men born in 1913. *J Chronic Dis* 1980;**33**:627–36.

18 **Landahl S, et al.** Age-related changes in blood pressure. *Hypertension* 1986;**8**:1044–9.

19 **Franklin SS, et al.** Hemodynamic patterns of age-related changes in blood pressure. The Framingham Heart Study. *Circulation* 1997;**96**:308–15.

20 **Safar ME, et al.** The data from an epidemiologic study on the Insulin Resistance Syndrome Study: the change and the rate of change of the age-blood pressure relationship. *J Hypertens* 2008;**26**:1903–11.

21 **Pearson JD, et al.** Age-associated changes in blood pressure in a longitudinal study of healthy men and women. *J Gerontol A Biol Sci Med Sci* 1997;**52**:M177–83.

22 **Singh GM, et al.** The age associations of blood pressure, cholesterol, and glucose: analysis of health examination surveys from international populations. *Circulation* 2012;**125**:2204–11.

23 **Wills AK, et al.** Life course trajectories of systolic blood pressure using longitudinal data from eight UK cohorts. *PLoS Med* 2011;**8**:e1000440.

24 **Bush TL, et al.** Blood pressure changes with aging: evidence for a cohort effect. *Aging (Milano)* 1989;**1**:39–45.

25 **Reitz C, Luchsinger JA.** Relation of blood pressure to cognitive impairment and dementia. *Curr Hypertens Rev* 2007;**3**:166–76.

26 **Wills AK, et al.** Population heterogeneity in trajectories of midlife blood pressure. *Epidemiology* 2012; **23**:203–11.

27 **Carvalho JJ, et al.** Blood pressure in four remote populations in the INTERSALT Study. *Hypertension* 1989;**14**:238–46.

28 **Stevenson DR.** Blood pressure and age in cross-cultural perspective. *Hum Biol* 1999;**71**:529–51.

29 **Gurven M, et al.** Does blood pressure inevitably rise with age? Longitudinal evidence among forager-horticulturalists. *Hypertension* 2012;**60**:25–33.

30 **Colhoun HM, et al.** Socio-economic status and blood pressure: an overview analysis. *J Hum Hypertens* 1998;**12**:91–110.

31 **Batty GD, Leon DA.** Socio-economic position and coronary heart disease risk factors in children and young people. Evidence from UK epidemiological studies. *Eur J Public Health* 2002;**12**:263–72.

32 **Lawlor DA, et al.** Childhood socioeconomic position, educational attainment and adult cardiovascular risk factors: findings from the Aberdeen childhren of the 1950s cohort study. *Am J Public Health* 2005;**95**:1245–51.

33 **Lawlor DA, Davey Smith G.** Early life determinants of adult blood pressure. *Curr Opin Nephrol Hypertens* 2005;**14**:259–64.

34 **Hardy R, et al.** Birthweight, childhood social class, and change in adult blood pressure in the 1946 British birth cohort. *Lancet* 2003;**362**:1178–83.

35 **Law CM, et al.** Initiation of hypertension in utero and its amplification throughout life. *BMJ* 1993;**306**: 24–7.

36 **Huxley R, et al.** Unravelling the fetal origins hypothesis: is there really an inverse association between birthweight and subsequent blood pressure? *Lancet* 2002;**360**:659–65.

37 **Tu YK, et al.** Why evidence for the fetal origins of adult disease might be a statistical artifact: the "reversal paradox" for the relation between birth weight and blood pressure in later life. *Am J Epidemiol* 2005;**161**:27–32.

38 **Leon DA, Koupilova I.** Birth weight, blood pressure, and hypertension. In: Barker DJP, editors. Fetal Origins of Cardiovascular Disease. New York: Marcel Dekker; 2000:23–48.

39 **Koupilova I, et al.** Size at birth and hypertension in longitudinally followed 50–70 year-old men. *Blood Pressure* 1997;**6**:223–8.

40 **Uiterwaal CS, et al.** Birth weight, growth, and blood pressure: an annual follow-up study of children aged 5 through 21 years. *Hypertension* 1997;**30**:267–71.

41 **Williams S, Poulton R.** Birth size, growth, and blood pressure between the ages of 7 and 26 years: failure to support the fetal origins hypothesis. *Am J Epidemiol* 2002;**155**:849–52.

42 **Chen W, et al.** Amplification of the association between birthweight and blood pressure with age: the Bogalusa Heart Study. *J Hypertens* 2010;**28**:2046–52.

43 **Langenberg C, et al.** Influence of short stature on the change in pulse pressure, systolic and diastolic blood pressure from age 36 to 53 years: an analysis using multilevel models. *Int J Epidemiol* 2005;**34**:905–13.

44 **Ferrie JE, et al.** Birth weight, components of height and coronary heart disease: evidence from the Whitehall II study. *Int J Epidemiol* 2006;**35**:1532–42.

45 **Gunnell DJ, et al.** Socio-economic and dietary influences on leg length and trunk length in childhood: a reanalysis of the Carnegie (Boyd Orr) survey of diet and health in prewar Britain (1937–39). *Paediatr Perinat Epidemiol* 1998;**12**:96–113.

46 **Wadsworth ME, et al.** Leg and trunk length at 43 years in relation to childhood health, diet and family circumstances; evidence from the 1946 national birth cohort. *Int J Epidemiol* 2002;**31**:383–90.

47 **Howe LD, et al.** Changes in ponderal index and body mass index across childhood and their associations with fat mass and cardiovascular risk factors at age 15. *PLoS ONE* 2010;**5**:e15186.

48 **Lawlor DA, et al.** Association between general and central adiposity in childhood, and change in these, with cardiovascular risk factors in adolescence: prospective cohort study. *BMJ* 2010;**341**:c6224.

49 **Hardy R, et al.** Birthweight, childhood growth, and blood pressure at 43 years in a British birth cohort. *Int J Epidemiol* 2004;**33**:121–9.

50 **Kramer MS, et al.** Long-term effects of prolonged and exclusive breastfeeding on child height, weight, adiposity, and blood pressure: new evidence from a large randomized trial. *Am J Clin Nutr* 2007;**86**:1717–21.

51 **Brion M-J, et al.** What are the causal effects of breastfeeding on IQ, obesity and blood pressure? Evidence from comparing high-income with middle-income cohorts. *Int J Epidemiol* 2011;**40**:670–80.

52 **Shankar RR, et al.** The change in blood pressure during pubertal growth. *J Clin Endocrinol Metab* 2005;**90**:163–7.

53 **Tu W, et al.** Synchronization of adolescent blood pressure and pubertal somatic growth. *J Clin Endocrinol Metab* 2009;**94**:5019–22.

54 **Lakshman R, et al.** Early age at menarche associated with cardiovascular disease and mortality. *J Clin Endocrinol Metab* 2009;**94**:4953–60.

55 **Jacobsen BK, et al.** Age at menarche, total mortality and mortality from ischaemic heart disease and stroke: the Adventist Health Study, 1976–88. *Int J Epidemiol* 2009;**38**:245–52.

56 **Widen E, et al.** Pubertal timing and growth influences cardiometabolic risk factors in adult males and females. *Diabetes Care* 2012;**35**:850–6.

57 **Hardy R, et al.** Age at puberty and adult blood pressure and body size in a British birth cohort study. *J Hypertens* 2006;**24**:59–66.

58 **Macdonald-Wallis C.** Maternal blood pressure change in pregnancy. PhD thesis. Bristol, UK: University of Bristol; 2012.

59 **Thompson ML, et al.** Construction and characterisation of a longitudinal clinical blood pressure database for epidemiological studies of hypertension in pregnancy. *Paediatr Perinat Epidemiol* 2007;**21**: 477–86.

60 **Gaillard R, et al.** Blood pressure tracking during pregnancy and the risk of gestational hypertensive disorders: the Generation R Study. *Eur Heart J* 2011;**32**:3088–97.

61 **Macdonald-Wallis C, et al.** Blood pressure change in normotensive, gestational hypertensive, preeclamptic, and essential hypertensive pregnancies. *Hypertension* 2012;**59**:1241–8.

62 **Macdonald-Wallis C, et al.** Established preeclampsia risk factors are related to patterns of blood pressure change in normal term pregnancy: findings from the Avon Longitudinal Study of Parents and Children. *J Hypertens* 2011;**29**:1703–11.

63 **Macdonald-Wallis C, et al.** Relationships of risk factors for pre-eclampsia with patterns of occurrence of isolated gestational proteinuria during normal term pregnancy. *PLoS ONE* 2011;**6**:e22115.

64 **Bellamy L, et al.** Pre-eclampsia and risk of cardiovascular disease and cancer in later life: systematic review and meta-analysis. *BMJ* 2007;**335**:974.

65 **Fraser A, et al.** Associations of pregnancy complications with calculated cardiovascular disease risk and cardiovascular risk factors in middle age: the Avon Longitudinal Study of Parents and Children. *Circulation* 2012;**125**:1367–80.

66 **Magnussen EB, et al.** Prepregnancy cardiovascular risk factors as predictors of pre-eclampsia: population based cohort study. *BMJ* 2007;**335**:978.

67 **Coylewright M, et al.** Menopause and hypertension: an age-old debate. *Hypertension* 2008;**51**:952–9.

68 **Matthews KA, et al.** Are changes in cardiovascular disease risk factors in midlife women due to chronological aging or to the menopausal transition? *J Am Coll Cardiol* 2009;**54**:2366–73.

69 **McCarron P, et al.** Blood pressure in young adulthood and mortality from cardiovascular disease. *Lancet* 2000;**355**:1430–1.

70 **Raitakari OT, et al.** Cardiovascular risk factors in childhood and carotid artery intima-media thickness in adulthood: the Cardiovascular Risk in Young Finns Study. *JAMA* 2003;**290**:2277–83.

71 **Allen N, et al.** Impact of blood pressure and blood pressure change during middle age on the remaining lifetime risk for cardiovascular disease: the cardiovascular lifetime risk pooling project. *Circulation* 2012;**125**:37–44.

72 **Ghosh AK.** Life course determinants of cardiac structure and function in the MRC National Survey of Health and Development 1946 birth cohort. PhD thesis. London, UK: Imperial College London; 2013.

73 **Jolliffe CJ, Janssen I.** Distribution of lipoproteins by age and gender in adolescents. *Circulation* 2006; **114**:1056–62.

74 **Dai S, et al.** Blood lipids in children: age-related patterns and association with body-fat indices: Project HeartBeat!*Am J Prev Med* 2009;**37**:S56–S64.

75 **Sniderman AD, Furberg CD.** Age as a modifiable risk factor for cardiovascular disease. *Lancet* 2008; **371**:1547–9.

76 **Mann D, et al.** Trends in statin use and low-density lipoprotein cholesterol levels among US adults: impact of the 2001 National Cholesterol Education Program guidelines. *Ann Pharmacother* 2008;**42**: 1208–15.

77 **Lawlor DA, et al.** Socioeconomic position in childhood and adulthood and insulin resistance: cross sectional survey using data from the British women's heart and health study. *BMJ* 2002;**325**:805–7.

78 Lawlor DA, et al. The association of childhood socioeconomic position with coronary heart disease risk in post-menopausal women: findings from the British Women's Heart and Health Study. *Am J Public Health* 2004;**94**:1386–92.

79 Howe LD, et al. Are there socioeconomic inequalities in cardiovascular risk factors in childhood, and are they mediated by adiposity? Findings from a prospective cohort study. *Int J Obes (Lond)* 2010;**34**:1149–59.

80 Pierce MB, Leon DA. Age at menarche and adult BMI in the Aberdeen children of the 1950s cohort study. *Am J Clin Nutr* 2005;**82**:733–9.

81 Kivimaki M, et al. Association of age at menarche with cardiovascular risk factors, vascular structure, and function in adulthood: the Cardiovascular Risk in Young Finns study. *Am J Clin Nutr* 2008;**87**: 1876–82.

82 Feng Y, et al. Effects of age at menarche, reproductive years, and menopause on metabolic risk factors for cardiovascular diseases. *Atherosclerosis* 2008;**196**:590–7.

83 Pierce MB, et al. Role of lifetime body mass index in the association between age at puberty and adult lipids: findings from men and women in a British birth cohort. *Ann Epidemiol* 2010;**20**:676–82.

84 Darmady JM, Postle AD. Lipid metabolism in pregnancy. *Br J Obstet Gynaecol* 1982;**89**:211–5.

85 Jimenez DM, et al. Longitudinal study of plasma lipids and lipoprotein cholesterol in normal pregnancy and puerperium. *Gynecol Obstet Invest* 1988;**25**:158–64.

86 Qureshi IA, et al. Hyperlipidaemia during normal pregnancy, parturition and lactation. *Ann Acad Med Singapore* 1999;**28**:217–21.

87 Sattar N, et al. Lipoprotein subfraction changes in normal pregnancy: threshold effect of plasma triglyceride on appearance of small, dense low density lipoprotein. *J Clin Endocrinol Metab* 1997;**82**:2483–91.

88 Sattar N, et al. Lipoprotein subfraction concentrations in preeclampsia: pathogenic parallels to atherosclerosis. *Obstet Gynecol* 1997;**89**:403–8.

89 Sattar N, et al. A longitudinal study of the relationships between haemostatic, lipid, and oestradiol changes during normal human pregnancy. *Thromb Haemost* 1999;**81**:71–5.

90 Gunderson EP, et al. Long-term plasma lipid changes associated with a first birth: the Coronary Artery Risk Development in Young Adults study. *Am J Epidemiol* 2004;**159**:1028–39.

91 Jensen J, et al. Influence of menopause on serum lipids and lipoproteins. *Maturitas* 1990;**12**:321–31.

92 Do KA, et al. Longitudinal study of risk factors for coronary heart disease across the menopausal transition. *Am J Epidemiol* 2000;**151**:584–93.

93 Derby CA, et al. Lipid changes during the menopause transition in relation to age and weight: the Study of Women's Health Across the Nation. *Am J Epidemiol* 2009;**169**:1352–61.

94 Strong JB, et al. Prevalence and extent of atherosclerosis in adolescents and young adults. *JAMA* 1999;**281**:727–35.

95 McGill HC, et al. Effects of serum lipoproteins and smoking on atherosclerosis in young men and women. *Arterioscler Thromb Vasc Biol* 1997;**17**:95–106.

96 Berenson GS, et al. Association between multiple cardiovascular risk factors and atherosclerosis in children and young adults. The Bogalusa Heart Study. *N Engl J Med* 1998;**338**:1650–6.

97 Juonala M, et al. Influence of age on associations between childhood risk factors and carotid intima-media thickness in adulthood: the Cardiovascular Risk in Young Finns Study, the Childhood Determinants of Adult Health Study, the Bogalusa Heart Study, and the Muscatine Study for the International Childhood Cardiovascular Cohort (i3C) Consortium. *Circulation* 2010;**122**:2514–20.

98 Magnussen CG, et al. Pediatric metabolic syndrome predicts adulthood metabolic syndrome, subclinical atherosclerosis, and type 2 diabetes mellitus but is no better than body mass index alone: the Bogalusa Heart Study and the Cardiovascular Risk in Young Finns Study. *Circulation* 2010;**122**:1604–11.

99 Morrison JA, et al. Pediatric triglycerides predict cardiovascular disease events in the fourth to fifth decade of life. *Metabolism* 2009;**58**:1277–84.

Chapter 12

A life course approach to healthy musculoskeletal ageing

Kate A Ward, Judith E Adams, Ann Prentice, Avan Aihie Sayer, and Cyrus Cooper

12.1 Introduction

A healthy bone is one that is fit for purpose and does not fail, i.e. fracture, under physiological loading. Fragility fractures are an important consequence of ageing in the developed world resulting in significant morbidity and mortality. In the UK one in two women and one in five men aged over 50 will suffer a fragility fracture during their remaining life [1]. Healthy musculoskeletal function is also essential for maintaining mobility and the ability to undertake the physical tasks of daily living and, preventing falls. For fracture prevention and subsequent reduction of morbidity and mortality, it is necessary to understand the life course determinants of musculoskeletal health.

Bone densitometry was developed to assess an individual's fracture risk through measurement of surrogates for bone strength, bone mineral content (BMC; amount of bone within a projected bone area) and areal bone mineral density (aBMD; amount of bone per unit projected area). These measures predict approximately 70% of variation in bone strength in populations at high fracture risk [2]. However, a paradox exists where a low aBMD or BMC do not necessarily predict fracture [3,4]. It has become increasingly clear that a more comprehensive assessment of bone strength is required to understand the pathogenesis of fracture and the prediction of risk. Such an assessment needs to include other components of bone strength, such as bone size, shape, internal architecture and loading conditions, rather than simply measuring the mineral mass contained within the bony envelope [5,6].

Figure 12.1 illustrates the life course progression of bone health and shows when, at each stage, key milestones are reached and when 'healthy' ageing and pre-disease states progress to an increased risk of fracture and associated consequences. The contribution to musculoskeletal ageing of factors in the internal and external environments at all stages of life is also represented. The internal environment consists of innate factors such as gender and genotype, and those factors which are, in part, dependent on external environmental factors such as growth rate, cognitive decline, and ethnicity. External environment describes those extrinsic factors related to lifestyle and social circumstances that have a key role in determining musculoskeletal health. These include nutrition, physical activity, and socioeconomic position. Muscle loading is the primary determinant of postnatal bone strength. The mechanostat is the regulatory mechanism that facilitates the modification of bone in response to muscular loading and/or environment throughout life [7,8]. The mechanostat may respond to changes in internal (e.g. hormone status) or external (e.g. physical activity) environments. Cross-sectional and longitudinal studies made at key life stages provide the majority of evidence on the indirect or direct relationships between muscle and bone, and for the contribution of the internal or external environment to bone health [9]. Studies

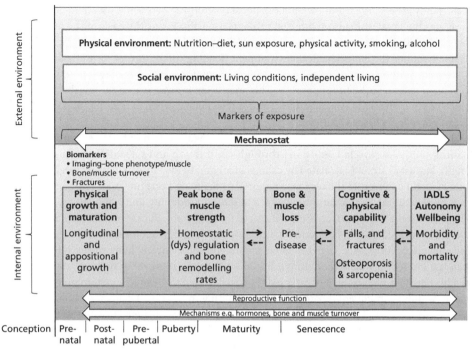

Figure 12.1 An integrated life course approach to musculoskeletal ageing. IADLS, instrumental activities of daily living.

of individuals in cohorts who have been followed from infancy and childhood into young adulthood provide valuable opportunities to investigate how the internal and external environments throughout life contribute to healthy musculoskeletal growth and ageing [10–13]. Cohorts have also shown the importance of growth during gestation, infancy and childhood for determining future fracture risk [14,15]. Data from birth cohorts such as the MRC National Survey for Health and Development (NSHD) provide the opportunity to extend the evidence by providing data on pre-pubertal and pubertal growth and environmental factors collected across life.

This chapter describes how an integrated approach to the study of bone and muscle can be applied to increase our understanding of musculoskeletal ageing. Key life stages are identified and we describe how early life (defined in this chapter as the pre-and postnatal period through to infancy), childhood, and adolescence are essential for bone health and for the prevention of skeletal disease in later life. The important factors in the internal and external environments are discussed. The focus for the external environment is on nutrition and physical activity, the two main modifiable factors known to influence bone health across life. The chapter also describes the role of quantitative imaging in providing measures that can act as biomarkers of a healthy musculoskeletal phenotype, with an overview of currently available techniques.

12.2 **Muscle and bone—an integrative approach**

Bone strength is determined by mass, material and structural properties, metabolism and loading conditions. Loading conditions are intrinsically related to body weight and body composition, but importantly are also related to the biomechanical relationship between muscle and bone. Muscle generates the greatest loads on bone and this relationship forms the basis of the mechanostat theory [7,8]. Postnatal bone development and ageing are driven in response to muscle loading [8]. Throughout life, the biomechanical environment (loading conditions) of the individual changes continuously. Bone must adapt to these changes in environment, to maintain functionality and to prevent failure, i.e. be fit for purpose. This adaptation is achieved via the 'mechanostat' [7,8], which controls alterations in longitudinal and appositional growth, in bone loss and in the repair of damage to bone tissue [7,8].

The mechanostat theory describes a negative feedback system of bone response to muscle loading [7,8]. As muscle loads bone through contraction and relaxation, bone changes in length, known as strain (calculated by change in length divided by original length). The magnitude of strain determines the response required to maintain bone integrity. Two processes may alter bone strength in response to changes in strain: modelling and remodelling. Modelling adds bone to the outer surfaces (apposition) of bone, thereby thickening, shaping and reshaping bone. Remodelling replaces and repairs bone and is important for maintenance of strength and calcium homeostasis. Depending on the magnitude of strain, bone strength is increased through modelling and remodelling, decreased through removal of bone or maintained at steady state with replacement of fatigued/damaged bone [8]. Beyond a certain point, overload occurs without subsequent repair, ultimately resulting in fracture. Characteristics of bone that may be modified are: (1) bone mass—the amount of bone within a specific volume; (2) material properties—the stiffness of bone, which is dependent on the ratio and arrangement of inorganic (hydroxyapatite) and organic (osteoid) matrix of bone; and (3) structural design—the shape, size and distribution of bone. Non—mechanical factors in the internal and external environment, such as sex hormones and factors secreted by adipose tissue (internal) and nutrition and physical activity (external) contribute to bone strength in two ways, either by altering loads generated by muscle or the capacity of bone to respond to changes in strain [9]. Together, the responses of the mechanostat to changes in muscle loading (internal environment) and/or non-mechanical factors (internal or external environment) form a functional model of bone across life [9].

12.3 Quantitative imaging of bone and muscle for determination of phenotype

12.3.1 Bone

The study of bone health requires the assessment of bone strength in children and adults. Direct measurement of bone strength, or fracture load, is not possible *in vivo*. Imaging techniques have been developed to quantify surrogate measures of bone strength (biomarkers), most commonly BMC and aBMD. In the 1960s, hand radiographs were used to measure cortical thinning in metacarpals [16]. This method was replaced by low radiation single- and dual-photon absorptiometry, which used radionuclides to quantify BMC and aBMD in the peripheral and central skeleton respectively [17]. In the late 1970s, single- and dual-energy X-ray absorptiometry (DXA) were introduced to replace single- and dual-photon absorptiometry through the use of X-radiation rather than isotope sources; X-rays are much more stable and do not decay, giving more stability and improved precision and accuracy to measurements [18]. At the same time, quantitative computed tomography (QCT), also based on X-ray technology, was introduced to provide three-dimensional images of bone.

12.3.1.1 Bone mineral density (BMD)

The term BMD has many different meanings depending on the measurement technique and it is important to understand the distinctions when interpreting BMD as a measure of bone strength. Bone densitometry either provides measures of bone as a whole organ or the cortical and trabecular compartments separately: BMD_{TOTAL} measures cortical and trabecular bone together; $BMD_{COMPARTMENT}$ measures the cortical compartment, including Haversian canals and pores, and the trabecular compartment, including bone marrow, separately; and BMD_{TISSUE} measures the two compartments separately but without inclusion of pores, canals or marrow [19]. Until recently only measures of BMD_{TOTAL} and $BMD_{COMPARTMENT}$ were possible. Newer high-resolution techniques (CT) offer measurement of cortical BMD_{TISSUE} and of cortical bone at fracture relevant sites [20]. Over the past 20 years we have moved from the ability to measure BMD_{TOTAL} to BMD_{TISSUE} in the peripheral skeleton—how these refinements improve prediction of fracture risk remains to be determined [9].

DXA measures a two-dimensional projection of bone giving an $aBMD_{TOTAL}$ (g/cm^2) measurement of integral (cortical and trabecular) bone, which is size dependent. The implication of measuring BMD_{TOTAL} is that the measure may not be sensitive enough to reflect differences or change in BMD in the cortical and/or trabecular compartments [9]. The only $BMD_{COMPARTMENT}$ measured by DXA is of femoral shaft cortical bone. QCT (peripheral and central) measures volumetric $BMD_{COMPARTMENT}$ (mg/cm^3) which is independent of size and gives separate measures of cortical and trabecular bone. High-resolution peripheral QCT allows the *in vivo* measurement of $BMD_{COMPARTMENT}$ and cortical BMD_{TISSUE} [19].

Whilst BMC and $aBMD_{TOTAL}$ have been used as surrogate measures of bone strength for many years, limitations of the measurements have become apparent. More than 50% of individuals with a low trauma fracture do not have low $aBMD_{TOTAL}$ and would therefore not have been predicted to be at increased fracture risk [3]. Similarly, a quarter of overweight/obese individuals suffer a fracture despite having normal $aBMD_{TOTAL}$ [21]. Studies from the Gambia have questioned the usefulness of BMC or $aBMD_{TOTAL}$ to define fracture risk in populations at low risk [4]. Despite low $aBMD_{TOTAL}$ and BMC, and similar rates of bone loss when compared to individuals in the UK, there are low rates of fracture in older Gambian women [22]. These observations demonstrate, therefore, the need to move beyond BMC and $aBMD_{TOTAL}$ to other measures of bone strength, such as bone shape, size and geometry, in order to fully describe how bone 'ages healthily'.

12.3.1.2 Bone shape, size, and geometry

DXA measurements of bone area and hip structural geometry, e.g. cross-sectional area, hip axis length and moment of inertia, extend 'phenotyping' beyond BMC and $aBMD_{TOTAL}$. These measurements are based on a two-dimensional image; assumptions are applied to express the data in 'three dimensions', which increases the need for careful interpretation. Lateral scanning of the lumbar and thoracic spine allows vertebral shape assessment and visual and semi-quantitative diagnosis of fractures [23]. This is one of the greatest advances in DXA in recent years, providing a low radiation method for diagnosis of vertebral fractures. QCT (peripheral or axial) measures a volume of tissue, using either a single- or multi-slice acquisition. Bone shape, geometry and distribution of mineral are measured in the cortical and trabecular compartments. From these, several measures of bone strength are derived, such as stress strain index and moment of inertia, measures that predict failure load (the point at which bone fractures) [24,25].

High resolution pQCT is the highest resolution *in vivo* scanning method available and is described as a non-invasive bone biopsy. Direct and indirect measures of trabecular and cortical microarchitecture of the distal radius and tibia are provided, such as cortical porosity and trabecular thickness, number and separation, and the ratio of trabecular bone volume to total volume [26–28].

12.3.1.3 Finite element modelling (FEM)

FEM simulates stress and strain distributions within bone based on pixel/voxel mineral density values. The method assumes bone is made of a connected number of elements, of given elasticity, to which loads are applied. The response of these elements to load is calculated to give measures of failure load, stress, and strain in bone compartments. The technique has been applied to DXA images and radiographs (two-dimensional images) and, more widely, to three-dimensional QCT. Failure load from FEM analysis of forearm, spine and hip scans is an independent predictor of fracture [29,30]. As with other methods, it is important to remember that FEM is based on a set of assumptions that require careful interpretation [20].

When the load applied to bone exceeds strength, a fracture will result and has been termed 'biomechanical fracture threshold' [31]. Fall or compressive loads are calculated from a subject's weight and height, measured directly or derived from body segment length and weight, respectively; for example the compressive loads on vertebrae are calculated from body segment length and segment weight, which are assumed to be a percentage of total height and weight [32]. A load-to-strength ratio is calculated as the ratio of fall, or vertebral, load to bone strength calculated from FEM. These ratios predict an individual's biomechanical fracture threshold and can be used to improve the prediction of hip or vertebral fracture risk [31–33]. This approach may provide greater understanding of why some people fracture and some people do not, even when they have the same $aBMD_{TOTAL}$ [32,33].

12.3.2 Muscle

Muscle strength is a term used to describe the force and power generating capacity of muscle. Sarcopenia is the age-related loss of muscle mass and function [34]; there is continuing debate about the quantitative definition of sarcopenia [35,36]. Quantitative imaging or functional tests are common ways to assess muscle mass and function.

12.3.2.1 Muscle mass

Lean tissue mass, measured by DXA, or cross-sectional muscle area (CSMA), measured by QCT or magnetic resonance imaging (MRI), are commonly used in studies of muscle–bone relationships. The advantage of these methods is that data are acquired on bone and muscle simultaneously. Visceral fat measurements by DXA are precise, involve a low exposure to ionizing radiation, and take less time than the more established techniques such as MRI. A disadvantage of DXA is the inability to separate the visceral organs from other lean tissue, which leads to inaccurate assessment of trunk lean mass. This leads to inaccurate and insensitive measures of whole body lean mass for the study of sarcopenia [37]. Appendicular lean tissue mass, the sum of arm and leg lean masses, is more commonly used than whole body lean mass to quantify age-related loss of muscle mass [37]. Cross-sectional muscle area by QCT or pQCT, and lean mass by DXA, do not decline with age as rapidly as muscle functional tests, such as chair rising time. This could be due to the greater declines in muscle strength and power which also influence test performance, but could also reflect a lack of sensitivity of the imaging techniques [37,38]. An advantage of obtaining quantitative measurements of mass and area at the same time as performing bone densitometry is that they are not limited by the ability or motivation of the individual to perform. Another advantage of imaging is the simultaneous measurement of fat mass. A major advance in DXA technology is the automated analysis of visceral fat mass, a risk factor for obesity-related disease [39,40]. Visceral fat measurements by DXA are precise, involve low exposure to ionizing radiation, and take less time than the more established techniques such as MRI.

Alternative approaches to the use of imaging for the study of muscle phenotype are being developed [41]. Measurements of muscle atrophy and the extent to which muscle tissue has been replaced by fatty and non-functional tissue may be important to help to understand age-related loss of muscle function. Fat infiltration (myosteosis) is an important contributor to decline in muscle function with age. Lean mass, measured by DXA, and CSMA, measured by QCT, do not quantify this fat infiltration. Measurements of muscle attenuation (a measure of how much of an X-ray beam is absorbed by tissues through which it passes) by QCT or pQCT reflect the degree of myosteosis in the muscle [41]. Muscle attenuation predicted hip fracture risk independently of volumetric BMD [42]. Magnetic resonance spectroscopy (MRS) is the gold standard technique to quantify myosteosis. It gives a direct measurement of the intra- and extra-cellular lipid content of muscle and may also measure muscle metabolism [41]. However, MRS is technically challenging, costly to acquire and is impractical for application in large population-based studies.

12.3.2.2 Muscle function

Muscle function includes muscle strength, force and power, measured using tests such as dynamometry or ground reaction force platforms, as well as physical performance, characterized by gait speed, chair rises and standing balance (Chapter 2) [43,44]. These measures appear to be more sensitive to the effects of advancing age than muscle mass. For example, grip strength and lower limb power showed greater decline with age than did measurements of CSMA or lean mass [38,42]. Another example of the greater sensitivity of functional measurements than mass is in response to vitamin D supplementation, where muscle power of the lower limb, but not CSMA, increased [45]. These observations could indicate the lack of sensitivity of CSMA to changes in muscle composition and intramuscular fat, and/or that global measures of lower limb function are a better reflection of a person's ability to perform a task. A more detailed discussion of physical capability is considered in Chapter 2.

12.4 **Musculoskeletal health across life**

An individual's fracture risk in later life is likely to depend on 'optimal' longitudinal and appositional bone growth until skeletal maturity, and subsequently on the ability to maintain and repair the skeleton during reproductive years and early to mid adulthood [5,6]. At the end of longitudinal growth and period of mineral accumulation no further net gain of bone occurs. To achieve and maintain the maximum genetic potential, adequate environmental factors must exist. These include nutrition, physical activity, maintenance of a healthy weight, normal muscle function and hormone status (Figure 12.1). As the mechanostat is central to bone development and ageing, the contribution of the environment to muscle mass and function is also important [9].

Most research is directed at studying the effects of environment on bone during a single life stage and whilst providing important insights into factors affecting bone health, this type of research sometimes yields conflicting or confusing results [4,9,46]. This is probably due to the fact that many studies are cross-sectional in design, or they are interventions or trials with only limited time of follow-up in which to assess the long-term effects on musculoskeletal health. Such studies also generally lack any consideration of the possibility that different populations respond differently to environmental factors [4,9,46]. Data from several longitudinal studies are becoming available for the study of bone development and ageing, and will be valuable for the identification of sensitive life stages for bone development and ageing [12,15,47–49]. Birth cohorts perhaps provide the best opportunity to understand how the internal and external environments influence bone health across life. A number of the oldest birth cohorts, such as the MRC NSHD, and historical cohorts, such as the Hertfordshire Cohort Study (HCS), are reaching older age, and provide an ideal opportunity to study how events or environmental factors earlier in life may influence healthy musculoskeletal ageing. In addition, it is possible to collect fracture incidence data prospectively in these older cohorts to enable more definitive descriptions of how factors earlier in life affect later fracture risk.

12.4.1 **Internal environment**

12.4.1.1 Developmental origins of musculoskeletal health

There is a strong basis for a model of osteoporosis and sarcopenia pathogenesis, based on the concepts of fetal programming and developmental plasticity. The intrauterine and postnatal periods are important for rapid mineral accretion and, combined with the relative plasticity of musculoskeletal development *in utero*, offer the possibility of important interactions between the genome and environment at this early stage of life. Evidence that musculoskeletal health might be modified by the intrauterine and early postnatal environment has emerged from two groups of studies: cohort studies of adults whose detailed birth and/or childhood records have been preserved and who have subsequently had BMC and $aBMD_{TOTAL}$ measurements and fracture risk ascertained; and secondly, mother–offspring cohorts in which nutrition, body build, and lifestyle of pregnant women have been related to the bone mass of their offspring [48]. The relationships between birthweight, weight in infancy, and adult BMC and bone area have been replicated in several adult cohort studies and confirmed in a recent meta-analysis and systematic review [11,50]. These observations have been replicated in societies at different points in the nutritional transition, as observed in cohorts from New Delhi and the Gambia [49,51]. Findings have been consistent for a relationship between intrauterine and early postnatal growth, and adult bone cross-sectional area, length and geometry, with a consequent potential impact on bone strength [51–54]. The lack of, or weak, associations between birthweight, or weight at one year, and aBMD, size-corrected BMC, or vBMD suggests that bone size, rather than mineralization, is driven by early growth. Finally, the influences of early growth on femur bone size, shape, geometry and mechanical strength, clearly translate into an impact on hip fracture [14,15].

Mother–offspring cohort studies have documented the impact of several maternal environmental factors on neonatal and childhood bone mineral accrual; these include maternal smoking, diet, and exercise [55]. Maternal vitamin D insufficiency has been identified as an important nutritional correlate of attenuated intrauterine mineral accrual and persisting deficits in BMC and lean mass in children measured at 9 years [56–58], though the largest study from the Avon Longitudinal Study of Parents and Children (ALSPAC) cohort failed to find an association between maternal vitamin D and offspring BMC at around age 10 years [59]. Detailed morphological study of the proximal femur during pregnancy using high resolution ultrasound scanning has demonstrated an impact of vitamin D insufficiency as early as the second trimester of pregnancy [58]. It is important to note, however, that associations between maternal vitamin D status and infant and child growth require confirmation in well-designed randomized controlled trials [46,59,60].

The mechanisms underlying the developmental origins of osteoporosis remain a subject for research. At the level of the whole organism, alterations in activity of the growth hormone, insulin-like growth factor and hypothalamic–pituitary–adrenal axis have been demonstrated in adult cohort studies (Chapter 10) [61,62]. At the molecular level, it is possible that these associations reflect epigenetic modification of gene expression during critical periods of early development. Epigenetic changes are stable and heritable and appear to last through multiple generations (Chapter 15). The most widely studied form of epigenetic marking is DNA methylation, and experimental data from animal models, as well as early studies in human cohorts, suggest that alterations in maternal diet might lead to reduced methylation of key CpG-rich islands (genomic areas rich in sequences of cytosine and guanine pairs) in the promoter region of various genes critical to the transduction of vitamin D signalling, and other important metabolic pathways in skeletal homeostasis [63,64]. Regardless of the underlying mechanism, strategies to improve human health in future generations, by modulating maternal environmental risk factors, are already being evaluated [59].

12.4.1.2 Childhood and adolescence

As growth proceeds from pre-puberty through to skeletal maturity, continuous modelling and remodelling ensures the bone remains fit for purpose in response to changing internal and external environments. The only time this is compromised is during early puberty when bone growth exceeds mineralization and a period of skeletal fragility ensues [65,66]. By the end of the second or early in the third decade, depending on sex and skeletal site, the skeletal reservoir for later life is fixed, and is known as peak bone mass—by definition the product of vBMD and volume. Thereafter, no net change in bone mass occurs until the menopause in females and with ageing in both sexes. There are three phases of bone acquisition in adolescence: firstly, an increase in height velocity marks accelerated longitudinal growth, followed by an increase in bone area (width), and subsequently peak mineral accretion when the skeletal envelope is mineralized [47,67]. There is asynchrony in the timing of these peak velocities: bone area increases up to 4 years after peak height velocity (PHV), and BMC increases for up to 6 years [47]. The timing of events from PHV is also site dependent, an important factor to consider when designing interventions to maximize bone accrual during adolescence [45,68]. Support for the importance of muscle accrual during growth is evident, with peak muscle mass accrual occurring between PHV and peak increase in bone area (appositional growth) [67].

Individuals gain up to 30–40% of total bone mass during puberty, making puberty a sensitive period for bone development. The majority of sexual dimorphism in bone phenotype emerges during the pubertal years [5,69,70]. Despite this, the evidence that the timing of puberty, e.g. early or late menarche in girls, has an influence on future bone health is inconclusive [71–73]. This may be due to lack of prospective data on pubertal timing, or to the possibility that other effects during adulthood override earlier events. Rising oestradiol concentrations in females drive accrual of bone mineral, thought to prepare the skeleton for pregnancy and lactation [74]. Testosterone in males is linked to increases in bone size and in muscle mass and strength, although oestradiol also has positive effects on bone in males [75]. At the end of skeletal growth there is no net change in bone until age- and menopause-related bone loss. It therefore follows, that healthy longitudinal and appositional growth rates are important for future bone health, and not just the amount of bone mineral accrued by skeletal maturity. Low rates of childhood growth were associated with hip fracture risk in the Helsinki cohort at age 50 and older, with height and weight increase between ages 7 and 15 being less in those who subsequently suffered a fracture than those who did not [14]. In females with fractures, the magnitude of weight gain was less than gain in height, indicating that reduced body mass index (BMI) during childhood was a risk factor for fracture in later life. This may be related to a slower rate of weight gain through growth and/or less loading to the skeleton from lower body weight [15]. These data suggest that fracture aetiology may be related to poor weight gain during childhood, and/or weight loss during ageing. Data from the NSHD are supportive of these observations with osteoporotic individuals having lower height and weight z-scores through the life course (unpublished findings). In the same cohort, greater weight gain was also associated with higher hip and spine $aBMD_{TOTAL}$, which may indicate lower fracture risk [76]. Bone size and strength, measured by pQCT, at age 60–64 were associated with height and weight change at most stages of growth [76]. There were weak or no associations between height and weight gain and $vBMD_{COMPARTMENT}$ or BMD_{TOTAL}. On the whole, these data from the NSHD support the early life data showing that childhood and adolescent growth influences shape and size of the bone envelope and has little or no influence on the amount of mineral within.

Whilst these life course data indicate that slow or inadequate weight gain during growth may be detrimental to future bone health, there is increasing evidence that overweight or obese children are at increased risk of fracture [77–79]. In a prospective study of girls with forearm fractures, high body weight significantly increased risk of future fracture [79]. Identification of when excess weight gain may be detrimental to bone health is crucial to help ensure bone health in later life for overweight or obese individuals.

12.4.1.3 Maturity and senescence

Pregnancy and lactation are associated with rapid changes in BMC during early to mid- adulthood, when the skeleton acts as a reservoir for calcium and other nutrients for the developing fetus and neonate. Decreases in BMC are observed in skeletal sites rich in trabecular bone during pregnancy and lactation, which are reversed after breastfeeding stops [80,81]. When pregnancy occurs before skeletal maturity this may compromise future bone health [82,83]. Pregnancy after skeletal maturity is not deleterious to bone; there are suggestions that the effects may be positive [84].

At the menopause the decrement in oestrogen levels results in rapid loss of 3–5% bone mass per year, and is greatest for the first 4 years following the menopause. Ageing, in both females and males, is associated with bone loss of 1–2% per year, with loss in males starting later than in females. Sex differences in fracture rates are thought to be due to different patterns of periosteal accrual and endosteal bone loss through ageing. In males proportional losses and gains on the endosteal and periosteal surfaces to maintain strength were observed, whereas less periosteal apposition relative to endosteal resorption was observed in females [5,26]. Reduced circulating testosterone and/or aromatization of testosterone to oestradiol are related to bone loss and fragility in males [85–87]. The study of different population groups and ethnicities with different fracture rates also contributes to our understanding of healthy musculoskeletal ageing [4]. However, there are currently limited life course data in these populations.

During ageing, the decline in muscle strength and reduced neuromuscular function and cognitive capacity (Chapters 2 and 3) increase the risk of falls, and therefore fracture. Muscle force generating capacity is reduced through loss of muscle mass, increased intramuscular fat and reduced physical activity. Consequently, these factors are likely to increase bone loss and thus reduce bone strength. For example, incident hip fracture was increased in individuals with low muscle attenuation which is indicative of more intramuscular fat [42,88]. Therefore, reductions in muscle mass and strength with ageing are likely to contribute directly or indirectly to bone loss.

12.4.2 External environment

The mechanostat is challenged to successfully modify bone phenotype in different ways at various life stages. Nutrition and physical activity are the most important modifiable external environmental factors influencing bone health. What is clear is that 'one rule does not fit all' and that different life stages and different populations/ethnicities must be considered separately rather than generically when making recommendations on nutrition and physical activity aimed at maintaining or optimizing muscle and bone health [4].

12.4.2.1 Nutrition

There are several ways in which nutrition contributes to musculoskeletal health: (1) provision of bone forming minerals; (2) ensuring healthy longitudinal growth; (3) supply of vitamins involved in calcium–phosphate homeostasis; (4) supply of energy, amino acids and ions; and (5) ensuring healthy muscle function. For example, during growth, protein intake has been shown to be positively associated with bone and muscle accrual [4]. Calcium and vitamin D are essential for longitudinal growth and bone mineralization; vitamin D is also required for protein synthesis in muscle. Associations have been reported suggesting that a higher calcium intake and vitamin D status in ranges above frank deficiency promote longitudinal growth and bone mineralization, although the effects of supplementation studies have not been consistent and appear to differ over the short- and the long-term; the 'positive' effects of supplementation are not always sustained or there may be unintended consequences in the long term [9,12]. During ageing, declining protein intake has been associated with loss of muscle mass, while calcium and vitamin D supplementation has been shown to reduce falls and fractures in some studies [89–91]. Low BMI and, as recent evidence also suggests, high BMI, are risk factors for fracture, indicating that maintenance of a healthy weight is important at all life stages [4,9,21,79]. There is also emerging evidence for possible interactions between adipose tissue and bone, and/or muscle [13,92]. Many studies of nutrition and bone fail to find strong associations with dietary intake of single nutrients or food groups [4]. There are perhaps multiple reasons for this: cross-sectional analyses of diet and bone do not take into account the cumulative effects of diet across life; it is difficult to consider potential synergies between nutrients and food groups; a single nutrient is a small part of total food intake; confounders such as socioeconomic position and lifestyle of the individual are also important to consider. Therefore consideration of the diet as a whole, through dietary pattern analysis, may be useful to increase understanding of the role of nutrition in musculoskeletal health [93,94]. For public health guidelines to be developed it is important to understand the relative contribution of diet across life, between genders and in different populations (Chapter 16) [4].

12.4.2.2 Physical activity

Physical activity is an important determinant of musculoskeletal health across life [95–97]. This is most clearly demonstrated when considering the effects of the removal of loading on bone [8], for example during spaceflight, when an individual can lose up to 3% of bone per month [98]. Further to this, weight-bearing exercise has a strong anabolic effect on bone, through activities such as jogging or racquet sports; tennis players have up to 20% more bone in the loaded, compared to unloaded, limbs [99]. Despite clear associations between physical activity and bone, data from exercise interventions are inconsistent and there are few data from life course studies. Difficulties in quantifying and documenting levels of activity (Chapter 17) are likely to be part of the reason for this lack of consistency. Whilst 'weight-bearing exercise' is a generic term used to describe an activity that generates higher than 'normal loads' in bone, it is difficult to quantify the amount of loading required to generate loads sufficient to increase bone strength and to translate this into recommendations for the amount and type of activity desirable for good bone health [10].

The most beneficial type of activity for bone accrual or maintenance differs depending on life stage. Weight-bearing exercise intervention trials indicate that the greatest effects on BMD or bone size are obtained in the years immediately pre- or early puberty [96]. The gains in BMD or bone size achieved during childhood exercise programmes appear to be maintained into adulthood, as shown in studies of retired gymnasts who had increased amounts of bone during adulthood, despite stopping training in late adolescence [95,100]. General population data from the Age, Gene/Environment Susceptibility-Reykjavik Study showed that continuation of exercise up to and over age 65 was beneficial for bone health [97]. During later life, other types of physical activity become important. Resistive exercise slows bone loss and balance, and postural exercises such as Tai-Chi have been shown to have a beneficial effect on fall prevention [101].

There are still unanswered questions regarding the effects of physical activity at different life stages. The nature and skeletal site of response appears to be dependent on activity type, timing, intensity and the populations being studied [10,96].

12.5 **Conclusions**

A healthy bone is fit for purpose and does not fail during physiological loading. Strategies to ensure healthy musculoskeletal ageing warrant a life course approach. It is essential to consider childhood and adolescence as vital periods for determinants of future bone health. Muscle and bone should be considered together as a functional unit, and studies are required to determine the nature and extent of the indirect and direct relationship between these tissues. The interaction of adipose tissue with this functional unit requires study. Quantitative skeletal imaging has progressed as a biomarker of skeletal health, with technological refinements now enabling a move beyond BMD_{TOTAL} to measurement of BMD_{TISSUE} and cross-sectional bone shape, size and geometry, the quantification of compartment microarchitecture and failure load in vivo, and the measurement of muscle function rather than mass. There are few data from studies exploiting new imaging techniques to gain a greater understanding of how the multiple components of bone strength develop. As with all measures of bone health, critical appraisal of the strengths and limitations of these new techniques is required to interpret the additional measurements correctly and to add to the definition of a healthy bone. Further work is required to determine how refining this definition ultimately improves our ability to predict fracture risk.

Longitudinal data are lacking that describe nutrition, physical activity, and other external environmental factors across life, and this has limited the understanding of how these interact with bone and muscle. Cohorts such as NSHD and ALSPAC have collected dietary and physical activity/functional capability data at several stages through life. Combined with skeletal assessment by DXA and pQCT, these data will allow a unique assessment of the contribution of factors in the internal and external environments to bone health at different life stages. In conclusion, cohort studies with long-term follow-up can provide valuable data for the identification of key stages in the life course for musculoskeletal health and for the investigation of how long-term exposures to external and internal environmental factors influence healthy musculoskeletal ageing.

References

1 van Staa TP, et al. Epidemiology of fractures in England and Wales. *Bone* 2001;**29**:517–22.

2 Marshall D, et al. Meta-analysis of how well measures of bone mineral density predict occurence of osteoporotic fractures. *BMJ (Clinical research ed)* 1996;**312**:1254–9.

3 Wainwright SA, et al. Hip fracture in women without osteoporosis. *J Clin Endocrinol Metab* 2005;**90**: 2787–93.

4 Prentice A. Diet, nutrition and the prevention of osteoporosis. *Public Health Nutr* 2004;**7**:227–43.

5 Seeman E. From density to structure: growing up and growing old on the surfaces of bone. *J Bone Miner Res* 1997;**12**:509–21.

6 Seeman E. An exercise in geometry. *J Bone Miner Res* 2002;**17**:373–80.

7 Frost H. Bone "mass" and the "mechanostat": a proposal. *Anat Rec* 1987;**219**:1–9.

8 Frost HM. The Utah Paradigm of Skeletal Physiology. vol. 1. Greece: International Society of Musculoskeletal and Neuronal Interactions; 2004.

9 Ward K. Musculoskeletal phenotype through the life course: the role of nutrition. *Proc Nutr Soc* 2012;**71**:27–37.

10 Deere K, et al. Habitual levels of high, but not moderate or low, impact activity are positively related to hip BMD and geometry: results from a population-based study of adolescents. *J Bone Miner Res* 2012;**27**:1887–95.

11 Baird J, et al. Does birthweight predict bone mass in adulthood? A systematic review and meta-analysis. *Osteoporos Int* 2011;**22**:1323–34.

12 Prentice A, et al. The effect of prepubertal calcium carbonate supplementation on the age of peak height velocity in Gambian adolescents. *Am J Clin Nutr* 2012;**96**:1042–50.

13 Timpson NJ, et al. How does body fat influence bone mass in childhood? A Mendelian randomization approach. *J Bone Miner Res* 2009;**24**:522–33.

14 Cooper C, et al. Maternal height, childhood growth and risk of hip fracture in later life: a longitudinal study. *Osteoporos Int* 2001;**12**:623–9.

15 Javaid MK, et al. Growth in childhood predicts hip fracture risk in later life. *Osteoporos Int* 2011;**22**: 69–73.

16 Barnett E, Nordin B. The radiological diagnosis of osteoporosis. *Clin Radiol* 1960;**11**:166–74.

17 Cameron J, Sorenson J. Measurement of bone mineral in vivo: an improved method. *Science* 1963;**142**:230–2.

18 Mazess RB, Barden HS. Measurement of bone by dual-photon absorptiometry (DPA) and dual-energy X-ray absorptiometry (DEXA). *Ann Chir Gynaecol* 1988;**77**:197–203.

19 Rauch F, Schonau E. Changes in bone density during childhood and adolescence: An approach based on bone's biological organization. *J Bone Miner Res* 2001;**16**:597–604.

20 Genant HK, et al. Advanced CT bone imaging in osteoporosis. *Rheumatology (Oxford)* 2008;**47**(Suppl 4): iv9–16.

21 Premaor MO, et al. Obesity and fractures in postmenopausal women. *J Bone Miner Res* 2010;**25**:292–7.

22 Aspray TJ, et al. Low bone mineral content is common but osteoporotic fractures are rare in elderly rural Gambian women. *J Bone Miner Res* 1996;**11**:1019–25.

23 Link TM, et al. Radiologic assessment of osteoporotic vertebral fractures: diagnostic and prognostic implications. *Eur Radiol* 2005;**15**:1521–32.

24 Augat P, Schorlemmer S. The role of cortical bone and its microstructure in bone strength. *Age Ageing* 2006;**35**:ii27–ii31.

25 Schiessl H, et al. Non-invasive bone strength index as analyzed by peripheral quantitative computed tomography (pQCT). In: E Schoenau, editor. Paediatric Osteology: New Developments in Diagnostics and Therapy. vol. 1105. International Congress Series. Amsterdam: Elsevier; 1996: 147–60.

26 Khosla S, et al. Effects of sex and age on bone microstructure at the ultradistal radius: a population-based noninvasive in vivo assessment. *J Bone Miner Res* 2006;**21**:124–31.

27 Nishiyama KK, et al. Cortical porosity is higher in boys compared with girls at the distal radius and distal tibia during pubertal growth: an HR-pQCT study. *J Bone Miner Res* 2012;**27**:273–82.

28 Burghardt AJ, et al. Reproducibility of direct quantitative measures of cortical bone microarchitecture of the distal radius and tibia by HR-pQCT. *Bone* 2010;**47**:519–28.

29 Keaveny TM. Biomechanical computed tomography—noninvasive bone strength analysis using clinical computed tomography scans. *Ann N Y Acad Sci* 2010;**1192**:57–65.

30 MacNeil JA, Boyd SK. Load distribution and the predictive power of morphological indices in the distal radius and tibia by high resolution peripheral quantitative computed tomography. *Bone* 2007;**41**:129–37.

31 Keaveny TM, Bouxsein ML. Theoretical implications of the biomechanical fracture threshold. *J Bone Miner Res* 2008;**23**:1541–7.

32 Melton LJ 3rd, et al. Relation of vertebral deformities to bone density, structure, and strength. *J Bone Miner Res* 2010;**25**:1922–30.

33 Orwoll ES, et al. Finite element analysis of the proximal femur and hip fracture risk in older men. *J Bone Miner Res* 2009;**24**:475–83.

34 Aihie Sayer A. Sarcopenia. *BMJ* 2010;**341**:c4097.

35 Cruz-Jentoft AJ, et al. Sarcopenia: European consensus on definition and diagnosis: report of the European Working Group on Sarcopenia in Older People. *Age Ageing* 2010;**39**:412–23.

36 Fielding RA, et al. Sarcopenia: an undiagnosed condition in older adults. Current consensus definition: prevalence, etiology, and consequences. International working group on sarcopenia. *J Am Med Dir Assoc* 2011;**12**:249–56.

37 Visser M, et al. Reexamining the sarcopenia hypothesis. Muscle mass versus muscle strength. Health, Aging, and Body Composition Study Research Group. *Ann N Y Acad Sci* 2000;**904**:456–61.

38 Runge M, et al. Is muscle power output a key factor in the age-related decline in physical performance? A comparison of muscle cross section, chair-rising test and jumping power. *Clin Physiol Funct Imaging* 2004;**24**:335–40.

39 Kaul S, et al. Dual-energy X-ray absorptiometry for quantification of visceral fat. *Obesity (Silver Spring)* 2012;**20**:1313–8.

40 Micklesfield LK, et al. Dual-energy X-ray performs as well as clinical computed tomography for the measurement of visceral fat. *Obesity (Silver Spring)* 2012;**20**:1109–14.

41 Lang T, et al. Sarcopenia: etiology, clinical consequences, intervention, and assessment. *Osteoporos Int* 2010;**21**:543–59.

42 Lang T, et al. Computed tomographic measurements of thigh muscle cross-sectional area and attenuation coefficient predict hip fracture: the health, aging, and body composition study. *J Bone Miner Res* 2010;**25**:513–9.

43 Martin HJ, et al. Is hand-held dynamometry useful for the measurement of quadriceps strength in older people? A comparison with the gold standard Bodex dynamometry. *Gerontology* 2006;**52**:154–9.

44 Roberts HC, et al. Finding the right outcome measures for care home research. *Age Ageing* 2010;**39**:517.

45 Ward KA, et al. A randomized, controlled trial of vitamin D supplementation upon musculoskeletal health in postmenarchal females. *J Clin Endocrinol Metab* 2010;**95**:4643–51.

46 Specker BL. Does vitamin D during pregnancy impact offspring growth and bone? *Proc Nutr Soc* 2012;**71**:38–45.

47 Baxter-Jones AD, et al. Bone mineral accrual from 8 to 30 years of age: an estimation of peak bone mass. *J Bone Miner Res* 2011;**26**:1729–39.

48 Cooper C, et al. Review: developmental origins of osteoporotic fracture. *Osteoporos Int* 2006;**17**:337–47.

49 Tandon N, et al. Growth from birth to adulthood and peak bone mass and density data from the New Delhi Birth Cohort. *Osteoporos Int* 2012;**23**:2447–59.

50 Schlussel MM, et al. Birth weight and adult bone mass: a systematic literature review. *Osteoporos Int* 2010;**21**:1981–91.

51 de Bono S, et al. Influence of birth weight on peripheral bone in young Gambian adults: a pQCT study. *J Musculoskelet Neuronal Interact* 2007;7:82.

52 Javaid MK, et al. Infant growth influences proximal femoral geometry in adulthood. *J Bone Miner Res* 2006;**21**:508–12.

53 Javaid MK, et al. Self-reported weight at birth predicts measures of femoral size but not volumetric BMD in eldery men: MrOS. *J Bone Miner Res* 2011;**26**:1802–7.

54 Oliver H, et al. Growth in early life predicts bone strength in late adulthood: the Hertfordshire Cohort Study. *Bone* 2007;**41**:400–5.

55 Godfrey K, et al. Neonatal bone mass: influence of parental birthweight, maternal smoking, body composition, and activity during pregnancy. *J Bone Miner Res* 2001;**16**:1694–703.

56 Javaid MK, et al. Maternal vitamin D status during pregnancy and childhood bone mass at age 9 years: a longitudinal study. *Lancet* 2006;**367**:36–43.

57 Ioannou C, et al. The effect of maternal vitamin D concentration on fetal bone. *J Clinical Endocrinol Metab* 2012;**97**:E2070–7.

58 Mahon P, et al. Low maternal vitamin D status and fetal bone development: cohort study. *J Bone Miner Res* 2010;**25**:14–9.

59 Lawlor DA, et al. Association of maternal vitamin D status during pregnancy with bone-mineral content in offspring: a prospective cohort study. *Lancet* 2013;**381**:2176–83.

60 Harvey NC, et al. MAVIDOS Maternal Vitamin D Osteoporosis Study: study protocol for a randomized controlled trial. The MAVIDOS Study Group. *Trials* 2012;**13**:13.

61 Dennison EM, et al. Growth hormone predicts bone density in elderly women. *Bone* 2003;**32**:434–40.

62 Dennison EM, et al. A study of relationships between single nucleotide polymorphisms from the growth hormone–insulin-like growth factor axis and bone mass: the Hertfordshire cohort study. *J Rheumatol* 2009;**36**:1520–6.

63 Gluckman PD, et al. Effect of in utero and early-life conditions on adult health and disease. *N Engl J Med* 2008;**359**:61–73.

64 Harvey NC, et al. Evaluation of methylation status of the eNOS promoter at birth in relation to childhood bone mineral content. *Calcif Tissue Int* 2012;**90**:120–7.

65 Cooper C, et al. Epidemiology of childhood fractures in Britain: a study using the general practice research database. *J Bone Miner Res* 2004;**19**:1976–81.

66 Khosla S, et al. Incidence of childhood distal forearm fractures over 30 years: a population-based study. *JAMA* 2003;**290**:1479–85.

67 Rauch F, et al. The 'muscle-bone unit' during the pubertal growth spurt. *Bone* 2004;**34**:771–5.

68 El-Hajj Fuleihan G, et al. Effect of vitamin D replacement on musculoskeletal parameters in school children: a randomized controlled trial. *J Clin Endocrinol Metab* 2006;**91**:405–12.

69 Ashby RL, et al. The muscle-bone unit of peripheral and central skeletal sites in children and young adults. *Osteoporos Int* 2011;**22**:121–32.

70 Gilsanz V, et al. Differential effect of gender on the sizes of the bones in the axial and appendicular skeletons. *J Clin Endocrinol Metab* 1997;**82**:1603–7.

71 Rauch F, et al. Age at menarche and cortical bone geometry in premenopausal women. *Bone* 1999;**25**:69–73.

72 Jackowski SA, et al. Maturational timing does not predict HSA estimated adult bone geometry at the proximal femur. *Bone* 2011;**49**:1270–8.

73 Kindblom JM, et al. Pubertal timing predicts previous fractures and BMD in young adult men: the GOOD study. *J Bone Miner Res* 2006;**21**:790–5.

74 Garn S, et al. Bone measurement in the differential diagnosis of osteopenia and osteoporosis. *Radiology* 1971;**100**:509–18.

75 Lorentzon M, et al. Free testosterone is a positive, whereas free estradiol is a negative, predictor of cortical bone size in young Swedish men: the GOOD study. *J Bone Miner Res* 2005;**20**:1334–41.

76 Kuh D, et al. Growth from birth to adulthood and bone phenotype in early old age: a British birth cohort study. *J Bone Miner Res* 2013. Epub ahead of print; doi: 10.1002/jbmr.2008.

77 Dimitri P, et al. Fat and bone in children: differential effects of obesity on bone size and mass according to fracture history. *J Bone Miner Res* 2010;**25**:527–36.

78 **Skaggs DL, et al.** Increased body weight and decreased radial cross-sectional dimensions in girls with forearm fractures. *J Bone Miner Res* 2001;**16**:1337–42.

79 **Goulding A, et al.** Bone and body composition of children and adolescents with repeated forearm fractures. *J Bone Miner Res* 2005;**20**:2090–6.

80 **Olausson H, et al.** Calcium economy in human pregnancy and lactation. *Nutr Res Rev* 2012;**25**:40–67.

81 **Laskey M, Prentice A.** Bone mineral changes during and after lactation. *Obstet Gynecol* 1999;**94**: 608–15.

82 **Chantry CJ, et al.** Lactation among adolescent mothers and subsequent bone mineral density. *Arch Pediatr Adolesc Med* 2004;**158**:650–6.

83 **Ward KA, et al.** Postpartum bone status in teenage mothers assessed using peripheral quantitative computed tomography. *J Clin Densitom* 2009;**12**:219–23.

84 **Specker B, Binkley T.** High parity is associated with increased bone size and strength. *Osteoporos Int* 2005;**16**:1969–74.

85 **Roura-Pascual N, et al.** Relative roles of climatic suitability and anthropogenic influence in determining the pattern of spread in a global invader. *Proc Natl Acad Sci USA* 2011;**108**:220–5.

86 **Khosla S, et al.** Relationship of volumetric BMD and structural parameters at different skeletal sites to sex steroid levels in men. *J Bone Miner Res* 2005;**20**:730–40.

87 **Vanderschueren D, et al.** Gonadal sex steroid status and bone health in middle-aged and elderly European men. *Osteoporos Int* 2010;**21**:1331–9.

88 **Schafer AL, et al.** Fat infiltration of muscle, diabetes, and clinical fracture risk in older adults. *J Clin Endocrinol Metab* 2010;**95**:E368–72

89 **Heaney RP, Layman DK.** Amount and type of protein influences bone health. *Am J Clin Nutr* 2008;**87**:1567S–70S.

90 **Lips P, et al.** Reducing fracture risk with calcium and vitamin D. *Clin Endocrinol (Oxf)* 2010;**73**: 277–85.

91 **DIPART.** Patient level pooled analysis of 68500 patients from seven major vitamin D fracture trials in US and Europe. *BMJ* 2010;**340**:b5463.

92 **Reid I.** Fat and Bone. *Arch Biochem Biophys* 2010;**503**:20–7.

93 **Tucker KL, et al.** Bone mineral density and dietary patterns in older adults: the Framingham Osteoporosis Study. *Am J Clin Nutr* 2002;**76**:245–52.

94 **Langsetmo L, et al.** Dietary patterns and incident low-trauma fractures in postmenopausal women and men aged >/= 50 y: a population-based cohort study. *Am J Clin Nutr* 2011;**93**:192–9.

95 **Bass S, et al.** Exercise before puberty may confer residual benefits in bone density in adulthood: studies in active prepubertal and retired female gymnasts. *J Bone Miner Res* 1998;**13**:500–7.

96 **Specker BL.** Influence of rapid growth on skeletal adaptation to exercise. *J Musculoskelet Neuronal Interact* 2006;**6**:147–53.

97 **Rianon NJ, et al.** Lifelong physical activity in maintaining bone strength in older men and women of the Age, Gene/Environment Susceptibility-Reykjavik Study. *Osteoporos Int* 2012;**23**:2303–12.

98 **Lang T, et al.** Cortical and trabecular bone mineral loss from the spine and hip in long-standing space-flight. *J Bone Miner Res* 2004;**19**:1006–12.

99 **Kannus P, et al.** The site-specific effects of long-term unilateral activity on bone mineral density and content. *Bone* 1994;**15**:279–84.

100 **Eser P, et al.** Skeletal benefits after long-term retirement in former elite female gymnasts. *J Bone Miner Res* 2009;**24**:1981–8.

101 **Clemson L, et al.** Integration of balance and strength training into daily life activity to reduce rate of falls in older people (the LiFE study): randomised parallel trial. *BMJ* 2012;**345**:e4547.

Chapter 13

A life course approach to biomarkers of ageing

Carmen Martin-Ruiz and Thomas von Zglinicki

13.1 Introduction

The challenge of devising a set of biomarkers capable of measuring the ageing rate in humans was articulated long ago. Despite major concerted efforts, progress so far has been limited. In recent years, developments in the basic biology of ageing reveal the possibility of pharmacological or gene therapeutic extension of healthy lifespan in mammals, as well as the increasing importance of frailty as a clinically relevant syndrome. This approach enhances the need for sensitive and specific biomarkers of ageing that are validated in both experimental animals and, importantly, in humans over the whole age range. In this chapter we will discuss present challenges in biomarker validation over the human life course.

13.2 Biomarkers and the stochastic nature of the ageing process

Over the last 30 years, biogerontology has moved from an observational to an interventional science with increasingly realistic potential for human interventions. This has generated an urgent need for markers that can precisely predict the biological age of populations, groups and individuals. Various approaches to define criteria for biomarkers of ageing have been published, either in conjunction with, or opposed to, biomarkers of age-related disease [1–4]. The essential feature of a biomarker of ageing was defined by Baker and Sprott as: 'a biological parameter that either alone or in some multivariate composite will . . . better predict functional capability at some late age, than will chronological age' [2]; although the impact of age-related disease as originally excluded by Baker and Sprott is still a matter of debate [1–7]. Extensive programmes to validate marker candidates for intervention testing in mice [5], and non-human primates [6], have been run, however, with limited success so far [7]. This is to a large extent due to our still insufficient mechanistic understanding of the ageing process. Ageing is immensely complex. It is to a significant extent governed by chance, leading to stochastic distributions of all parameters that define the rate of ageing even in genetically identical individuals under (as much as possible) identical environmental influences [8]. While we know many of the gene products and environmental influences and their principal routes of interactions that determine the rate of ageing, the impact of any of these on the ageing process in a given individual can vary greatly due to chance events that may occur already during early development. In some cases, this will be 'true' chance that is by its nature unpredictable (as described by the uncertainty principle in particle physics). In other cases, it will be randomness that arises from the sheer number of interactions, each of which is essentially deterministic (and so can, in principle, be measured and assessed). Finally, experimental ignorance, not having discovered the relevance of a gene or the existence of a pathway, is still a major cause of unexplained variance in ageing. For all these reasons, we are yet far from understanding ageing mechanistically. This is reflected by the fact that there is no definition of ageing as a process that occurs in an individual. Rather, the best available definition of biological ageing is a probabilistic one, by which ageing is identified by an ever increasing intrinsic probability of death with progressing time.

Accordingly, the perfect biomarker would allow the precise measurement of the probability of death at any given time. It is immediately clear from the above that a truly perfect biomarker of ageing cannot exist, because there will always be true or apparent chance events in the future that change the ageing trajectory of an individual. In other words, biomarkers of ageing are by their nature probabilistic, with a limited precision of a prediction at the level of the individual. On the other hand, every improvement of biomarker prediction contributes to the reduction of apparent randomness and ignorance. Therefore, biomarkers of ageing not only have a utilitarian value, but do contribute greatly to the conceptual understanding of the ageing process.

13.3 **Use of birth cohorts for biomarker validation**

Chronologic age is the most universally available 'biomarker' of ageing (forensics being a notable exception). However, it is also a weak marker—the differences in survival between the longest and the shortest living member of a cohort are typically greater than mean or median lifespan of the cohort, even in genetically and environmentally homogeneous cohorts under protected conditions with very little impact of external causes of death (Figure 13.1). Therefore, the first requirement for a candidate biomarker of ageing is that it needs to have better predictive power than chronological age. Many population-based studies include participants over a wide age range, and associations are adjusted for age. This might not always be a robust procedure, given that biomarker candidates and their predictive power are often non-linearly associated with chronologic age. This problem is circumvented if associations between marker candidates and ageing 'outcomes' are analysed in birth cohorts, in which all cohort members fall within a narrow age

Figure 13.1 Survival curve (right censored) of a long-lived mouse strain (IRCFa substrain of C57Bl/6; see [90]) under optimal housing conditions. Median survival was 29.4 ± 0.2 months (middle arrow) and mean survival was 29.1 ± 0.2 months. However, the variation in lifespan for 99% of the cohort (range within arrows either side) was 31.9 months.

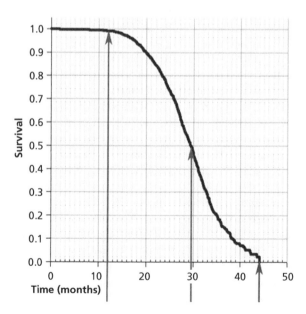

range. This approach addresses directly the relevant question, namely: are (groups of) individuals that are of the same chronological age different in their 'biological age' and, if so, by how much?

The limitation of the birth cohort approach is that, even if the study group was representative of the whole population at that age, it answers the question only for a narrow age group. There is now ample evidence that the predictive power of multiple candidate biomarkers of ageing varies with age group. For instance, up to an age of about 70 years systolic blood pressure (SBP) increases continuously with age [9], and high SBP is a well recognized risk factor for cardiovascular disease and associated mortality [10–12]. At higher ages, however, SBP decreases rather than increases with age [9], and higher blood pressure becomes protective in terms of all-cause mortality and cognition, while low SBP confers increased risks for mortality, cognitive impairment and disability [13–18]. Similarly, short peripheral blood telomere length is recognized as a risk factor for both mortality and (multi-) morbidity [19–24]. These associations are strongest in the age group up to about 75 years but tended to disappear in older populations [21,25]. Similar decreases of predictive power at higher age have been noted for other potential biomarkers [26,27], although often there are not sufficient data on multiple age cohorts, especially the oldest old, available. Cohort and/or period effects may be partially responsible if there is a trend reversal or loss of predictive power at old age. Typically, later born cohorts show extended life expectancy as compared to earlier born cohorts at the same chronological age, and there is some evidence that they are physically and cognitively healthier [26]. Increasingly widespread use of certain medication in older populations will influence biomarker associations. For instance, we found an association between high levels of vitamin D and cognitive impairment in a population-based study of 85 year-olds, which is most probably explained by vitamin D supplementation specifically in care homes [17]. An increased use of antihypertensive medication in this age group may partially explain the decrease of SBP. However, the general pattern remained even for participants not on antihypertensive medication and after adjustment for survivor bias [9]. Moreover, low SBP predicted increased mortality in 90 year-olds without heart failure, defined by low levels of N-terminal prohormone of brain natriuretic peptide (NT-proBNP) [18,28].

13.4 **Longitudinal and life history cohorts**

The general assumption that biomarkers of ageing, measuring accruing deficits, will monotonously change with age is not true. Intervention studies show that physiological or cognitive function can be temporally improved and reversed to more youthful values. For example, muscular and cardiovascular training in older adults will improve a range of the most predictive biomarkers of ageing up to and over their previous levels. A similar improvement might be achieved by short-term treatment with, for example, somatotropic hormones like growth hormone or IGF-1. In both examples, a simple before-and-after biomarker assessment would conclude apparent rejuvenation. Only continuous follow-up would show whether there was a long-term benefit resulting in delayed ageing (as might be expected in the trained individuals), or whether the intervention induced faster decline, resulting in accelerated ageing (which might be the outcome in the second group) [29]. This exemplifies the importance of long-term follow-up, ideally in life history cohorts, to improve predictive power of biomarkers of ageing. Life history cohorts are birth cohorts for which candidate marker information is available longitudinally over a large fraction of the complete life history, and which have reached a sufficient age to be informative about age-related outcomes. Such cohorts are also the ideal test bed to establish the age dependency of candidate biomarkers of ageing. There are at least 60 to 70 human ageing cohorts that have been studied longitudinally worldwide [30,31]; however, few of these qualify as life history cohorts.

Examples of the latter from the UK include the MRC National Survey of Health and Development (NSHD) [32], and the Lothian Birth Cohorts of 1921 and 1936 [33,34]; see also <http://www.halcyon.ac.uk>. Some candidate biomarkers of physical capability (grip strength), cardiovascular function (SBP) and cognition have in fact been longitudinally assessed for long periods of time, with follow-ups spanning in some cases over 50 years in the same participants, enabling comprehensive validation of their predictive power of the life course [9,35–44]. However, for the vast majority of biomarker candidates, life course longitudinal data are not available and will not be for a long while, if at all. For instance, telomere length as a biomarker of ageing was only introduced in 2000 [20]. In this case, the best validation strategy follows the biomarker criteria derived by Nakamura and colleagues [3,6], by combining longitudinal analyses in multiple birth cohorts, in which the longitudinal change with age is expected to be consistent with the cross-sectional differences between the cohorts. However, differences between cross-sectional and longitudinal results might still be found. These might be caused by 'true' cohort effects, relevant parameter differences between cohorts (e.g. health differences), or methodological problems. For instance, in their analysis of SBP in eight longitudinal UK cohorts, Wills and colleagues [9] noticed lower SBP in the included occupational 'white-collar' cohort as compared to population-based cohorts. As suggested, this might be indicative of better health and, by extension, lower biological age in this cohort. Nonetheless, even with a biomarker as simple as SBP, there are variations in measurement technology between cohorts and, as pointed out [9], a contribution of technical variation to the observed cohort effect cannot be ruled out. For most known candidate biomarkers of ageing, technical variation between labs might be larger than for SBP and so far, longitudinal biomarker studies have seldom if ever been done in multiple cohorts performed by a single laboratory with no variation in methodology. For instance, we measured peripheral blood cell telomere length in about 7000 participants of six UK cohorts with consistent methodology (unpublished). However, technical variation in blood sampling and DNA extraction could not be avoided, and the observed cohort-specific differences could thus not definitely be attributed to variation of average biological age between cohorts. It should be noted that Nakamura's criteria [3] also request the rates of age-related change of a potential biomarker to be proportional to differences in ageing rate or lifespan among related species. It might be concluded that most ageing marker candidates in present use have not been sufficiently validated.

13.5 **The missing gold standard**

In terms of biomarker development and validation, the main problem arising from the complex and stochastic nature of the ageing process is that there is no good single process or parameter to test biomarker prediction against. In other words, there is no gold standard. In most animal and a large number of human ageing biomarker studies, survival or lifespan is used as the closest approximation to an estimate of ageing rates. While this is in keeping with the definition of biological ageing, it has two major disadvantages: (1) it rapidly loses power in small cohorts and cannot logically be applied as a biomarker to individuals; and (2) especially in the context of human interventions, measures of 'health span' rather than lifespan are required. There has been a longstanding debate as to whether and to what extent the two co-vary [45–47]. While recent data show clear compression of mortality in super–centenarians [47], it is also clear that (multi-)morbidity, disability, and mortality are at best loosely associated even in octa- and nonagenarians. It has often been proposed that ageing, being a basic process underlying the development of disease and frailty, should be researched (and biomarkers of ageing should be validated) in disease-free subjects (see [48] for review). In contrast, there is increasing evidence for positive feedback loops between age-related disease and basic ageing processes. For instance, chronic inflammation, which is strongly associated with most age-related chronic diseases, including dementias, depression, atherosclerosis, cancers, and diabetes, aggravates cellular senescence, which in turn reduces tissue regenerative potential and enhances pro-inflammatory signals, potentially increasing the risk for additional diseases [49,50]. Thus, both from an opportunistic and a conceptual point of view it seems appropriate to view 'basic' ageing and age-related multi-morbidity and disability as a continuum, especially with respect to bio-marker development and validation. Accordingly, in a recent competitive biomarker candidate validation study, we used four separate 'outcomes' or endpoint measures, namely survival, cognitive decline, disability, and multi-morbidity, and accepted as informative only those biomarker candidates that were associated with at least two of these four endpoint measures [17]. To better capture the multi–dimensionality of the ageing process, additional endpoint measures, prominently including measures of psychological and mental wellbeing, need to be considered for biomarker validation, as these deteriorate in significant subgroups of the population, with important consequences for physiology and perception of the ageing process.

The concept of frailty requires special consideration in the context of ageing biomarker validation. Frailty is characterized by increased vulnerability to stress, resulting in an increased risk of adverse health outcomes including disability, hospitalization, institutionalization, and death. There is as yet no universally accepted definition of frailty. The two leading concepts are frailty as a clinical syndrome—a cluster of specific symptoms and signs including weight loss, exhaustion, low physical activity, muscle weakness, and slow walking speed, as developed by Fried [51], or as a cumulative index of health deficits and indicator of biological age as proposed by Rockwood [52,53]. These individual deficits can include diseases, symptoms, signs, function tests, and laboratory tests. Provided enough deficits are included in the index, their exact nature seems unimportant [54]. Thus, frailty can be regarded as a complex biomarker of ageing (the Rockwood model) or as a clinical definition of an ageing syndrome (the Fried model), clearly illustrating the ambivalence between endpoints and biomarkers in ageing research. Application of both models to the same population shows that they measure overlapping but not identical concepts, with significant fractions of participants falling in one but not the other frailty category. Interestingly, on a cohort level, associations to a large number of biomarker candidates, especially inflammation markers, were very similar for both frailty models [55].

13.6 **Some illustrative examples**

The following examples illustrate the state-of-the-art with respect to biomarker of ageing validation and application in longitudinal studies. It should be noted that forced expiratory volume in the first second (FEV1) and hand grip strength are regarded not only as the best validated markers in the domains of physical and physiological function, but also as some of the strongest (in terms of predictive power) biomarkers of ageing over a wide range of age groups. Further information on hand grip strength is available in Chapter 2, and on cognitive decline (our third example) in Chapter 3.

13.6.1 **FEV1**

Several authors have suggested that FEV1 is a strong marker of biological ageing [56]. It is related to cardiovascular fitness [57], and to environmental/lifestyle factors such as smoking or exercise [58,59], and declines with age with a rate of about 1% a year. It correlates with all-cause mortality [60], and is a long-term predictor of lung function [61], and survival [62]. FEV1 is associated with life course cognitive abilities [63–65], as well as with measures of cognitive intra-individual variability [66]. Low FEV1 is a predictor of poor cognitive performance as well as disability [17]. However, the possibility of large cohort and methodological effects has been noted, and there are wide discrepancies between cross-sectional and longitudinal estimates of the decline of FEV1 with age [67].

13.6.2 **Hand grip strength**

Hand grip strength is probably the best characterized biomarker of mortality so far. The prognostic relevance of this test (originally designed to assess upper extremities muscle strength) has been proven in many clinical and epidemiologic studies. In healthy adults, low grip strength predicts increased risk of functional limitations and disability in later life as well as all-cause mortality through a wide age range [68–74], with a clear potential as a screening tool because of its simplicity and consistently strong association with premature mortality, disability development, and risk of post–surgery complications or longer hospitalization (Chapter 2) [73]. It has, however, been found that the association between grip strength and mortality becomes weaker in cohorts with ages above 60 years at baseline. Moreover, cohort effects were noted in studies with long-term (20 years or longer) follow-up [74].

13.6.3 **Memory and global cognitive decline**

Ageing is associated with diminishing cognitive function (including memory) associated with relatively subtle alterations of specific synaptic connections in the hippocampus and prefrontal cortex rather than neuronal loss *per se* in the forebrain (for review see [75] and Chapter 3). Already in young adulthood [76], the brain is affected by changes including thinning of white matter tracts, volumetric declines in frontal cortex, and hippocampus, as well as reductions in neurotransmitter production and receptors; these changes are especially important in regions intimately related to memory encoding processes [77–80]. Thus, it is no surprise that all measurements of memory function show a consistent decline from an early age in cross-sectional studies, although results from longitudinal studies confirm this decline only after age 55 [80–84]. On average, longitudinal cognitive decline is faster in older persons when compared to younger ones, although wide inter–individual differences in rates of decline appear at all ages [76,85]. Moreover, rates of cognitive decline show different trends with age when comparing longitudinal and cross-sectional estimates [84]. The predictive potential of measures of cognitive decline to assess mortality risk has been shown in several studies [26,86]. An increase of the rate of memory decline was measurable already up to 6 years before death, and in one study the rate of global cognitive decline increased by six-fold beginning at about 43 months prior to death [86]. A meta–analysis showed that an increase in intelligence test scores by one standard deviation conveys a 24% lower risk of death for both men and women [41]. However, the evaluation of longitudinal cognitive decline is complicated by re-test effects (for review see [84]), and the presence of cohort effects on the association between survival and cognitive decline remains disputed [26,84].

13.7 **Conclusions**

A candidate biomarker of ageing should only be regarded as fully validated, if:

1 Its longitudinal change with age has been measured in multiple birth cohorts and cohort effects are either absent or can be attributed to corresponding differences in average biological age between cohorts; and

2 Predictive power better than chronological age has been demonstrated for multiple 'outcomes' of ageing, at least for a limited age range.

As shown by the examples above, these are very stringent criteria that are only just met by some of the longest established biomarkers of ageing. Many candidate biomarkers, especially those measuring molecular or cellular properties of the ageing body, have simply not been around for long enough. For instance, the use of pro-inflammatory cytokines as biomarkers of ageing in humans was first proposed in 1993 [87], peripheral blood telomere length followed in 2000 [20], while p16 expression was first suggested as a biomarker of ageing in mice in 2004 [88], and first applied to humans in 2006 [89]. Such marker candidates still need to be more rigorously tested with the above criteria in mind.

There is increasing evidence for a major impact of early life events on ageing trajectories (Chapter 1), making a strong case for preventive public health interventions to be started as early as possible. To assess the impact of preventive interventions, especially at an early age, biomarkers of ageing that fulfil these criteria and thus are validated over the whole life course will be essential.

References

1 **Reff ME, Schneider EL.** Biological Markers of Aging. Washington, DC: US Department of Health and Human Sciences; 1992.

2 **Baker GT, 3rd, Sprott RL.** Biomarkers of aging. *Exp Gerontol* 1988;**23**:223–39.

3 **Nakamura E, et al.** Evaluating measures of hematology and blood chemistry in male rhesus monkeys as biomarkers of aging. *Exp Gerontol* 1994;**29**:151–77.

4 **Butler RN, et al.** Biomarkers of aging: from primitive organisms to humans. *J Gerontol A Biol Sci Med Sci* 2004;**59**:B560–7.

5 **Warner HR.** Current status of efforts to measure and modulate the biological rate of aging. *J Gerontol A Biol Sci Med Sci* 2004;**59**:692–6.

6 **Ingram DK, et al.** Strategy for identifying biomarkers of aging in long-lived species. *Exp Gerontol* 2001;**36**:1025–34.

7 **Sprott RL.** Biomarkers of aging and disease: introduction and definitions. *Exp Gerontol* 2010;**45**:2–4.

8 **Finch CE, Kirkwood TBL.** Chance, Development, and Aging. New York: Oxford University Press; 2000.

9 **Wills AK, et al.** Life course trajectories of systolic blood pressure using longitudinal data from eight UK cohorts. *PLoS Med* 2011;**8**:e1000440.

10 **Borghi C, et al.** The relationship between systolic blood pressure and cardiovascular risk—results of the Brisighella Heart Study. *J Clin Hypertens* 2003;**5**:47–52.

11 **Paultre F, Mosca L.** The relation of blood pressure to coronary heart mortality in different age groups varies by ethnicity. *Am J Hypertens* 2006;**19**:179–83.

12 **Kannel WB, et al.** Systolic versus diastolic blood pressure and risk of coronary heart disease: the Framingham study. *Am J Cardiol* 1971;**27**:335–46.

13 **Euser SM, et al.** The effect of age on the association between blood pressure and cognitive function later in life. *J Am Geriatr Soc* 2009;**57**:1232–7.

14 **Blom JW, et al.** Changing prediction of mortality by systolic blood pressure with increasing age: the Rotterdam study. *Age (Dordr)* 2013;**35**:431–8.

15 **Sabayan B, et al.** High blood pressure, physical and cognitive function, and risk of stroke in the oldest old: the Leiden 85-plus Study. *Stroke* 2013;**44**:15–20.

16 **Sabayan B, et al.** High blood pressure and resilience to physical and cognitive decline in the oldest old: the Leiden 85-plus Study. *J Am Geriatr Soc* 2012;**60**:2014–9.

17 **Martin-Ruiz C, et al.** Assessment of a large panel of candidate biomarkers of ageing in the Newcastle 85+ study. *Mech Ageing Dev* 2011;**132**:496–502.

18 Poortvliet RK, et al. Blood pressure trends and mortality: the Leiden 85-plus Study. *J Hypertens* 2013; **31**:63–70.

19 von Zglinicki T, Martin-Ruiz CM. Telomeres as biomarkers for ageing and age-related diseases. *Curr Mol Med* 2005;**5**:197–203.

20 von Zglinicki T, et al. Short telomeres in patients with vascular dementia: an indicator of low antioxidative capacity and a possible risk factor? *Lab Invest* 2000;**80**:1739–47.

21 Cawthon RM, et al. Association between telomere length in blood and mortality in people aged 60 years or older. *Lancet* 2003;**361**:393–5.

22 Hoffmann J, Spyridopoulos I. Telomere length in cardiovascular disease: new challenges in measuring this marker of cardiovascular aging. *Future Cardiol* 2011;**7**:789–803.

23 Mather KA, et al. Is telomere length a biomarker of aging? A review. *J Gerontol A Biol Sci Med Sci* 2011; **66**:202–13.

24 von Zglinicki T. Will your telomeres tell your future? *BMJ* 2012;**344**:e1727.

25 Martin-Ruiz CM, et al. Blood cell telomere length is not associated with morbidity or mortality in the oldest old. *Aging Cell* 2005;**4**:287–90.

26 Gerstorf D, et al. Cohort differences in cognitive aging and terminal decline in the Seattle Longitudinal Study. *Dev Psychol* 2011;**47**:1026–41.

27 Nybo H, et al. Predictors of mortality in 2,249 nonagenarians—the Danish 1905-cohort survey. *J Am Geriatr Soc* 2003;**51**:1365–73.

28 Poortvliet RK, et al. Low blood pressure predicts increased mortality in very old age even without heart failure: the Leiden 85-plus Study. *Eur J Heart Fail* 2013;**15**:528–33.

29 Cohen E, Dillin A. The insulin paradox: aging, proteotoxicity and neurodegeneration. *Nat Rev Neurosci* 2008;**9**:759–67

30 Birnie K, et al. Childhood socioeconomic position and objectively measured physical capability levels in adulthood: a systematic review and meta-analysis. *PloS One* 2011;**6**:e15564.

31 Seematter-Bagnoud L, Santos-Eggimann B. Population-based cohorts of the 50s and over: a summary of worldwide previous and ongoing studies for research on health in ageing. *Eur J Ageing* 2006;**3**:41–59.

32 Wadsworth M, et al. Cohort profile: the 1946 National Birth Cohort (MRC National Survey of Health and Development). *Int J Epidemiol* 2006;**35**:49–54.

33 Gow AJ, et al. Mental ability in childhood and cognitive aging. *Gerontology* 2008;**54**:177–86.

34 Deary IJ, et al. The Lothian Birth Cohort 1936: a study to examine influences on cognitive ageing from age 11 to age 70 and beyond. *BMC Geriatr* 2007;**7**:28.

35 Stenholm S, et al. Long-term changes in handgrip strength in men and women—accounting the effect of right censoring due to death. *J Gerontol A Biol Sci Med Sci* 2012;**67**:1068–74.

36 Stenholm S, et al. Long-term determinants of muscle strength decline: prospective evidence from the 22-year mini-Finland follow-up survey. *J Am Geriatr Soc* 2012;**60**:77–85.

37 Xue QL, et al. Heterogeneity in rate of decline in grip, hip, and knee strength and the risk of all-cause mortality: the Women's Health and Aging Study II. *J Am Geriatr Soc* 2010;**58**:2076–84.

38 Hart CL, et al. Childhood IQ and all-cause mortality before and after age 65: prospective observational study linking the Scottish Mental Survey 1932 and the Midspan studies. *Br J Health Psychol* 2005;**10**:153–65.

39 Holsinger T, et al. Intelligence in early adulthood and life span up to 65 years later in male elderly twins. *Age Ageing* 2007;**36**:286–91.

40 Deary IJ, et al. The impact of childhood intelligence on later life: following up the Scottish mental surveys of 1932 and 1947. *J Pers Soc Psychol* 2004;**86**:130–47.

41 Calvin CM, et al. Intelligence in youth and all-cause-mortality: systematic review with meta-analysis. *Int J Epidemiol* 2011;**40**:626–44.

42 Andersen UO, et al. Decreasing systolic blood pressure and declining mortality rates in an untreated population: results from the Copenhagen City Heart Study. *Eur J Cardiovasc Prev Rehabil* 2011;**18**:248–53.

43 **Arbeev KG, et al.** Age trajectories of physiological indices in relation to healthy life course. *Mech Ageing Dev* 2011;**132**:93–102.

44 **Andersen UO, Jensen GB.** Trends and determinant factors for population blood pressure with 25 years of follow-up: results from the Copenhagen City Heart Study. *Eur J Cardiovasc Prev Rehabil* 2010;**17**: 655–9.

45 **Fries JF.** Aging, natural death, and the compression of morbidity. *New Engl J Med* 1980;**303**:130–5.

46 **Crimmins EM, Beltran-Sanchez H.** Mortality and morbidity trends: is there compression of morbidity? *J Gerontol B Psychol Sci Soc Sci* 2011;**66**:75–86.

47 **Andersen SL, et al.** Health span approximates life span among many supercentenarians: compression of morbidity at the approximate limit of life span. *J Gerontol A Biol Sci Med Sci* 2012;**67**:395–405.

48 **Holloszy JO.** The biology of aging. *Mayo Clin Proc* 2000;**75**:S3–8.

49 **Salminen A, et al.** Emerging role of NF-κB signaling in the induction of senescence-associated secretory phenotype (SASP). *Cell Signal* 2012;**24**:835–45.

50 **Freund A, et al.** Inflammatory networks during cellular senescence: causes and consequences. *Trends Mol Med* 2010;**16**:238–46.

51 **Fried LP, et al.** Frailty in older adults: evidence for a phenotype. *J Gerontol A Biol Sci Med Sci* 2001;**56**: M146–56.

52 **Rockwood K, Mitnitski A.** Frailty in relation to the accumulation of deficits. *J Gerontol A Biol Sci Med Sci* 2007;**62**:722–7.

53 **Searle SD, et al.** A standard procedure for creating a frailty index. *BMC Geriatr* 2008;**8**:24.

54 **Rockwood K, et al.** Long-term risks of death and institutionalization of elderly people in relation to deficit accumulation at age 70. *J Am Geriatr Soc* 2006;**54**:975–9.

55 **Collerton J, et al.** Frailty and the role of inflammation, immunosenescence and cellular ageing in the very old: cross-sectional findings from the Newcastle 85 + Study. *Mech Ageing Dev* 2012;**133**:456–66.

56 **Singh-Manoux A, et al.** Association of lung function with physical, mental and cognitive function in early old age. *Age (Dordr)* 2011;**33**:385–92.

57 **Sin DD, et al.** The relationship between reduced lung function and cardiovascular mortality: a population-based study and a systematic review of the literature. *Chest* 2005;**127**:1952–9.

58 **Anstey KJ, et al.** Measuring human functional age: a review of empirical findings. *Exp Aging Res* 1996; **22**:245–66.

59 **Emery CF, et al.** Longitudinal and genetic effects in the relationship between pulmonary function and cognitive performance. *J Gerontol B Psychol Sci Soc Sci* 1998;**53**:P311–7.

60 **Sabia S, et al.** Why does lung function predict mortality? Results from the Whitehall II Cohort Study. *Am J Epidemiol* 2010;**172**:1415–23.

61 **Kalhan R, et al.** Lung function in young adults predicts airflow obstruction 20 years later. *Am J Med* 2010;**123**:468.e1–7.

62 **Schunemann HJ, et al.** Pulmonary function is a long-term predictor of mortality in the general population: 29-year follow-up of the Buffalo Health Study. *Chest* 2000;**118**:656–64.

63 **Corley J, et al.** Smoking, childhood IQ, and cognitive function in old age. *J Psychosom Res* 2012;**73**:132–8.

64 **Deary IJ, et al.** Physical fitness and lifetime cognitive change. *Neurology* 2006;**67**:1195–200.

65 **Richards M, et al.** Lung function and cognitive ability in a longitudinal birth cohort study. *Psychosom Med* 2005;**67**:602–8.

66 **Anstey KJ, et al.** Biomarkers, health, lifestyle, and demographic variables as correlates of reaction time performance in early, middle, and late adulthood. *Q J Exp Psychol A* 2005;**58**:5–21.

67 **Kerstjens HA, et al.** Decline of FEV1 by age and smoking status: facts, figures, and fallacies. *Thorax* 1997;**52**:820–7.

68 **Rantanen T, et al.** Muscle strength and body mass index as long-term predictors of mortality in initially healthy men. *J Gerontol A Biol Sci Med Sci* 2000;**55**:M168–73.

69 **Rantanen T, et al.** Muscle strength as a predictor of onset of ADL dependence in people aged 75 years. *Aging Clin Exp Res* 2002;**14**(3 Suppl):10–15.

70 **Gale CR, et al.** Grip strength, body composition, and mortality. *Int J Epidemiol* 2007;**36**:228–35.

71 **Sasaki H, et al.** Grip strength predicts cause-specific mortality in middle-aged and elderly persons. *Am J Med* 2007;**120**:337–42.

72 **Newman AB, et al.** Strength, but not muscle mass, is associated with mortality in the health, aging and body composition study cohort. *J Gerontol A Biol Sci Med Sci* 2006;**61**:72–7.

73 **Bohannon RW.** Hand-grip dynamometry predicts future outcomes in aging adults. *J Geriatr Phys Ther* 2008;**31**:3–10.

74 **Cooper R, et al.** Objectively measured physical capability levels and mortality: systematic review and meta-analysis. *BMJ* 2010;**341**:c4467.

75 **Morrison JH, Baxter MG.** The ageing cortical synapse: hallmarks and implications for cognitive decline. *Nat Rev Neurosci* 2012;**13**:240–50.

76 **Tucker-Drob EM.** Global and domain-specific changes in cognition throughout adulthood. *Dev Psychol* 2011;**47**:331.

77 **Raz N, et al.** Regional brain changes in aging healthy adults: general trends, individual differences and modifiers. *Cereb Cortex* 2005;**15**:1676–89.

78 **Raz N.** Aging of the brain and its impact on cognitive performance: integration of structural and functional findings. In: Craik FIM, Salthouse TA, editors. The Handbook of Aging and Cognition. 2nd, illustrated ed. Mahwah, New Jersey: Lawrence Erlbaum Associates; 2000:1–90.

79 **Giorgio A, et al.** Age-related changes in grey and white matter structure throughout adulthood. *NeuroImage* 2010;**51**:943–51.

80 **Park DC, Reuter-Lorenz P.** The adaptive brain: aging and neurocognitive scaffolding. *Ann Rev Psychol* 2009;**60**:173–96.

81 **Hedden T, Gabrieli JD.** Insights into the ageing mind: a view from cognitive neuroscience. *Nat Rev Neurosci* 2004;**5**:87–96.

82 **Schaie KW.** Intellectual Development in Adulthood: The Seattle Longitudinal Study. New York: Cambridge University Press; 1996.

83 **Salthouse TA.** When does age-related cognitive decline begin? *Neurobiol Aging* 2009;**30**:507–14.

84 **Salthouse TA, Warner Schaie, K.** Developmental Influences on Adult Intelligence: The Seattle Longitudinal Study. Oxford: Oxford University Press; 2005. *Intelligence* 2005;**33**:551–4.

85 **Wilson RS, et al.** Individual differences in rates of change in cognitive abilities of older persons. *Psychol Aging* 2002;**17**:179–93.

86 **Wilson RS, et al.** Terminal decline in cognitive function. *Neurology* 2003;**60**:1782–7.

87 **Fagiolo U, et al.** Increased cytokine production in mononuclear cells of healthy elderly people. *Eur J Immunol* 1993;**23**:2375–8.

88 **Krishnamurthy J, et al.** Ink4a/Arf expression is a biomarker of aging. *J Clin Invest* 2004;**114**:1299–307.

89 **Ressler S, et al.** p16INK4A is a robust in vivo biomarker of cellular aging in human skin. *Aging Cell* 2006;**5**:379–89.

90 **Rowlatt C, et al.** Lifespan, age changes and tumour incidence in an ageing C57BL mouse colony. *Lab Anim* 1976;**10**:419–42.

Chapter 14

Genetic aspects of ageing

Teri-Louise Davies, Tamuno Alfred, and Ian NM Day

14.1 Introduction

Most people, at some point in their lives, have looked at their older relatives and wondered wheth-er they will age as well or as badly in comparison. If your great, great grandmother lived to the ripe old age of 98 then is there something in the family genes? So what can we learn about and from genetic factors? This chapter gives an overview of the plethora of genetic insights into ageing.

14.2 Traits of human ageing—what is the phenotype of interest?

The accurate determination of the role of genetics in ageing firstly requires appropriate outcome measures. The way that we choose to measure ageing is a contentious issue, which is underpinned by how we choose to define ageing in the first place. For example, it has been suggested [1] that ageing is one of four characteristics of the 'finitude of life', the remaining three being the determi-nants of longevity, age-associated diseases, and death. Although defined separately from ageing here, mortality (i.e. longevity or death) is often used as an outcome measure in ageing research, while chronic disease studies will always have an ageing theme (Martin and colleagues [2] provide a useful table of geriatric disorders). In fact, Hayflick [1] has posited that ageing *per se* is a random process which can no longer be suppressed by natural selection after reproductive maturity and hence is not genetically driven, while longevity, which relates to the amount of reserve an organ-ism accumulates up to the point of reproductive maturity, is. We return to evolutionary theories of ageing in Section 14.3.

Studies investigating the role of genetics in ageing try to find associations between genet-ic markers (e.g. single nucleotide polymorphisms; SNPs) and ageing phenotypes. This can be implemented on a refined scale using candidate genotyping with *a priori*, biologically moti-vated hypotheses (Section 14.9) or in an exploratory fashion testing for associations throughout the genome between hundreds of thousands of SNPs and one or more phenotypes. This latter approach, termed a genome-wide association study (GWAS), will be discussed in Section 14.8.

Longevity is a popular outcome measure in ageing research. Although the length of life does not necessarily reflect quality of living, it is generally assumed when using this measure that individu-als who live longer age 'better' than those with shorter lifespans. Younger chronological age (at death) is therefore used as a surrogate marker of accelerated ageing. This is considered acceptable given that the individual who ages faster will normally be the individual with the higher prema-ture mortality risk. Geneticists are therefore interested in finding associations between genes and longevity to identify novel pathways related to ageing. Martin and colleagues [2], however, have stressed the difference between lifespan and health span; the latter they define as 'the period of life during which an individual is free of chronic illness and substantial functional decrements.' Perhaps health span, as opposed to lifespan, would be a more appropriate outcome measure in ageing research. Undeniably, longevity is a much easier outcome to define than health span. Baudisch, however, describes ageing by pace and shape [3]. This, for example, shows that the African buffalo may have a lower life expectancy compared to Swedish females (a faster pace of ageing), but the shape of ageing suggests stronger senescence in Swedish females after 80% adult life expectancy (the increase of mortality with age is steeper for humans). Thus the conventional view that longevity is the best measure of 'ageing' *per se* may not necessarily be true.

Cancer is probably the most well recognized ageing disease and is a key biomarker for ageing. Mutations which cause cancer have been labelled as either 'gatekeepers' or 'caretakers', according to whether they control cellular proliferation or DNA integrity, respectively [4]. As noted by Campisi [5], gatekeepers act at the tissue and organism level while caretakers act at the cellular level. Campisi [5] provides a detailed review of the complex relationship between cancer and ageing phenotypes. As she explains, unmutated caretaker variants can serve to suppress cancer and ageing phenotypes, while unmutated gatekeeper variants which induce apoptosis or senescence in cancerous cells will prevent cancer at the expense of causing age-related phenotypes later in life in an antagonistic pleiotropic manner.

Physical and cognitive capability will decline in the ageing individual and are thus candidate outcome measures in the genetics of ageing research. Physical capability is measured via tests such as assessment of grip strength or timed chair rises (Chapter 2). Cognitive function is similarly assessed through a different suite of measures; for example, measures of verbal fluency and word recall ability (Chapter 3). It is of great interest to ascertain the degree of influence our genome has over physical capability and/or cognition in later life. Understandably, environmental factors like smoking history are likely to play a key role (for example, see the recent work of Dregan and colleagues [6] for cognitive function) and the goal is made even more difficult given that these phenotypes are 'complex'. We discuss Mendelian and complex traits in Sections 14.6 and 14.8 respectively.

14.3 **Evolutionary models**

Antagonistic pleiotropy [7] underpins one of the several evolutionary theories of ageing. This theory posits that later acting deleterious traits remain in the population because the causal variants have early acting advantageous effects which are selected for by natural selection. A mutation in a gene with harmful effects later in life is more likely to be passed to the next generation than a gene with harmful effects early in life, because the latter would confer a reproductive disadvantage. From a life course perspective, we might therefore expect mutations which cause more rapid growth (a reproductive advantage) to additionally cause faster ageing. Other evolutionary theories of ageing exist, but will not be discussed in detail here. For example, the disposable soma theory [8] and the mutation accumulation theory [9].

Budovsky and colleagues [10] have considered the relationship between longevity-associated and cancer-associated genes. From an evolutionary perspective, they found evidence to suggest that longevity-associated genes in model organisms including yeast, fly, worm, and mouse are highly conserved, with a significantly greater proportion of such genes having an orthologous human gene (i.e. a human gene with the same ancestor) compared with all types of gene. By considering the intersect set between animal longevity-associated genes and animal genes orthologous to human cancer-associated genes, they found evidence to suggest that pro-longevity genes are enriched for tumour suppressors and anti-longevity genes are enriched for oncogenes. They also found that more than one quarter of the human orthologues to animal longevity genes were also human cancer-associated genes, and that human tumour suppressors were enriched for pro-longevity orthologues while human oncogenes were enriched for anti-longevity orthologues. Using protein network analyses they found evidence to suggest that human proteins classified as both cancer-associated and longevity-associated are highly connected.

Motivated by the hypothesis that cancer and ageing are traded off against one another, Christensen and colleagues [11] used data on 4354 pairs of same-sex monozygotic and dizygotic twins to establish the relationship between age at death in one twin with cancer occurrence in the other. Their results went against the prediction that age at death in one twin would positively correlate with cancer occurrence in the co-twin (i.e. that longevity and cancer occurrence exist as a trade-off). They actually found that higher age at death in one twin correlated with lower cancer incidence in the other. Their initial analyses included both twins for cancer occurrence and death (when possible), but the finding was generally robust to random allocation of a twin to cancer occurrence or death information, in addition to stratifications by zygosity and sex. One might argue that this study and that of Budovsky and colleagues [10] is against the view that ageing and cancer are antagonistic. However, confounding by shared environment (e.g. both twins are non-smokers) is an alternative explanation for the correlation in the former study. In addition, given that cancer is a leading cause of death, one might anyway predict a close relationship between cancer and longevity traits. Budovsky and colleagues [10] address this issue, for example highlighting that the lower organisms studied rarely develop tumours, while Christensen and colleagues [11] recognize these caveats.

14.4 **Animal studies**

Animal models have provided important insights into the genetics of ageing. The results are often used to motivate hypotheses in studies on humans; for example by taking identified genes from a particular study of an organism and identifying the homologous genes in humans to test whether the results are the same or different. Similar molecular mechanisms across organisms suggest evolutionary conservation which, in turn, provides evidence of natural selection and effects on reproductive fitness.

One of the key (non-genetic) findings from animal models is that the lifespan of an organism can be manipulated by dietary restriction (e.g. see the work of Masoro and colleagues [12]). This field of study has been critically reviewed by Piper and Partridge [13] in the context of Drosophila melanogaster. Piper and Partridge [13] also discuss the growing body of evidence that autophagy might be the underlying mechanism that drives the relationship between protein restriction and longevity. As explained by the authors, longevity could be enhanced as a by-product of autophagy removing certain damaged molecules. It has been noted that the influence of growth factor gene mutants may represent a 'genocopy' of the 'phenocopy' generated by dietary restriction. That is, these gene mutants produce the same effects as dietary restriction.

Caenorhabditis elegans (C. elegans), which are very small nematode worms, are a popular animal model in ageing research as non-mutant strains have a short lifespan of just a few weeks. Over 20 years ago, Friedman and Johnson [14] conducted experiments using C. elegans to investigate the effects of the *age-1* gene on longevity and fertility. They found evidence for the antagonistic pleiotropic theory of ageing, whereby a recessive *age-1* allele increased lifespan and decreased the self-fertility of hermaphrodites. It has since been suggested [15] that if antagonistic pleiotropy does exist in terms of a trade-off between reproduction and longevity, then it is likely to be a complex relationship affected by metabolism and diet also. Kenyon and colleagues [16] used C. elegans to discover that two genes, *daf-2* and *daf-16*, are instrumental in longevity pathways and *daf-2* mutants can more than double the lifespan of hermaphrodites—an action which was independent of reproductive potential.

As outlined by Antebi in a 2007 review [17], the work of Friedman and Johnson [14] and Kenyon and colleagues [16], in addition to several other seminal works, paved the way for researchers to converge on the discovery that longevity can be enhanced by the downregulation of insulin/insulin-like growth factor-1(IGF-1) signalling. For example, Holzenberger and colleagues [18] proved that what had been previously shown in invertebrates was in fact a phenomenon that extended into the vertebrates. Kimura and colleagues [19] had shown that the *daf-2* gene in C. elegans is the nematode equivalent of the insulin receptor family in humans. Tatar and colleagues [20] were one of the groups who analysed the Drosophila *InR* gene. *InR* to Drosophila is the *daf-2* to C. elegans. They found that the heteroalleleic combination of the *InR*[p5545] mutant and the *InR*[E19] mutant in females resulted in 85% lifespan extension, and that this lifespan effect can be removed by administering methoprene, a surrogate to the Drosophila juvenile hormone. In addition, Clancy and colleagues [21] found that a mutation in the *chico* gene in Drosophila, which encodes the insulin receptor substrate CHICO, extended lifespan in heterozygotes and female homozygotes. Building on this evidence, studies in mice implicated IGF-1 levels in lifespan determination. For example, Coschigano and colleagues [22] disrupted the *GHR/BP* gene in mice and found that homozygous disruptions resulted in longer lifespan for both males and females. Motivated by the above studies and others, Holzenberger and colleagues [18] inactivated *IGF-1R* in mice. Although the homozygotes for the null allele died at birth, the heterozygous females lived on average 33% longer than the controls and were more resistant to oxidative stress.

These comparative studies across multiple organisms have collectively illustrated the importance of some specific growth factor pathways in longevity, and invite similar studies in humans. It has been noted [15], however, that identifying ageing genes in the manner described above does not prove that these exact mutants are those responsible for longevity variance in the wild.

Antebi [17] summarizes some of the classes of gene that have been associated with lifespan in C. elegans since the breakthrough insulin/IGF-1 research. These include sensory perception, signal transduction, and genes encoding transcription factors/cofactors, microRNAs, and checkpoint proteins. An understanding of the complex pathways controlling longevity has made much progress over the last few decades.

The most important biological pathway in ageing research is arguably the insulin/IGF-1 signalling pathway. Ageing research has evolved by considering environmental effects on longevity in addition to pathway molecular mechanisms, and trying to determine whether effects are independent, analogous or synergistic. Certain environmental stresses induce changes within organisms which promote longevity. 'Stress' can be imposed in diverse ways, for example calorie restriction. A classic paper by Sohal and Weindruch [23] examined the link between the calorie restriction model and the oxidation model. In brief, calorie restriction reduces metabolism which should, in turn, reduce the production of deleterious reactive oxygen metabolites by the mitochondria. These metabolites can accumulate in cells and react with important molecules, resulting in a cumulative ageing phenotype.

Shore and colleagues [24] considered the association between longevity and cytoprotective pathway induction using C. elegans. Their research was motivated by the fact that lifespan extension in C. elegans can be induced by interventions such as calorie restriction and xenobiotics; stressful environments which induce cytoprotective responses which in turn, may be the causes of increased longevity. They found, by testing gene inactivations which increase longevity to see whether they induced stress-responsive fusion genes, that those longevity genes which induce at least one fusion gene had a significantly higher mean increase in longevity than those which did not. They also performed a test via RNAi screening to identify gene inactivations which inhibited expected cytoprotective responses. They established a set of 29 genes which are necessary for the induction of cytoprotective genes, which they subsequently tested for effects on lifespan extension. Overall these authors found that, following certain interventions, genes which are required for cytoprotective response induction are additionally required for longevity extension. Studies such as these show that insight into the molecular mechanisms of ageing can be drawn from model organisms such as C. elegans and importantly, there exists potential for transferability to a human context.

C. elegans has also been used in ageing research to engineer organisms with extended lifespan. Sagi and Kim [25] aimed to genetically engineer strains with otherwise normal phenotypes but improved longevity. They used four approaches to achieve this goal, namely: (1) selecting genes with *a priori* known associations with longevity extension in this organism; (2) a candidate gene approach; (3) using orthologous genes from zebrafish and human ageing pathways; and (4) trying to introduce biological mechanisms novel to this organism, again using a transgenic approach with zebrafish genes. They converged on a set of four artificially over-expressed C. elegans genes and three artificially expressed zebrafish genes. These seven strains increased lifespan between 20–50%. By gradually combining the separate genetic modifications, they created a quadruple strain with four modifications. Overall, the authors found a monotonic increase in lifespan with number of genetically modified components, and that the worms remained mobile up to the median lifespan of 40 days for the quadruple strains, compared with impaired mobility at the median age of 18 days for the control strain. This 2012 study demonstrates the current 'state of the art' and the potential for lifespan extension apparently without a cost to quality of life.

Genetic studies of ageing in both animals and humans have also been focused on telomeres. Hayflick [26] first made the observation that cells taken directly from a fetus into cell culture could only divide about 40 to 60 times (the 'Hayflick limit') before entering a senescent phase. The molecular basis of this has turned out to be that the repeating sequence that cap structures at the end of chromosomes ('telomeres') get shorter on each cell cycle, until the telomere and consequently chromosome fails. Telomere length maintenance requires telomerase activity [27], but this enzyme is only active in some specialized cells such as embryonic stem cells and immune cells which need to retain high replication potential.

Bernardes de Jesus and colleagues [28] used mouse models to test whether telomerase gene therapy administered later in life can be used to extend lifespan and reduce ageing without increasing risk of cancer. They used AAV9 vectors to express *TERT* in 420 day-old and 720 day-old mice. They found, for example, that the gene therapy improved femoral bone mineral density for both classes of age, and additionally that the treated at 2 years mice had an increased subcutaneous fat layer compared with age-matched controls. The authors also considered various behavioural assays and obtained some evidence of a beneficial effect in the *TERT*-treated mice. As well as increasing survival in both age classes, the gene therapy did not increase cancer incidence as ascertained at time of death. In addition, the results suggested that the treated mice had longer telomeres and a smaller percentage of cells in differentiated tissues with short telomeres (although they highlight other possible explanations for this finding). The study showed that telomerase activity can be 'reactivated' to ameliorate ageing effects without causing cancer. Since inherited telomerase mutations cause pulmonary fibrosis, this would represent a first context in which to consider gene therapy.

14.5 **Heritability studies in humans**

Insight from studies of twins, family members, adoptees, and migrants can help to unravel the true extent of inheritance of the ageing phenotype. Indeed these have long formed the mainstay for attempting to determine the overall genetic contribution to specific traits and diseases. A study of same-sex Danish twin pairs estimated the heritability of human longevity to be 26% in males and 23% in females [29].

Comparing separate studies, Perls and colleagues showed that siblings of supercentenarians (over 110 year-olds) and siblings of centenarians seem to have similar likelihoods of lifespan over 90 years, this likelihood being 10–20% greater than that observed for the general population [30]. The authors note that such 'familial aggregation for exceptional longevity' is not only attributable to the heritability of longevity, but common environmental and behavioural variables could also be in force.

14.6 Natural genetic experiments—Mendelian disorders

Most human traits are complex; that is, they are determined by more than one gene or locus. A trait is subjected to Mendelian inheritance if it is genetically governed by one locus. A trait is dominant if inheritance of the trait-determining allele from one parent causes the phenotype. A trait is recessive if the trait-determining allele must be inherited in two copies, one from each parent. Co-dominant traits present a continuum, with increasing severity as the number of causal loci increase (from 0 to 2). There are not many true dominant Mendelian traits; most are co-dominant.

There exists a class of Mendelian inherited genetic disorders called 'progeroid syndromes' [31,32]. Individuals who are affected present with ageing-like phenotypes at a much younger age. Perhaps the most well known of these is Werner Syndrome. We now know that the chromosome 8 *WRN* gene is responsible for this disorder. *WRN* encodes an ATP-dependent DNA helicase necessary for DNA replication and repair. Strikingly, other Mendelian genes causing similar syndromes also seem to be important in DNA and nuclear events (Table 14.1). *BANF1* and *LMNA* both localize to the nucleus, lamin A forming part of the nuclear lamina and playing a role in chromatin structure and gene expression. *BANF1* shows nuclear envelope and mitotic chromosome interactions. A further progeroid gene *ZMPSTE24* encodes a metalloproteinase involved in *LMNA* processing. Overall, these syndromes suggest that DNA replication and repair represent an important factor in premature ageing, and hence possibly in ageing generally.

14.7 Linkage studies of human longevity

As noted by Kerber and colleagues [33], GWASs for longevity are faced with the problem of electing appropriate controls, given that they have to be at least one generation younger than the cases. This can bias the analysis due to the intergenerational implications on allele frequencies and

Table 14.1 Genes causing progeroid syndromes*

Disease	Gene	OMIM number
Werner syndrome	*WRN*	#277700
Hutchinson-Gilford progeria syndrome	*LMNA*	#176670
Nestor-Guillermo progeria syndrome	*BANF1*	#614008
Restrictive dermopathy	*ZMPSTE24, LMNA*	#275210
Mandibuloacral dysplasia	*ZMPSTE24, LMNA*	#248370, #608612

*Source: data from Kudlow BA, et al. Werner and Hutchinson-Gilford Progeria Syndromes: mechanistic basis of human progeroid diseases, *Nature Reviews Molecular Cell Biology*, Volume **8**, pp. 394–404, Copyright © 2007 Nature Publishing Group and McKusick-Nathans Institute of Genetic Medicine, Johns Hopkins University, Online Mendelian Inheritance in Man, OMIM®, available at http://omim.org/, Copyright © 1966–2013 Johns Hopkins University.

behavioural differences, when controls are selected from the current population. These authors conducted a genome-wide genetic linkage study (i.e. a family based linkage study, not a GWAS) of familial exceptional longevity (the 'Fertility, Longevity and Aging' study). Results suggested a locus at 3p22–24. A study of 2118 nonagenarian sibling pairs [34] confirmed by linkage the role of *APOE* (which encodes a protein expressed in the brain and is a major influence on late onset Alzheimer's disease as well as influencing lipoproteins and cardiovascular risk) in longevity. Additional loci were suggested at 14q11.2, 17q12-q22, and 19p13.3-p13.11.

14.8 **Genome-wide association studies of ageing**

GWAS analyses involve genotyping large numbers of individuals for hundreds of thousands of genetic loci and testing for associations with one or more phenotypes. The sample sizes have to be large to detect the small effects which are analogous with complex traits. (Traits which are not Mendelian, that is, traits which are not governed by the presence or absence of a single inherited locus, are termed 'complex traits'). In addition, because the analysis involves multiple tests for association, statistical corrections have to be made to adjust the results for false positive associations which arise by chance. In recent years, genetic research has moved towards whole-genome sequencing and greater coverage of the genome. With the birth of the 1000 Genomes Project [35] researchers are gaining access to dense genetic data which will increase the likelihood of uncovering true causal loci. As they are now an established analytical approach and are less expensive than the more cutting edge techniques, GWASs continue to be widely used. Although their ability to explain the entire heritability of most complex traits is limited, the results of studies which detect signals of association can be combined retrospectively with the results of previous studies and meta-analysed. This increases the power to detect effects.

Perusal of the NGHRI GWAS Catalog [36] reveals that at the time of writing this chapter, genome-wide association studies have been conducted against ageing, longevity, and cognition. Newman and colleagues [37] performed a meta-analysis of four GWASs for survival to 90 years and older in Caucasians. Although no SNPs reached genome-wide significance in the meta-analysis, a SNP near to *MINPP1* emerged as a potential candidate following the inclusion of results from a second discovery phase. Interestingly another SNP that was a potential candidate was found in pregnancy-associated plasma protein A2 (PAPPA2) which is a metalloproteinase that regulates local IGF pathway action. A single GWAS by Nebel and colleagues [38] confirmed *APOE* as the major gene influencing survival in long-lived individuals.

14.9 **Selected SNP and gene studies**

In 2008, Willcox and colleagues [39] published their findings of an association between polymorphisms in the *FOXO3A* gene and longevity in humans, after conducting a nested case-control study on a cohort of Japanese–American ageing males. Incidentally, *FOXO3A* is a human *daf-16* homologue (*daf-16* being a C. elegans gene). They defined cases as those individuals who reached 95 years by 2007 and controls as those who had died before reaching 81 years. One study to replicate this finding was that of Flachsbart and colleagues [40], who demonstrated that SNPs in this gene are associated with longevity in both male and female Germans.

Kleindorp and colleagues [41] were motivated by previous *FOXO3A* results to test for an association between three other genes in the *FOXO* family and longevity. They considered haplotype-tagging SNPs for *FOXO1*, *FOXO4*, and *FOXO6* in German individuals comprising cases of 1447 centenarians/nonagenarians and 1029 controls. The authors found no associations between these genes and longevity. Pooling of data with an Italian cohort of females also failed to detect an association for two specific SNPs. These are just three examples of the diverse literature on *FOXO* genes and longevity.

Alfred and colleagues [42] tested for an association between the *TERT-CLPTM1L* SNP rs401681 and physical and cognitive function in a multi-cohort analysis of 25,774 individuals as part of the HALCyon research collaboration. This was motivated by the hypothesis that this SNP, which had been previously linked with various cancers, might also be associated with additional ageing phenotypes. The results of the research indicate that this SNP is not associated with physical or cognitive capability in middle-aged to older individuals.

Alfred and colleagues [43] have also tested for an association between the *ACTN3* rs1815739 SNP and physical capability in 17,835 individuals, again as part of the HALCyon research collaboration. This was motivated by evidence from the literature that the C allele is more common in sprinters/power athletes compared with controls or endurance athletes, combined with evidence that physical capability demonstrates some heritability. They found weak evidence for an association between the C allele and grip strength in males ($p = 0.09$), but all other physical capability measures demonstrated a null association.

Animal genetic models have suggested that the insulin/IGF-1 signalling pathway is implicated in ageing. In 1990, Rudman and colleagues [44] conducted a study in older males with low IGF-1 levels which showed that administering replacement doses of biosynthetic human growth hormone over a period of 6 months replenished the IGF-1 levels to that of younger individuals. They demonstrated that low growth hormone in these males was responsible for low IGF-1 levels. Physiological measurements of the treated and control groups suggested that the increase in lean body mass was greater in the growth-hormone treated men. Although not genetic, this was an interesting study because it supported the notion that therapeutic interventions of growth hormone might serve to reverse some ageing phenotypes (like decreased lean body mass). The Rudman study provided some of the stimulus for a recent HALCyon analysis which tested for associations between several SNPs in the growth hormone/insulin-like growth factor axis and anthropometric measures and physical capability in 13,364 individuals [45]. This meta-analysis identified an association between the *GH1* SNP rs2665802 and ability to balance, although the overall study results suggest that the six variants tested do not influence physical capability in later life. As highlighted in the paper, given that associations with physical capability were largely absent in this study, any real associations must relate to very small effect sizes as the HALCyon collaboration is so well powered.

Alfred and colleagues [46] recently considered whether SNPs associated with serum calcium, bone mineral density or osteoarthritis risk, are associated with physical capability in older age in the HALCyon cohorts. They found that a SNP previously associated with increased serum calcium levels was associated with weaker grip strength ($p = 0.05$).

Selected SNP studies such as those carried out by the HALCyon research collaboration are post-GWAS, biologically motivated and avoid the problem of multiple testing and 'fishing' for association. However, they do rely on the intersection of disease-specific GWAS SNP hits with plausibly ageing-related biological pathways. In addition, physical and cognitive capability are clearly complex traits (Chapters 2 and 3) which are likely associated with hundreds of genetic loci. The effect sizes are thus very small and can only be detected using vast sample sizes. This is not a problem restricted to candidate SNP studies, nor is it restricted to ageing phenotypes. All genetic research today is burdened by the problem of 'missing heritability' [47], whereby the gap between accountable heritability and estimated heritability is large. Ultimately, very large scale GWASs of ageing traits are still awaited, potentially to identify relevant new pathways.

14.10 **Other aspects and the future of ageing genetics**

We have not touched on epigenetic changes (Chapter 15) but note that secondary modifications of DNA and of its associated nucleoproteins represent a layer of biochemical regulation which may propagate during cell division, as well as interact with germline variation. Neither have we focused on mitochondrial genetics. The mitochondrion contains its own genome and the mitochondrion, through the generation of free radicals, may profoundly influence oxidation and mutation events. Wallace [48] considers the complexity of mitochondrial genetics. However, as yet, there is no compelling evidence that mitochondrial haplogroups influence ageing traits. A further topic not covered here is therapeutics, which is relevant to the genetics of ageing because the discovery of genes affecting lifespan reveals potential for therapeutic intervention. Lastly, Mendelian randomization (MR) and its role in genetics of ageing research deserves more discussion than we have been able to provide here. MR [49] uses genotype as an instrument to determine causation in epidemiological associations. An example has been using genetic determinants of high density lipoprotein cholesterol (HDLc) level to test whether HDLc level is a causal factor in myocardial infarction, with the possibly surprising finding that it may not be [50]. The MR approach may have potential for relating nutritional, lifestyle and other factors to traits of ageing [51].

The field of genetics is fast moving with novel research methods continuously outdating previous methodology. Next generation sequencing (NGS), which provides whole genome coverage, may unearth some of the missing heritability of phenotypic traits and potentially expose the action of rarer variants. In the context of ageing, this may provide further insight into the genetic components of longevity, frailty in later life, and ageing disease. As with GWAS in the early years, next generation sequencing is currently too expensive for wide application. However costs are falling rapidly and widespread development of NGS can be anticipated over the next decade. As discussed elsewhere [15], it is also important to amalgamate knowledge from evolutionary ageing theory with molecular ageing studies, to ascertain both why and how we age. The parallel progress in comprehensive approaches in animal models, in metabolomics, transcriptomics, epigenomics (chromatin structure and regulation), and cellular and organismal imaging, seems likely to increase our insights into biological ageing: and with that, potential to develop novel interventions.

References

1 Hayflick L. Entropy explains aging, genetic determinism explains longevity, and undefined terminology explains misunderstanding both. *PLoS Genet* 2007;3:e220.

2 Martin GM, et al. Genetic determinants of human health span and life span: progress and new opportunities. *PLoS Genet* 2007;3:e125.

3 Baudisch A. The pace and shape of ageing. *Methods Ecol Evol* 2011;2:375–82.

4 Kinzler KW, Vogelstein B. Gatekeepers and caretakers. *Nature* 1997;386:761–3.

5 Campisi J. Cancer and ageing: rival demons? *Nat Rev Cancer* 2003;3:339–49.

6 Dregan A, et al. Cardiovascular risk factors and cognitive decline in adults aged 50 and over: a population-based cohort study. *Age Ageing* 2013;42:338–45.

7 Williams GC. Pleiotropy, natural selection, and the evolution of senescence. *Evolution (NY)* 1957;11:398–411.

8 Kirkwood TBL. Evolution of ageing. *Nature* 1977;270:301–4.

9 Medawar PB. An Unsolved Problem of Biology. London: HK Lewis; 1951.

10 Budovsky A, et al. Common gene signature of cancer and longevity. *Mech Ageing Dev* 2009;130:33–9.

11 Christensen K, et al. Cancer and longevity—is there a trade-off? A study of cooccurrence in Danish twin pairs born 1900–1918. *J Gerontol A Biol Sci Med Sci* 2012;**67A**:489–94.

12 Masoro EJ, et al. Action of food restriction in delaying the aging process. *Proc Natl Acad Sci USA* 1982;**79**:4239–41.

13 Piper MDW, Partridge L. Dietary restriction in *Drosophila*: delayed aging or experimental artefact? *PLoS Genet* 2007;**3**:e57.

14 Friedman DB, Johnson TE. A mutation in the *age-1* gene in *Caenorhabditis elegans* lengthens life and reduces hermaphrodite fertility. *Genetics* 1988;**118**:75–86.

15 Flatt T, Schmidt PS. Integrating evolutionary and molecular genetics of aging. *Biochim Biophys Acta* 2009;**1790**:951–62.

16 Kenyon C, et al. A *C. Elegans* mutant that lives twice as long as wild type. *Nature* 1993;**366**:461–4.

17 Antebi A. Genetics of aging in *Caenorhabditis elegans*. *PLoS Genet* 2007;**3**:e129.

18 Holzenberger M, et al. IGF-1 receptor regulates lifespan and resistance to oxidative stress in mice. *Nature* 2003;**421**:182–7.

19 Kimura KD, et al. *daf-2*, an insulin receptor-like gene that regulates longevity and diapause in *Caenorhabditis elegans*. *Science* 1997;**277**:942–6.

20 Tatar M, et al. A mutant *Drosophila* insulin receptor homolog that extends life-span and impairs neuroendocrine function. *Science* 2001;**292**:107–10.

21 Clancy DJ, et al. Extension of life-span by loss of CHICO, a *Drosophila* insulin receptor substrate protein. *Science* 2001;**292**:104–6.

22 Coschigano KT, et al. Assessment of growth parameters and life span of GHR/BP gene-disrupted mice. *Endocrinology* 2000;**141**:2608–13.

23 Sohal RS, Weindruch R. Oxidative stress, caloric restriction, and aging. *Science* 1996;**273**:59–63.

24 Shore DE, et al. Induction of cytoprotective pathways is central to the extension of lifespan conferred by multiple longevity pathways. *PLoS Genet* 2012;**8**:e1002792.

25 Sagi D, Kim SK. An engineering approach to extending lifespan in *C. elegans*. *PLoS Genet* 2012;**8**:e1002780.

26 Hayflick L. The limited *in vitro* lifetime of human diploid cell strains. *Exp Cell Res* 1965;**37**:614–36.

27 Greider CW, Blackburn EH. Identification of a specific telomere terminal transferase activity in tetrahymena extracts. *Cell* 1985;**43**:405–13.

28 Bernardes de Jesus B, et al. Telomerase gene therapy in adult and old mice delays aging and increases longevity without increasing cancer. *EMBO Mol Med* 2012;**4**:691–704.

29 Herskind AM, et al. The heritability of human longevity: a population-based study of 2872 Danish twin pairs born 1870–1900. *Hum Genet* 1996;**97**:319–23.

30 Perls T, et al. Survival of parents and siblings of supercentenarians. *J Gerontol A Biol Sci Med Sci* 2007;**62**:1028–34.

31 Kudlow BA, et al. Werner and Hutchinson-Gilford progeria syndromes: mechanistic basis of human progeroid diseases. *Nat Rev Mol Cell Biol* 2007;**8**:394–404.

32 McKusick-Nathans Institute of Genetic Medicine. Online Mendelian Inheritance in Man, OMIM®. Baltimore, MD: Johns Hopkins University. Available at: <http://omim.org/> (accessed 30 January 2013).

33 Kerber RA, et al. A genome-wide study replicates linkage of 3p22–24 to extreme longevity in humans and identifies possible additional loci. *PLoS ONE* 2012;**7**:e34746.

34 Beekman M, et al. Genome-wide linkage analysis for human longevity: genetics of Healthy Ageing study. *Aging Cell* 2013;**12**:184–93.

35 The 1000 Genomes Project Consortium. A map of human genome variation from population-scale sequencing. *Nature* 2010;**467**:1061–73.

36 Hindorff LA, et al. A Catalog of Published Genome-Wide Association Studies. Available at: <http://www.genome.gov/gwastudies> (accessed 27 November 2012).

37 **Newman AB, et al.** A meta-analysis of four genome-wide association studies of survival to age 90 years or older: the cohorts for heart and aging research in genomic epidemiology consortium. *J Gerontol A Biol Sci Med Sci* 2010;**65A**:478–87.

38 **Nebel A, et al.** A genome-wide association study confirms *APOE* as the major gene influencing survival in long-lived individuals. *Mech Ageing Dev* 2011;**132**:324–30.

39 **Willcox BJ, et al.** FOXO3A genotype is strongly associated with human longevity. *Proc Natl Acad Sci USA* 2008;**105**:13987–92.

40 **Flachsbart F, et al.** Association of *FOXO3A* variation with human longevity confirmed in German centenarians. *Proc Natl Acad Sci USA* 2009;**106**:2700–5.

41 **Kleindorp R, et al.** Candidate gene study of *FOXO1, FOXO4*, and *FOXO6* reveals no association with human longevity in Germans. *Aging Cell* 2011;**10**:622–8.

42 **Alfred T, et al.** Absence of association of a single-nucleotide polymorphism in the *TERT-CLPTM1L* locus with age-related phenotypes in a large multicohort study: the Halcyon programme. *Aging Cell* 2011;**10**:520–32.

43 **Alfred T, et al.** ACTN3 genotype, athletic status, and life course physical capability: meta-analysis of the published literature and findings from nine studies. *Hum Mutat* 2011;**32**:1008–18.

44 **Rudman D, et al.** Effects of human growth hormone in men over 60 years old. *N Engl J Med* 1990;**323**: 1–6.

45 **Alfred T, et al.** A multi-cohort study of polymorphisms in the GH/IGF axis and physical capability: the Halcyon Programme. *PLoS ONE* 2012;**7**:e29883.

46 **Alfred T, et al.** Genetic markers of bone and joint health and physical capability in older adults: the Halcyon programme. *Bone* 2013;**52**:278–85.

47 **Manolio TA, et al.** Finding the missing heritability of complex diseases. *Nature* 2009;**461**:747–53.

48 **Wallace DC.** Mitochondrial DNA mutations in disease and aging. *Environ Mol Mutagen* 2010;**51**: 440–50.

49 **Davey Smith G, Ebrahim S.** 'Mendelian randomization': can genetic epidemiology contribute to understanding environmental determinants of disease? *Int J Epidemiol* 2003;**32**:1–22.

50 **Voight BF, et al.** Plasma HDL cholesterol and risk of myocardial infarction: a Mendelian randomisation study. *Lancet* 2012;**380**:572–80.

51 **Alfred T, et al.** Genetic variants influencing biomarkers of nutrition are not associated with cognitive capability in middle-aged and older adults *J Nutr* 2013;**143**:606–12.

Chapter 15

Life course epigenetics and healthy ageing

Paul Haggarty and Anne C Ferguson-Smith

15.1 Introduction

Human life expectancy is increasing. In developed countries life expectancy at birth has risen by approximately 3 months per year over the past 150 years [1] but this success comes at a cost. Poor health in later life is putting an increasing strain on health and social care budgets and there is a need to ensure that physical and mental health is maintained as long as possible into old age. A growing body of evidence indicates that factors acting across life shape health risks for older people and that earlier, more vigorous, and longitudinally maintained management of risk factors is required. Strategies designed to promote healthy ageing need to take account of heightened physiological or behavioural plasticity throughout life and particularly at the key biological and social transition points; from birth, adolescence, pregnancy, becoming a parent, menopause, through to retirement [2].

Key challenges for any mechanistic explanation of the observations in life course epidemiology are (1) the delay, often of decades, between the exposure and the effect on health, and (2) the apparent transmission of health and healthy ageing between the generations. The characteristics of epigenetics make it a good candidate to explain these phenomena. Epigenetics refers to the information in the genome over and above that contained in the DNA sequence (Figure 15.1). This information can be heritable in the sense that it may be passed from one generation to another during reproduction or it may persist within a lifetime in tissues and organs, even as the constituent cells are replenished. The former is relevant to the transgenerational transmission of health and the latter to the time delay between exposure and later health within a lifetime. Even this definition fails to capture the enormous range of biological phenomena now considered to involve epigenetics. There is an increasing understanding of the way in which epigenetic processes control the genome, how the genome is able to respond to the environment, and even potentially the way in which the genome can influence its own environment via effects on behaviour. Recent developments in the ENCODE (encyclopaedia of DNA elements) project have highlighted the importance of epigenetic control of the genome at large scale and the interaction between epigenetics and genetics [3].

Epigenetic control is potentially influenced by two opposing forces relevant to healthy ageing (Figure 15.2). The first is a gradual relaxation of epigenetic control and the fidelity of epigenetic copying with age, which may result in loss of integrity and function, leading to morbidity and early death. The second is the way in which environmental factors at key life stages may result in relatively stable epigenetic marks that can persist over decades, or potentially even more than one lifetime, with possible consequences for health and longevity (Figure 15.2).

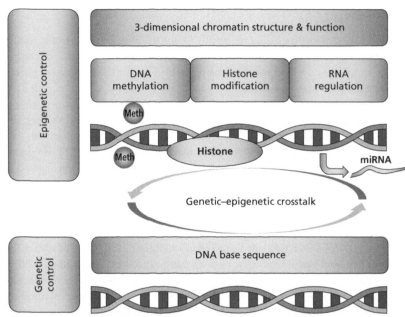

Figure 15.1 Processes influencing genome structure and function. Genetic control results from variation in the base sequence within DNA. Epigenetic control mechanisms include: modification of DNA by methylation; modification of histone proteins by acetylation and methylation; and regulation via microRNAs (miRNA). There is crosstalk between genetic and epigenetic regulation allowing feedback and interaction.

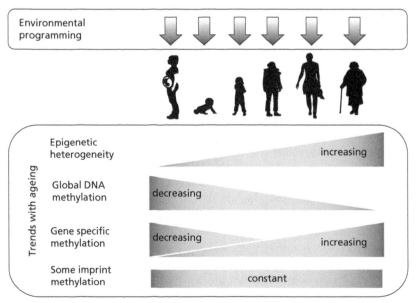

Figure 15.2 Trends in epigenetic status (DNA methylation) with age. Different regions, genes, and functional groups within the genome may change in different ways with age. Epigenetic status is also influenced by environmental exposures at different stages in life. Programmed epigenetic states may persist over decades, be modified by subsequent exposures, or relax over time.

15.2 **Epigenetics**

Epigenetic mechanisms involve chemical modifications to DNA and chromatin, and these are well-established regulators of genome function. Such epigenetic modifications are important for chromosome architecture and segregation during mitosis, for the silencing of repetitive elements that have the potential to disrupt genome integrity, and the regulation of gene activity and repression. Epigenetic modifications can be stably maintained or dynamic in nature. Perhaps the best studied epigenetic modification is DNA methylation which in mammals usually occurs on cytosines at CpG dinucleotides [4]. Importantly, DNA methylation is heritable in somatic lineages upon DNA replication because the DNA methyltransferase DNMT1 recognizes hemimethylated DNA (an old methylated strand and the newly synthesized unmethylated one) and places new methyl groups on the new strand. Thus there exists an inherent mechanism that faithfully retains the memory of methylation state—be it normal or abnormal—from one cell division to another during the lifetime of the individual. DNA methylation can also be acquired *de novo* by the enzymes DNMT3A and DNMT3B, which generate new methyl groups where there were none. DNA methylation can also be removed by both active and passive mechanisms [5]. Recently it has been noted that active demethylation can occur through an oxidation step that converts methyl-C to hydroxymethyl-C via the TET enzymes [6]. As hydroxymethyl-C is not recognized by DNMT1, the memory imposed by methyl-C is not retained upon cell division. Removal of DNA methylation is an important step during the two known phases of genome-wide epigenetic reprogramming that occur during primordial germ cell development and then after fertilization in the pre-implantation embryo. These genome-wide reprogramming events are also accompanied by changes in histone modifications. Reprogramming is important for re-setting primordial germ cell epigenetic states, thus providing totipotency to the developing germ cells in male and female offspring, and for programming the early blastomeres in preparation for the earliest stem cell decisions that they must make after fertilization and prior to implantation.

Approximately 45% of the human genome is made up of transposable repeat elements such as the long interspersed nuclear element (LINE-1) and Alu elements [7–9]. These transposable elements can generate insertions, mutations, and genomic instability resulting in pathology [8], notably in relation to neural development and some forms of cancer [7]. Transposable elements are frequently found in or near genes and the chromatin conformation at retrotransposons may spread and influence the transcription of nearby genes [7,8]. Methylation is a key process regulating the function of the transposable elements [7–9].

Imprinted genes are epigenetically regulated and expressed according to parental origin. Hence, in this category of genes, the methylation marks, which act as the memory of parental origin, are more constant across the life course. These genes make up only around 1% of all human genes but they have important roles throughout the life course, primarily influencing prenatal growth and placental function in addition to critical postnatal adaptations, brain function, and behaviour [10–14]. In the mouse, methylation imprints are established in the germline, maintained during the pre-implantation reprogramming phase and then passed on through the somatic cell lineages where they impact gene expression [15–17]. Despite the stable germline-derived methylation marks in all somatic cells, some imprinted genes exhibit tissue- and stage-specific expression indicating that other factors, in addition to the imprinting control regions, can influence their expression. Transposable elements that flank imprinted genes also demonstrate parent-of-origin effects characteristic of imprinting [18], such as the ability to be refractory to epigenetic reprogramming [19].

15.3 **Epigenetic change across the life course**

Epigenetic changes with age can occur in response to both genetic and environmental effects and the study of genetically identical twins is a useful way to examine the influence of environment in isolation. In a study of global and locus-specific differences in DNA methylation and histone acetylation, Fraga and colleagues found that monozygotic twins are epigenetically very similar during the early years of life [20]. Modest differences begin to develop in childhood [21] and accumulate over time such that, by the age of 30, even monozygotic twins exhibit significant epigenetic differences, with the magnitude of these being dependent on age and discordance in lifestyle [20].

Because the repeat elements make up such a large proportion of the genome, the average (global) methylation over all potentially methylated sites is sometimes equated with that in the repeat elements, but this may not always be valid. Ageing is characterized by loss of global DNA methylation [22,23] and a fall in methylation in some repeat elements; Alu sequences [23–25] and human endogenous retrovirus K[25]. However, there is no corresponding fall in LINE-1; indeed Alu and LINE1 are negatively correlated, particularly over age 49 [25], emphasizing the heterogeneity and specificity of the changes that occur with age.

The biological processes that contribute to ageing are complex and involve a large number of genes, with some becoming up-regulated and others down-regulated with age. It is not surprising therefore that age-related changes in gene specific methylation are similarly complicated. Christensen and colleagues reported that that CpG island methylation increased with age in parallel with decreases in methylation in regions outwith CpG islands in a range of solid tissues and blood-derived DNA [26]. Others have reported age-related increases in DNA methylation linked to genes involved in the development of anatomical structures and transcriptional control [23], and in promoter methylation within CpG islands in prostate tissue [27]. Heyn et al. observed a fall in methylation with age across all genomic categories; promoters, exonic, intronic, and intergenic regions [24]. Madrigano and colleagues reported that ageing was associated with decreases in the methylation of some genes and increased methylation of others in a large elderly cohort in the US [28]. Methylation within the estrogen receptor-α gene in human vasculature increases with age [29].

The functional implications of age-related changes in methylation are generally unknown and indeed, changes in methylation are difficult to interpret. Age-related effects on methylation are often assumed to cause changes in expression but may also be secondary effects of the ageing genome occurring in response to local changes in transcription.

The fidelity of copying of epigenetic states across the life course may also play a role in ageing. Methylation status within adjacent CpG sites is highly correlated [30] and the correlation in the methylation status of neighbouring CpG sites is lower in centenarian compared to newborn DNA [24].

Taken as a whole the available evidence suggests that:

- epigenetic variation increases with age
- global methylation falls with age
- gene specific methylation may increase or decrease with age
- some repeat elements decrease in methylation with age but this is not universal
- the methylation status of a number of imprinted regions is relatively stable across life
- the pattern of coherent blocks of DNA methylation breaks down with age.

15.4 **Health consequences of epigenetic variation**

Some have tried to link human longevity to epigenetic status. Madrigano and colleagues have suggested that blood DNA methylation may be a useful marker of biological rather than chronological age [28], and there are reports of a reduced rate of decline in age-related global DNA methylation in the offspring of centenarians [23]. These differences may also be linked to healthy ageing, as individuals who live longest also have a fundamentally different health trajectory; they stay healthier longer and their susceptibility to disease appears to be shifted to later life in a phenomenon termed 'compression of morbidity' [31].

Historically, cancer is the disease in which epigenetics has been studied most extensively. Tumours exhibit epigenetic abnormalities in virtually every component of chromatin involved in the regulation of the human genome [32]. However, it has been proposed that more subtle epigenetic changes could play a seminal role in the earliest steps in cancer initiation [32–34]. Large scale hypomethylation in particular has been proposed as an early trigger in non-tumour tissue that may bring about genome-wide changes in the structure of the epigenome and predispose cells to genomic instability and cancer [32,33]. Epigenetic mechanisms have also been implicated in Alzheimer's disease [35], mental impairment, and normal cognitive function [12,36,37]. Altered methylation of the estrogen receptor-α gene has been observed in coronary atherosclerotic plaques compared to normal proximal aorta [29]. Elevated global DNA methylation in blood is positively associated with the prevalence of cardiovascular disease and predisposing conditions such as diabetes and hypertension [38]. Epimutation at the well-established epigenetically regulated imprinted genes is known to be important for a number of health outcomes [39] including imprinting disorders, where the imprint is disrupted or absent. Perturbations of epigenetic state in these syndromes, which can also have an underlying genetic aetiology, can lead to diabetes [40], cancer risk [41], impaired cognitive development, and obesity [42].

The biochemical and physiological processes thought to underpin healthy ageing have also been linked to epigenetic change. The methyl and acetyl groups that constitute the main epigenetic marks are at the heart of nutritional metabolism and energy flux [43] and there is growing interest in the potential for chronic nutrient and energy restriction to delay the onset of ageing and extend the life span [44]. The methyl groups which epigenetically modify DNA and histones are produced by the methylation pathway, involving nutrients such as the B vitamins and methionine, whilst histone acetylation uses acetyl groups produced in the metabolism of carbohydrate, fat, and some amino acids [43]. The important redox metabolite nicotinamide adenine dinucleotide (NAD) is a cofactor for the sirtuins (a group of protein deacetylases) and it has been suggested that they may play a role in sensing metabolic flux [45,46]. The accumulation of damage to DNA, and the ability to repair this, are also thought to be important factors in biological ageing, and DNA methylation plays an important role in this process [47].

15.5 **Early life exposures and epigenetic programming**

Events during the early years, starting before birth, have been linked to aspects of health and wellbeing throughout life—from obesity, heart disease, diabetes, cancer, and mental health, to educational achievement and economic status [48]. Marmot has argued that the close links between early disadvantage and poor outcomes throughout life can only be broken if action to reduce health inequalities starts before birth and is followed through the life of the child [48]. In order to develop effective strategies we need to understand the causal links between key early exposures and subsequent health.

The period before birth, and even before conception, is characterized by intense epigenetic activity, with waves of methylation and demethylation closely linked in time to critical developmental windows and processes [5,16]. This suggests that there may be windows of epigenetic vulnerability when environmental factors might have greater impact. Imprinted genes have been proposed as genes that might be particularly susceptible to environmental modulation of the developmental programme with an impact on later health. This is because many important imprinted genes are exquisitely dosage sensitive and function to regulate many of the developmental and metabolic pathways that impact health in adult life [13,39,49]. Recent work in humans suggests that many imprinted genes maintain their allele specific methylation signal in a wide range of adult somatic tissues, independent of the absolute levels of expression [50], and that many parent of origin specific epigenotypes remain stable over decades [51–53]. However, individuals vary in their level of imprinting methylation [51,54–56], and there is interest in the extent to which this variability may be influenced by early environmental factors, such as nutrition, and its effect on human health throughout life [39,49].

Since 1992 in the UK, the periconceptional use of folic acid supplements has been recommended to reduce the risk of neural tube defect. This nutrient is metabolized through the pathway that provides methyl groups for DNA methylation and its use in human pregnancy has been reported to influence methylation of the imprinted genes, insulin like growth factor 2 (IGF2) [56,57] and paternally expressed gene 3 (PEG3), and the repeat element LINE-1 [56] in the offspring. Altered IGF2 methylation has also been observed in women decades after prenatal exposure to famine during the Dutch Hunger Winter of 1944–45 [58]. Little is known about the health consequences of these epigenetic changes but the epigenetic regulation of imprinted genes and retrotransposons is thought to influence function. IGF2 methylation has been linked to cancer risk [34,58] whilst methylation of LINE-1 inhibits transposition which has the potential to cause abnormal function and disease [7,8]. Much of the work on imprint programming in pregnancy has focused on maternal nutrition but the paternal contribution could also be important [59].

A number of studies in animal models have also demonstrated effects on offspring phenotype and epigenotype of the maternal diet (particularly the content of methyl donors) in pregnancy [39,49]. The hypothesis that imprinted genes as a class might be more or less vulnerable than other genes to environmental modulation was also recently tested in an intergenerational mouse model of undernutrition [60]. In this model, pregnant female mice fed a 50% calorically restricted diet, give birth to small offspring which, though fed *ad libitum* themselves, go on to develop adult onset obesity and metabolic disease. Interestingly, these phenotypes are transmitted to a second generation upon both male and female transmission [61]. Radford et al. studied the tissue-specific expression and methylation at imprinted genes in the fetuses of the undernourished mothers and also at the same developmental stage in the grandchildren of these mothers. These levels were compared with the wider transcriptome. In this model imprinted genes were neither more nor less susceptible than randomly selected genes and in particular, as a class, were not directly environmentally modulated. Some individual imprinted genes, such as Peg3, showed perturbed expression in a tissue specific manner; however whether these were causal or a consequence of defective metabolism could not be determined. Where it was possible to assess, loss of imprinting was not observed [60]. More such mechanistic studies would help in the interpretation of the observations in human populations.

15.6 **Epigenetic heritability**

There is significant heritable variation in the way individuals respond to the environment. Such differences are at some level coded in the genome; either within the DNA sequence itself (Chapter 14) or at the level of epigenetic control. Many human diseases have a significant component of heritability and this is also true of longevity. Around 25% of human life expectancy can be ascribed to heritable factors but this component only becomes significant over about 60 years of age, with the contribution of this heritable component becoming stronger with increasing age thereafter [62]. Epigenetic factors are also relevant to the heritable components of health and longevity in two ways: (1) as the mechanism through which genetic variation might exert its effect; and (2) as heritable factors in themselves (both as drivers of change in genomic activity and as maintenance factors stabilizing long-term effects as a consequence of age). There is also an increasing awareness of the interplay between genetic and epigenetic control of biological function (Figure 15.1). Significant heritability of epigenetic status has been demonstrated in human twin studies [20,21,55,63]. Non-twin family studies have also highlighted familial clustering of DNA methylation and the change in methylation over time [53]. Even in imprinted genes the methylation status is more similar between genetically identical individuals [52]. Specific genetic variants have been linked to changes in methylation; e.g. a single polymorphism within the imprinting control region of the imprinted gene H19 is associated with altered methylation within the gene [52].

15.7 **Socioeconomic and lifestyle links to epigenetic states**

Health and longevity are strongly related to socioeconomic position (SEP). People living in the poorest neighbourhoods in England die on average 7 years earlier than people living in the richest neighbourhoods [48]. They also spend more of their shorter lives with a disability; the average difference in disability-free life expectancy between the richest and poorest neighbourhoods is 17 years [48]. Lower levels of global DNA methylation have been reported in the most socioeconomically deprived individuals, with manual workers having a lower level of DNA methylation than non-manual [64]. More detailed genome-wide methylation analysis of blood DNA from adult males from the 1958 British Birth Cohort Study has identified over 1000 gene promoters where the level of methylation was associated with childhood SEP [65]. Around half that number were linked to adult SEP and these authors concluded that childhood SEP was more important in determining adult blood DNA methylation profiles than adult SEP [65].

Inequalities in health arise because of inequalities in the conditions in which people are born, grow, live, work, and age (Chapter 18) [48]. Many of the environmental factors that co-vary with SEP—such as diet, alcohol consumption, physical activity, health related behaviours, have been linked to epigenetic status. The methyl and acetyl groups that constitute the key epigenetic marks are at the heart of nutritional metabolism [43], and there is a growing body of empirical evidence demonstrating an effect of individual nutrients on epigenetic status. These include folic acid, niacin, biotin, protein, phytoestrogens, sulforaphane, and polyphenols [43]. Alcohol influences DNA methylation in animal models [66], and in humans [67]. Smoking has also been linked to epigenetic states [68,69].

15.8 **Epigenetics and behaviour**

Like the heart, liver, and other organs and systems, the brain has its own biological disease mechanisms (e.g. stroke and dementia). However, the brain is different in that it can also influence the internal and external exposures which it and all the other body systems experience in the course of life (Figure 15.3). Such effects may help explain a component of the linkage between cognitive ability and intelligence and a wide range of health outcomes across the life course including cardiovascular disease, stroke, and respiratory disease [70]. The causal links between these factors are difficult to tease out but there is increasing interest in the concept of epigenetic programming

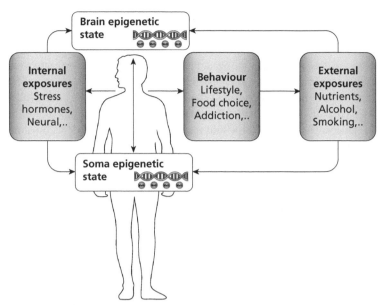

Figure 15.3 The central role of brain epigenetic state at the heart of a series of feedback loops that influence external and internal exposures relevant to brain and soma-wide epigenetic states.

operating in the brain in ways that predispose to particular behaviours and the psychological response to the environment throughout life. Epigenetic factors have been implicated in brain function, cognition and cognitive ageing [35,36], and numerous lines of evidence point to the importance of the correct epigenetic control of the imprinted genes for normal brain function and postnatal neurogenesis [12,71,72]. There is also a rapidly expanding literature on repetitive elements in the brain [73,74], though the biological significance of these is not yet clear.

Neural function and behaviour are also influenced by the early physical, emotional, and nutritional environment and there is evidence suggesting that this might operate through an epigenetic mechanism. The offspring of dams fed a high-fat/high-sugar diet during pregnancy and lactation have global and gene-specific changes in DNA methylation in the brain associated with long-term alterations in dopamine and opioid gene expression [75]. These epigenetic changes were also associated with the offspring's own preference for palatable foods [75]. Alcohol exposure during early neural development also results in changes in DNA methylation and gene expression in the brain [76]. Much of the research on the early physical and emotional environment has focused on the stress response, its regulation by the hypothalamic–pituitary–adrenal (HPA) axis, and the role of cortisol in particular (Chapter 10). Cortisol is a glucocorticoid hormone, released in response to stress, that influences the brain (e.g. memory formation and retrieval) and numerous organ systems within the body. In animals, maternal stress during pregnancy and increased glucocorticoid exposure are associated with reduced birth weight, a higher risk of hypertension and hyperglycemia, and altered brain HPA activity and behaviour in the offspring after birth [77,78]. High levels of maternal stress are associated with low birth weight in humans [79,80]. Cortisol levels of low birthweight babies are higher throughout life and neuropsychiatric disorders in later life have been linked to maternal stress in pregnancy, with some of these behavioural effects apparently being passed to subsequent generations [77]. These factors are also linked to SEP. Psychosocial stress and the physiological responses to stress are patterned by social class [81] and low birth weight is more common in deprived areas of Britain [82]. Some of the associations in the human studies could also have a genetic interpretation and this remains to be tested. The early postnatal environment also appears to influence brain epigenetic states and HPA function. In animal studies maternal care (grooming and licking) influences histone acetylation and transcription factor (nerve growth factor-inducible protein-A) binding to the glucocorticoid receptor promoter [78,83–85]. Children experiencing abuse or neglect in early life have an altered pattern of blood DNA methylation across a wide range of genes and regions [86], and there are epigenetic changes in the glucocorticoid receptor within the hippocampus of suicide victims with a history of childhood abuse [87].

15.9 **The importance of life course study designs**

Establishing the full pathway of epigenetic causality—exposure/event → epigenetic state → later health/longevity—is challenging and most research carried out in the field to date has attempted only to address the individual components of this sequence: (1) exposure/event → epigenetic state and (2) epigenetic state → later health/longevity.

Exposures are often difficult to quantify using traditional epidemiological techniques, particularly when they may have occurred many years previously or in a complex way. Epigenetic states have the potential to act as markers of exposure; e.g. in response to individual nutrients [43], alcohol [67], cigarette smoke [68,69], SEP [65], early emotional environment [86,87], and even exposure to maternal famine before birth [58]. Epigenetic markers may be particularly useful when the relevant exposure results from both external and internal factors; e.g. age at menarche, age at menopause, use of contraception and hormone replacement therapy, in the case of lifetime exposure to estrogen.

For the second component of epigenetic causality (epigenetic state → later health/longevity) most studies have reported association close to the time of appearance of the disease rather than demonstrate cause and effect separated in time. Fortunately, there is a growing availability of large birth cohorts, and other longitudinal study designs, with good event/exposure/phenotype data, and DNA collections taken at different life stages [88]. These offer the possibility of detection of epigenetic change in response to an exposure, prior to the overt development of pathology, and the linking of that change to the biological process leading to later health and disease. However, even with the availability of such valuable resources, epigenetic studies in human populations are still subject to a number of practical difficulties that must be addressed [43,88–90].

15.10 **Practical considerations**

One of the most important practical problems in this field results from differences in the epigenetic status of different tissues. In most large human cohorts appropriate to life course studies, typically only peripheral blood or buccal cell DNA may be available. The rationale for blood and buccal cell sampling is that epigenetic status within these cells is either indicative of key epigenetic events in the tissues and organs of interest or that it is simply a useful biomarker. Different tissues have different epigenetic profiles but in human cohort studies it is not necessary for them to be the same. It is sufficient that they are influenced in a similar way by the genetic/environmental exposure of interest and that the population ranking of epigenetic status in the peripheral cells is indicative of the ranking in the target organ. Genotype is common to all tissues and many environmental exposures, such as alcohol or nutrition, typically tend to reach similar concentrations in all tissues, or at least rank in a similar way. There are also specific types of epigenetic mark that are more likely to occur in multiple tissue types [50]. The setting of imprints early in development makes these potentially useful in the study of the epigenetic effects of early exposures [58]. There are now many studies demonstrating that epigenetic states in peripheral tissues such as blood and buccal cells can reflect genetic and/or environmental exposures in a wide range of tissues, but this is not universal and it is necessary to establish in advance the validity of each epigenetic study design and make explicit any underpinning assumptions.

Evidence for the involvement of epigenetic processes may also be obtained from genetic association studies. Genetic variants within the genes involved in epigenetic control have been implicated in a wide range of biological functions and health outcomes [91–93]. However, the conclusions that can be drawn from such genetic association studies are quite general. An extension of the standard genetic association model has been proposed that may allow inference of the full pathway of causality between an exposure and an epigenetic effect on health by exploiting genetic variants thought to influence specific methylation sites [90]. A general problem in applying genetic associations to life course studies is the fact that genotype is invariant throughout life and associations with disease provide little or no information on the period(s) when the implicated environmental exposure may have been critical [94]. With phenomena that are potentially transgenerational, such as epigenetics, this uncertainty may even extend to whether the relevant exposure may have occurred in the parent as the genotype of the offspring is highly correlated with that of the parents [94].

In any epigenetic study a decision has to be made about which epigenetic signal to measure. The most commonly studied is DNA methylation and, depending on the hypothesis, this can be investigated in individual methylation sites, specific genes, regions of the genome, or functional groups (e.g. gene promoters). An increasing number of human studies use array based technologies to measure a great many methylation sites in a single sample (e.g. over 480,000 methylation sites in the case of the Illumina 450k array, covering almost all known human genes) and the trend is towards larger arrays. This scanning approach is often used to gather information on which to base future hypotheses and it has the same advantages and disadvantages of genome wide association studies (GWAS); the equivalent epigenetic approach is sometimes referred to as epigenome wide association studies (EWAS). Traditional methods of statistical analysis struggle to cope with such large data sets and it is likely that innovative multidimensional statistical approaches, similar to those developed for GWAS data [95], will also allow EWAS data to take into account our emerging understanding of the way in which epigenetic control may be distributed across the genome [3].

15.11 **Conclusions**

Epigenetics has emerged in recent years as one of the most promising biological explanations linking exposures across the life course to long-term health. Epigenotype is influenced by genotype but, unlike genotype, there is the potential for modification. This leaves open the intriguing possibility that adverse epigenetic states, resulting from events/exposures at earlier life stages, may be reversible. One example is the nutritional reprogramming of brain epigenetic states created by adverse physical and emotional events in early life. In animal models central infusion of the nutrient methionine (involved in DNA methylation) appears to reverse the effect of maternal behaviour on the epigenetic changes that result in altered glucocorticoid receptor expression and HPA function and the responses to stress [96]. Chronic methionine administration also reverses the changes in prefrontal cortex DNA methylation and DNMT3b expression that occur in response to cocaine addiction [97].

Epigenetic states change with age and they may provide useful markers of biological ageing but the picture is not yet clear and it is likely that combinations of multiple epigenetic marks may be may be needed to fully define the heterogeneous biological processes that contribute to ageing. The sirtuins have been identified as possible epigenetic targets to counteract aspects of biological ageing [45,46]. In addition, the field of epigenetics has the potential to improve traditional life course study designs by providing objective markers of complex exposures based on the accumulation of epigenetic change.

The field of epigenetics is of increasing interest to policy makers searching for explanations for epidemiological observations and conceptual models on which to base interventions. The Chief Medical Officer for Scotland recently suggested that 'the persistence of health inequalities across the social spectrum, particularly in West Central Scotland, may be associated with such (epigenetic) effects' [98]. Human epigenetic studies are already providing evidence relevant to public health debates, including the use of folic acid supplements in pregnancy and fortification of foods with folic acid [56,57]. The epigenetic paradigm has the potential to explain a great many phenomena in human biology and the biology of ageing but the field is relatively new and in many cases we do not have a complete understanding of the biological significance of the epigenetic observations in human populations. Life course studies provide a good framework and discipline within which to study the role of epigenetics in human ageing.

Acknowledgements

Paul Haggarty acknowledges the support of Scottish Government. Anne C Ferguson-Smith is grateful to the MRC, Wellcome Trust, and the EU-FP7 programmes of EpiHealth and EpigeneSys for support in this area.

References

1 Scully T. Demography: to the limit. *Nature* 2012;**492**:S2–S3.

2 Kuh D, et al. Life course epidemiology. *J Epidemiol Community Health* 2003;**57**:778–83.

3 Bernstein BE, et al. An integrated encyclopedia of DNA elements in the human genome. *Nature* 2012;**489**:57–74.

4 Deaton AM, Bird A. CpG islands and the regulation of transcription. *Genes Dev* 2011;**25**:1010–22.

5 Hackett JA, Surani MA. DNA methylation dynamics during the mammalian life cycle. *Phil Trans R Soc Lond B Biol Sci* 2013;**368**:20110328. <http://dx.doi.org/10.1098/rstb.2011.0328>

6 Branco MR, Ficz G, Reik W. Uncovering the role of 5-hydroxymethylcytosine in the epigenome. *Nat Rev Genet* 2012;**13**:7–13.

7 Cordaux R, Batzer MA. The impact of retrotransposons on human genome evolution. *Nat Rev Genet* 2009;**10**:691–703.

8 Levin HL, Moran JV. Dynamic interactions between transposable elements and their hosts. *Nat Rev Genet* 2011;**12**:615–27.

9 Waterland RA, Jirtle RL. Transposable elements: targets for early nutritional effects on epigenetic gene regulation. *Mol Cell Biol* 2003;**23**:5293–300.

10 Reik W, et al. Imprinted genes and the coordination of fetal and postnatal growth in mammals. *Novartis Found Symp* 2001;**237**:19–31.

11 Tycko B, Morison IM. Physiological functions of imprinted genes. *J Cell Physiol* 2002;**192**:245–58.

12 Wilkinson LS, et al. Genomic imprinting effects on brain development and function. *Nat Rev Neurosci* 2007;**8**:832–43.

13 **Charalambous M, et al.** Genomic imprinting, growth control and the allocation of nutritional resources: consequences for postnatal life. *Curr Opin Endocrinol Diabetes Obes* 2007;**14**:3–12.

14 **Charalambous M, et al.** Imprinted gene dosage is critical for the transition to independent life. *Cell Metab* 2012;**15**:209–21.

15 **Ferguson-Smith AC, Surani MA.** Imprinting and the epigenetic asymmetry between parental genomes. *Science* 2001;**293**:1086–9.

16 **Ferguson-Smith AC.** Genomic imprinting: the emergence of an epigenetic paradigm. *Nat Rev Genet* 2011;**12**:565–75.

17 **Reik W, Walter J.** Genomic imprinting: parental influence on the genome. *Nat Rev Genet* 2001;**2**:21–32.

18 **Walter J, et al.** Repetitive elements in imprinted genes. *Cytogenet Genome Res* 2006;**113**:109–15.

19 **Seisenberger S, et al.** The dynamics of genome-wide DNA methylation reprogramming in mouse primordial germ cells. *Mol Cell* 2012;**48**:849–62.

20 **Fraga MF, et al.** Epigenetic differences arise during the lifetime of monozygotic twins. *Proc Natl Acad Sci USA* 2005;**102**:10604–9.

21 **Mill J, et al.** Evidence for monozygotic twin (MZ) discordance in methylation level at two CpG sites in the promoter region of the catechol-O-methyltransferase (COMT) gene. *Am J Med Genet B Neuropsychiatr Genet* 2006;**141**:421–5.

22 **Fraga MF, et al.** Cross-talk between aging and cancer: the epigenetic language. *Ann N Y Acad Sci* 2007; **1100**:60–74.

23 **Gentilini D, Mari D, et al.** Role of epigenetics in human aging and longevity: genome-wide DNA methylation profile in centenarians and centenarians' offspring. *Age* (Dordr) 2012; doi:10.1007/s11357-012-9463-1.

24 **Heyn H, et al.** Distinct DNA methylomes of newborns and centenarians. *Proc Natl Acad Sci USA* 2012; **109**:10522–7.

25 **Jintaridth P, Mutirangura A.** Distinctive patterns of age-dependent hypomethylation in interspersed repetitive sequences. *Physiol Genomics* 2010;**41**:194–200.

26 **Christensen BC, et al.** Aging and environmental exposures alter tissue-specific DNA methylation dependent upon CpG island context. *PLoS Genet* 2009;**5**:e1000602.

27 **Kwabi-Addo B, Chung W, Shen L, Ittmann M, Wheeler T, Jelinek J, et al.** Age-related DNA methylation changes in normal human prostate tissues. *Clin Cancer Res* 2007;**13**:3796–802.

28 **Madrigano J, et al.** Aging and epigenetics: longitudinal changes in gene-specific DNA methylation. *Epigenetics* 2012;**7**:63–70.

29 **Post WS, et al.** Methylation of the estrogen receptor gene is associated with aging and atherosclerosis in the cardiovascular system. *Cardiovasc Res* 1999;**43**:985–91.

30 **Eckhardt F, et al.** DNA methylation profiling of human chromosomes 6, 20 and 22. *Nat Genet* 2006;**38**: 1378–85.

31 **Andersen SL, et al.** Health span approximates life span among many supercentenarians: compression of morbidity at the approximate limit of life span. *J Gerontol A Biol Sci Med Sci* 2012;**67**:395–405.

32 **Jones PA, Baylin SB.** The epigenomics of cancer. *Cell* 2007;**128**:683–92.

33 **Robertson KD.** DNA methylation and human disease. *Nat Rev Genet* 2005;**6**:597–610.

34 **Feinberg AP, et al.** The epigenetic progenitor origin of human cancer. *Nat Rev Genet* 2006;**7**:21–33.

35 **Mattson MP.** Methylation and acetylation in nervous system development and neurodegenerative disorders. *Ageing Res Rev* 2003;**2**:329–42.

36 **Levenson JM, Sweatt JD.** Epigenetic mechanisms in memory formation. *Nat Rev Neurosci* 2005;**6**: 108–18.

37 **Tsankova N, et al.** Epigenetic regulation in psychiatric disorders. *Nat Rev Neurosci* 2007;**8**:355–67.

38 **Kim M, et al.** DNA methylation as a biomarker for cardiovascular disease risk. *PLoS One* 2010;**5**:e9692.

39 **Jirtle RL, Skinner MK.** Environmental epigenomics and disease susceptibility. *Nat Rev Genet* 2007;**8**:253–62.

40 **Temple IK, Shield JP.** Transient neonatal diabetes, a disorder of imprinting. *J Med Genet* 2002;**39**: 872–5.

41 **Rump P, et al.** Tumor risk in Beckwith-Wiedemann syndrome: a review and meta-analysis. *Am J Med Genet A* 2005;**136**:95–104.

42 **Horsthemke B, Buiting K.** Genomic imprinting and imprinting defects in humans. *Adv Genet* 2008;**61**: 225–46.

43 **Haggarty P.** Nutrition and the epigenome. *Prog Mol Biol Transl Sci* 2012;**108**:427–46.

44 **Anderson RM, Weindruch R.** The caloric restriction paradigm: implications for healthy human aging. *Am J Hum Biol* 2012;**24**:101–6.

45 **Baur JA, et al.** Are sirtuins viable targets for improving healthspan and lifespan? *Nat Rev Drug Discov* 2012;**11**:443–61.

46 **Cosentino C, Mostoslavsky R.** Metabolism, longevity and epigenetics. *Cell Mol Life Sci* 2013;**70**:1525–41.

47 **Jin B, Robertson KD.** DNA methyltransferases, DNA damage repair, and cancer. *Adv Exp Med Biol* 2013;**754**:3–29.

48 **Marmot M.** Fair society, healthy lives. In: Strategic Review of Health Inequalities in England Post-2010. London: The Marmot Review; 2010.

49 **Waterland RA, Jirtle RL.** Early nutrition, epigenetic changes at transposons and imprinted genes, and enhanced susceptibility to adult chronic diseases. *Nutrition* 2004;**20**:63–68.

50 **Woodfine K, et al.** Quantitative analysis of DNA methylation at all human imprinted regions reveals preservation of epigenetic stability in adult somatic tissue. *Epigenetics Chromatin* 2011;**4**:1.

51 **Sandovici I, et al.** Familial aggregation of abnormal methylation of parental alleles at the IGF2/H19 and IGF2R differentially methylated regions. *Hum Mol Genet* 2003;**12**:1569–78.

52 **Coolen MW, et al.** Impact of the genome on the epigenome is manifested in DNA methylation patterns of imprinted regions in monozygotic and dizygotic twins. *PLoS One* 2011;**6**:e25590.

53 **Bjornsson HT, et al.** Intra-individual change over time in DNA methylation with familial clustering. *JAMA* 2008;**299**:2877–83.

54 **Heijmans BT, et al.** Heritable rather than age-related environmental and stochastic factors dominate variation in DNA methylation of the human IGF2/H19 locus. *Hum Mol Genet* 2007;**16**:547–54.

55 **Kaminsky ZA, Tang T, Wang SC, Ptak C, Oh GH, Wong AH, et al.** DNA methylation profiles in monozygotic and dizygotic twins. *Nat Genet* 2009;**41**:240–5.

56 **Haggarty P, et al.** Folate in pregnancy and imprinted gene and repeat element methylation in the offspring. *Am J Clin Nutr* 2013;**97**:94–9.

57 **Steegers-Theunissen RP, et al.** Periconceptional maternal folic acid use of 400 microg per day is related to increased methylation of the IGF2 gene in the very young child. *PLoS ONE* 2009;**4**:e7845.

58 **Heijmans BT, et al.** Persistent epigenetic differences associated with prenatal exposure to famine in humans. *Proc Natl Acad Sci USA* 2008;**105**:17046–9.

59 **Ferguson-Smith AC, Patti ME.** You are what your dad ate. *Cell Metab* 2011;**13**:115–7.

60 **Radford EJ, et al.** An unbiased assessment of the role of imprinted genes in an intergenerational model of developmental programming. *PLoS Genet* 2012;**8**:e1002605.

61 **Jimenez-Chillaron JC, et al.** Intergenerational transmission of glucose intolerance and obesity by in utero undernutrition in mice. *Diabetes* 2009;**58**:460–8.

62 **Herskind AM, et al.** The heritability of human longevity: a population-based study of 2872 Danish twin pairs born 1870–1900. *Hum Genet* 1996;**97**:319–23.

63 **Wong CC, et al.** A longitudinal study of epigenetic variation in twins. *Epigenetics* 2010;**5**:516–26.

64 **McGuinness D, et al.** Socio-economic status is associated with epigenetic differences in the pSoBid cohort. *Int J Epidemiol* 2012;**41**:151–60.

65 **Borghol N, et al.** Associations with early-life socio-economic position in adult DNA methylation. *Int J Epidemiol* 2012;**4**:62–74.

66 **Garro AJ, et al.** Ethanol consumption inhibits fetal DNA methylation in mice: implications for the fetal alcohol syndrome. *Alcohol Clin Exp Res* 1991;**15**:395–8.

67 **Bonsch D, et al.** DNA hypermethylation of the alpha synuclein promoter in patients with alcoholism. *Neuroreport* 2005;**16**:167–70.

68 **Shenker NS, et al.** Epigenome-wide association study in the European Prospective Investigation into Cancer and Nutrition (EPIC-Turin) identifies novel genetic loci associated with smoking. *Hum Mol Genet* 2013;**22**:843–51.

69 **Suter M, et al.** Maternal tobacco use modestly alters correlated epigenome-wide placental DNA methylation and gene expression. *Epigenetics* 2011;**6**:1284–94.

70 **Deary IJ.** Intelligence. *Annu Rev Psychol* 2012;**63**:453–82.

71 **Kopsida E, et al.** The role of imprinted genes in mediating susceptibility to neuropsychiatric disorders. *Horm Behav* 2011;**59**:375–82.

72 **Ferron SR, et al.** Postnatal loss of Dlk1 imprinting in stem cells and niche astrocytes regulates neurogenesis. *Nature* 2011;**475**:381–5.

73 **Kan PX, et al.** Epigenetic studies of genomic retroelements in major psychosis. *Schizophr Res* 2004;**67**: 95–106.

74 **Singer T, et al.** LINE-1 retrotransposons: mediators of somatic variation in neuronal genomes? *Trends Neurosci* 2010;**33**:345–54.

75 **Vucetic Z, et al.** Maternal high-fat diet alters methylation and gene expression of dopamine and opioid-related genes. *Endocrinology* 2010;**151**:4756–64.

76 **Liu Y, et al.** Alcohol exposure alters DNA methylation profiles in mouse embryos at early neurulation. *Epigenetics* 2009;**4**:500–11.

77 **Seckl JR, Meaney MJ.** Glucocorticoid 'programming' and PTSD risk. *Ann N Y Acad Sci* 2006;**1071**:351–78.

78 **Meaney MJ, et al.** Epigenetic mechanisms of perinatal programming of hypothalamic–pituitary–adrenal function and health. *Trends Mol Med* 2007;**13**:269–77.

79 **Borders AE, et al.** Chronic stress and low birth weight neonates in a low-income population of women. *Obstet Gynecol* 2007;**109**:331–8.

80 **Paarlberg KM, et al.** Psychosocial predictors of low birthweight: a prospective study. *Br J Obstet Gynaecol* 1999;**106**:834–41.

81 **Muennig P, et al.** Socioeconomic status as an independent predictor of physiological biomarkers of cardiovascular disease: evidence from NHANES. *Prev Med* 2007;**45**:35–40.

82 **Dibben C, Sigala M, Macfarlane A.** Area deprivation, individual factors and low birth weight in England: is there evidence of an "area effect"? *J Epidemiol Community Health* 2006;**60**:1053–9.

83 **Meaney MJ, Szyf M.** Environmental programming of stress responses through DNA methylation: life at the interface between a dynamic environment and a fixed genome. *Dialogues Clin Neurosci* 2005;**7**:103–23.

84 **Weaver IC, et al.** The transcription factor nerve growth factor-inducible protein a mediates epigenetic programming: altering epigenetic marks by immediate-early genes. *J Neurosci* 2007;**27**:1756–68.

85 **Zhang TY, Meaney MJ.** Epigenetics and the environmental regulation of the genome and its function. *Annu Rev Psychol* 2010;**61**:439–3.

86 **Yang BZ, et al.** Child abuse and epigenetic mechanisms of disease risk. *Am J Prev Med* 2013;**44**:101–7.

87 **McGowan PO, et al.** Epigenetic regulation of the glucocorticoid receptor in human brain associates with childhood abuse. *Nat Neurosci* 2009;**12**:342–8.

88 **Ng JW, et al.** The role of longitudinal cohort studies in epigenetic epidemiology: challenges and opportunities. *Genome Biol* 2012;**13**:246. doi:10.1186/gb-2012-13-6-246.

89 **Heijmans BT, Mill J.** Commentary: the seven plagues of epigenetic epidemiology. *Int J Epidemiol* 2012;**41**:74–8.

90 **Relton CL, Davey Smith G.** Two-step epigenetic Mendelian randomization: a strategy for establishing the causal role of epigenetic processes in pathways to disease. *Int J Epidemiol* 2012;**41**:161–76.

91 **Cebrian A, et al.** Genetic variants in epigenetic genes and breast cancer risk. *Carcinogenesis* 2006;**27**: 1661–9.

92 **Shen H, et al.** A novel polymorphism in human cytosine DNA-methyltransferase-3B promoter is associated with an increased risk of lung cancer. *Cancer Res* 2002;**62**:4992–5.

93 **Haggarty P, et al.** Human intelligence and polymorphisms in the DNA methyltransferase genes involved in epigenetic marking. *PLoS One* 2010;**5**:e11329.

94 **Haggarty P.** B-vitamins, genotype and disease causality. *Proc Nutr Soc* 2007;**66**:539–47.

95 **Yang J, et al.** Genome partitioning of genetic variation for complex traits using common SNPs. *Nat Genet* 2011;**43**:519–25.

96 **Weaver IC, et al.** Reversal of maternal programming of stress responses in adult offspring through methyl supplementation: altering epigenetic marking later in life. *J Neurosci* 2005;**25**:11045–54.

97 **Tian W, et al.** Reversal of cocaine-conditioned place preference through methyl supplementation in mice: altering global DNA methylation in the prefrontal cortex. *PLoS One* 2012;**7**:e33435.

98 **Chief Medical Officer. Health in Scotland** 2011. Transforming Scotland's health. Annual Report of the Chief Medical Officer. Edinburgh: Scottish Government; 2012.

Part IV

The way we live

Chapter 16

Lifetime lifestyles I: diet, the life course, and ageing

Gita Mishra, Marcus Richards, Seema Mihrshahi, and Alison Stephen

16.1 Introduction

Diet is recognized as an important modifiable factor that in combination with other aspects of lifestyle, such as physical activity, can reduce the risk of various chronic diseases in later life. In this chapter we explore dietary patterns that may maximize the probability of healthy ageing. We briefly outline the use of guidelines for dietary patterns and describe the broader context of a life course approach to dietary choices. Current evidence for the influence of diet on healthy ageing in terms of physical and cognitive capability is then reviewed. We also discuss the main methodological challenges for research, seeking to identify and unravel the complex relationships involved, and conclude with recommendations for improving the way that current and future cohort studies can advance research in this field.

16.2 Diet, dietary patterns, and dietary guidelines: a life course perspective

Diet refers to the foods typically consume to provide energy, macronutrients (protein, fat and carbohydrate) and a range of micronutrients, that are essential to maintain health. Diet represents a key modifiable lifestyle factor that can have long-term health implications [1]. Dietary patterns, which refer to the combinations of foods that characterize an individual's diet, often reflect cultural or social norms and tend to be more aligned to the way people perceive their diet. They also better capture the potential for interactions or synergistic effects of these combinations of foods, than diet as individual food or nutrient intakes [2].

Over recent decades public health authorities have produced dietary guidelines to reflect recommendations for optimum intakes of nutrients based on available evidence. There has been an increasing focus on providing guidelines in ways that can influence dietary patterns, providing guidance on numbers and sizes of portions for different food groups. From 1992 until 2011 the US based their 'Dietary Guidelines for Americans' on the Food Guide Pyramid, the last of which had eight categories of food types and recommended servings of each [3]. In 2011 the guidance changed to MyPlate which is divided into sections which recommend 30% grains, 30% vegetables, 20% fruits and 20% protein, with a smaller circle representing dairy [4]. Other countries have had similar developments for representing dietary guidelines to the populace. The UK recently adopted the 'Eatwell' plate, which depicts the various proportions of different food groups, such as fruit and vegetables or milk and dairy products, that can provide a balanced healthy diet [5]. Australia also has its guidelines in a round plate-like format [6]. Canada's 'Food Guide for Healthy

Eating' depicts a rainbow with the outer bands being larger to indicate more servings [7]. Some countries also provide specific guidance for different populations and age groups, such as infants, children, pregnant or post-menopausal women, or for different ethnic groups.

In terms of evaluating the relative health benefits of dietary patterns, the Mediterranean diet stands out as the focus of considerable research. The Mediterranean diet is characterized by high consumption of vegetables, legumes, fruits and nuts, cereals and olive oil with low intake of saturated fat, moderately high intake of fish, low to moderate intake of dairy products, and low intake of meat [8]. The definition varies somewhat across studies, and in some includes a regular but moderate intake of alcohol during meals, primarily as red wine. A meta-analysis using data from more than a million healthy subjects and 40,000 fatal and non-fatal medical events, concluded that an increase of two points in the score used to measure the adherence to a Mediterranean diet was associated with 9% lower risk in both overall mortality and cardiovascular mortality, a 6% reduction in cancer incidence and mortality, and a 13% decline in the incidence of Parkinson's disease and Alzheimer's disease [9].

A life course approach recognizes that dietary patterns reflect a range of social and economic conditions that influence the availability and popularity of particular foods, as well as changing dietary requirements across life. Influences *in utero* and during early life, of which a major determining factor is maternal diet, both during pregnancy and after birth through breastfeeding, play critical roles in the subsequent healthy development of the child [10], and may well impact on adult health and disease risk [11]. In older age groups, numerous studies of diet indicate that between the ages of 40 and 70 years mean food intake levels fall by around 25% [12].

The foods that make up an individual's dietary intake are the result of choices based on a large number of factors related to the personal traits of the individual, which in turn are modified by influences of various types; these vary in impact across life depending on the circumstances and conditions in which the individual is living. Several models encompassing the many factors associated with food choice have been developed, one such originating from Cornell University (Figure 16.1). This model was the result of qualitative in-depth interviews which sought to clarify the interactions between personal and environmental influences [13].

The Food Choices Process model identifies an individual's 'personal system', which is made up of characteristics such as sensory perceptions, monetary considerations, convenience, health and nutrition, and personal relationships. The factors within this personal system contribute to the choices that a person makes when choosing foods to eat. The personal system is influenced by external factors, the social framework, the food context, other personal factors and ideals, all providing symbolic meaning that people associate with food. These influences are developed across life and influence the personal system in any food choice situation [13].

Of all the factors that influence the personal system those which have been found to be the most dominant and which are most stable across life are 'ideals'; those food habits and behaviours that are learned as people grow up and which provide their traditions, often dictated by their culture, religion or ethnicity, which they perceive to be the way 'things should be'. When applying the model to an older population, this characteristic was the most important of all influences [14]. Experiences across life were major factors in shaping food choices, but the most significant were those created in childhood [14,15]. These imprinted ideals remained important throughout life and into old age. For example, if childhood was associated with eating specific sit-down meals at certain times, then this would be a characteristic that would be dominant in food choice decisions. Similarly, cultural characteristics such as large family gatherings for Italians, even when relocated to other countries, remain from childhood into old age [16], in spite of major life events occurring in the intervening period [15]. It was only if a major turning point occurred that had

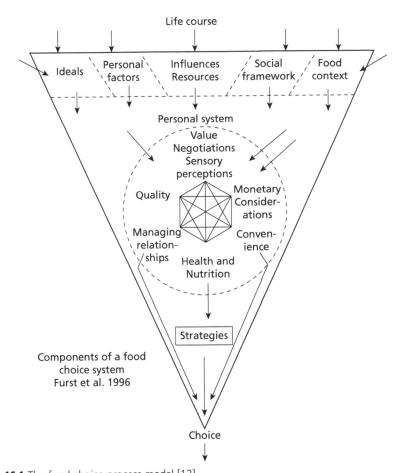

Figure 16.1 The food choice process model [13].

Reprinted from *Appetite*, Volume **26**, Issue 3, Furst T, et al., Food choice: A conceptual model of the process, pp. 247–65, Copyright © 1996, with permission from Elsevier.

such a dramatic impact on the way life was lived, that the pattern and influences on food choice made a major shift.

This conceptual research, when applied to the real world, indicates that many major food choice influences are developed early in life and are maintained throughout life and into older age. If early life is when ideals are developed, then this is the key time to influence food choice behaviour; and if those ideals are not conducive to a healthy diet early on, it is difficult to shift the ideals to one where healthier dietary choices will be made. In recent decades, the arrival of more convenient ways of eating, such as eating outside the home or buying takeaway meals to eat at home, have resulted in a gradual change in the norms of eating and the ideals adopted by many children and young adults. Given the dominance of ideals in determining food choice across life, these new ideals are likely to be maintained, with the likelihood that they will be difficult to change as future generations age.

The predominance of ideals driving food choices is challenged when major turning points occur. This can happen at any point in life, but in older age, major life changing events can have a dramatic influence on eating patterns and subsequently on health. A major problem which can lead to poor health and increased risk in older people is under-eating. Factors that lead to this include medical conditions, often including physical disability, oral health, depression, and reduced economic circumstances, often as a result of retirement, resulting in anxiety about the future. In a study of homebound older people, Locher and colleagues identified through interview that not being able to shop for food was a major barrier to adequate eating [17]. Being on a special diet because of a health condition led to lack of enthusiasm to eat, especially if the diet clashed with their normal eating pattern [16]. Problems with teeth and gums made eating difficult, often those foods that would normally be chosen, which took longer to eat [17].

Depression can have a major influence on food intake, even in otherwise healthy eaters, and can be brought on by loneliness and isolation, often the result of bereavement, or through a reduced sense of purpose following retirement or because of inability to carry out physical activities that were commonplace in earlier years [17]. Women appear to fare better than men, with their lifetime experience of preparing and caring about food [18], and a tendency to consume a healthier diet [18]. Older people with more social contacts tend to eat more and to have better quality diets, with more fruit and vegetables, especially if others actually eat with them [19].

16.3 Physical capability and lifetime diet and nutrition

This section highlights the role of lifetime diet and key nutrients for maintaining physical capability (the capacity to undertake the physical tasks of daily living; see Chapter 2) at older ages and reducing the loss of muscle mass and function (sarcopenia) that increases in prevalence with age [20,21].

16.3.1 Key nutrients associated with physical capability

Important nutrients shown to have an influence on physical capability include protein, omega-3 fatty acids, a range of antioxidant vitamins and vitamin D. In older populations, protein intake is hypothesized to be a key determinant of muscle strength, since amino acids from dietary protein are a stimulant of muscle protein synthesis [22,23]; and the type of protein may also be important [24–27]. Several population studies have found that dietary protein intake is associated with increased muscle mass and a lower rate of muscle loss after 3 years of follow-up [28]. However, findings from clinical trials on the use of protein supplementation in older populations to improve muscle mass and strength in combination with exercise have been mixed [29,30]. Protein intake has also been associated with grip strength and standing balance, but in one study this was mostly attenuated after adjustment for total energy intake [31]. Energy intake was also found to have a clear and consistent association with grip strength but no effect on standing balance. These findings also highlight the potential differential role of macronutrients on various aspects of physical capability, which are themselves differentiated by their varied requirements for balance, motor control, and mental concentration.

The manner in which protein is eaten through the day may also be important. Arnal and colleagues have identified that a 'pulse' or large dose of protein may be needed in older people to raise circulating amino acid concentration high enough to optimize uptake into muscle, an effect not seen in younger individuals [32–34]. Hence larger meals containing protein may be beneficial to maintain muscle mass in ageing, rather than smaller amounts of protein more often through the day.

Strong evidence exists for the beneficial effects of supplementation with omega-3 long-chain polyunsaturated fatty acids (n-3 LCPs), which are usually administered in the form of fish oil, on some inflammatory chronic diseases such as rheumatoid arthritis and other chronic inflammatory diseases [35,36].

Excessive oxidative stress is caused by the accumulation of reactive oxygen species and leads to macromolecular damage to cells and tissues, and thus is thought to be a causal factor in sarcopenia [37]. The Hertfordshire Cohort study examined consumption of a range of antioxidants and identified positive associations for β-carotene intakes with grip strength for both men and women, and for vitamin C intake for women [38]. The Invecchiare in Chianti (InCHIANTI) study of Italians aged 65 years and over found dose–response associations of vitamin C with knee extension strength and summary physical performance, and of β-carotene with knee extension strength [39] and reduced decline in muscular skeletal strength in men and women over 6 years of follow-up [40]. Antioxidant estimates obtained from self-reported food intakes may be subject to sizeable measurement error, whereas serum concentration of carotenoids provides an objective biomarker for fruit and vegetable consumption.

Findings from the Hertfordshire Cohort study also found links between selenium intake and grip strength in men and women, but not with other measures of physical capability [38], and a study from the US has shown similar results [41]. In the InCHIANTI study [39,40], there were relationships between serum concentrations of α-tocopherol on summary physical performance and γ-tocopherol on knee extension strength.

While only a small proportion of vitamin D is obtained from diet, its role is well established for bone health and hence is indirectly linked with physical capability. A meta-analysis of clinical trials concluded that supplementation of 700 to 800 IU/d appeared to reduce non-vertebral fractures among older people [42]. There is also evidence for its effect on muscle strength in the general population [43]. However, a recent meta-analysis of 17 randomized controlled trials mainly on older adults questioned the efficacy of supplementation to improve muscular strength for those who are not vitamin D deficient [44].

16.3.2 Foods, food groups, and dietary patterns associated with physical capability

With respect to findings from observational studies, the Hertfordshire Cohort study provides evidence for the influence of oily fish intake, as this was found to have both a strong cross-sectional association and a dose response [38]. It was estimated that, after adjusting for height, age and birthweight, each additional portion of oily fish consumed per week resulted in an increase in grip strength in men and women. No relationships were found between the consumption of white fish and shellfish and grip strength. While the effect sizes were markedly smaller than from oily fish, the Hertfordshire Cohort study also found that higher fruit and wholemeal cereal consumption was associated with higher grip strength for men and women, while vegetable consumption was similarly associated with grip strength for women [38].

In terms of dietary patterns, the InCHIANTI study showed that high adherence to a Mediterranean style diet was associated with slower decline of mobility over time in community-dwelling older persons [45].

Studies examining the long-term effects of diet and dietary patterns across life on physical capability are scarce. However some cohort studies suggest that similar relationships for dietary patterns can be identified in midlife and earlier. For instance, findings from the US Study of Women Across the Nation show that women with diets characterized by higher saturated and total fat intakes and lower fruit and vegetable consumption at age 42 to 52 years were more likely to have greater functional limitations [46]. This is consistent with an earlier study; the Whitehall II study found that among women, 'healthier' diets and greater fruit and vegetable consumption were associated with higher self-reported physical function in midlife [47].

16.4 Cognitive capability and lifetime diet and nutrition

Cognitive capability describes the capacity to undertake the mental tasks of daily living (Chapter 3) and provides another integrated marker for healthy ageing alongside physical capability. There is wide variation in the detailed objective metrics used for measuring cognitive capability; however they typically involve tests in the domains of memory, orientation, language, executive function, and praxis. A decline in all of these cognitive domains is expected with age, but the diagnostic threshold remains imprecise between this and pathological cognitive decline [48].

16.4.1 Key nutrients associated with cognitive capability

The main nutrients thought to be important for cognitive capability include n-3 LCPs, B vitamins, and antioxidants. One longitudinal study reported slower cognitive decline for diets high in unsaturated fat, and increased risk for those with high intakes of saturated fat [49]. However, in a recent systematic review, Plassman concluded that the evidence is currently inadequate to justify additional dietary recommendations to reduce the rate of cognitive decline [48].

The interest in n-3 LCPs and cognitive health is underscored by their presence in relatively high concentrations in the brain [50]. Numerous mechanisms for protective effects have been hypothesized, ranging from contributing to structural properties and functions of the neural membrane, to protecting against oxidative damage, as well as improved vascular function [51]. Reviews have pointed to the balance of evidence from observational studies indicating that n-3 LCPs, usually measured by dietary intake of oily fish, are associated with slower cognitive decline in older individuals, with two studies reporting a dose response for protective associations of n-3 LCPs on cognitive performance. A large French study of older people found that those who had a high intake of long-chain n-3 fatty acids and fish consumption reported fewer cognitive complaints 13 years later, after adjustment for socioeconomic and lifestyle factors, and depressive symptoms [52]. In contrast, a study from the UK found that such a link was greatly attenuated by other factors, including reported age at leaving full-time education [50,51]. Similarly, the US Veterans Affairs Normative Ageing study was unable to detect associations between n-3 LCPs and cognitive performance in older men over a 6-year follow-up, after adjustment for a range of confounders [53]. A recent systematic review of findings from seven randomized clinical trials of n-3 LCP supplementation among cognitively healthy and cognitively impaired older people concluded that the lack of consistent association does not support the use on n-3 LCPs for slowing the rate of cognitive decline [51].

While there has been a long held hypothesis that antioxidants can have protective effects against the oxidative damage that is thought to play a role in cognitive ageing, clear evidence from detailed studies to support their efficacy has been elusive. As a recent review on vitamin C points out [54], consideration of the digestion, metabolism, and excretion of micronutrients is essential and supplementation should not be assumed to result in markedly higher plasma concentrations. Estimating intakes is prone to greater measurement error than assessment of plasma concentrations. Harrison concluded that the evidence suggests some beneficial effects of a diet with adequate Vitamin C intake in reducing the rate of cognitive decline, rather than there being additional benefits from supplementation. A recent study of older people in the Oregon Brain Ageing study found that higher plasma concentrations of the biomarkers for vitamins B (B1, B2, B6, folate, and B12), C, D, and E were associated with healthier magnetic resonance imaging

(MRI) measures and better global cognitive function scores [55]. However, a systematic review that examined a comprehensive range of factors, including intake of the antioxidants vitamins C and E and beta-carotene in eight observational studies and clinical trials, concluded that the association with cognitive function was not consistently evident to recommend widespread supplementation among older people [48,56].

16.4.2 Food groups and dietary patterns associated with cognitive capability

In marked contrast to studies focusing on the role of a specific nutrient and cognitive outcomes, research on the role of food groups and dietary patterns remains scarce. This is critical when considering potential factors affecting the various domains of cognitive performance, which may involve synergistic effects between several or more nutrients. In a systematic review that focussed on nine cohort studies from the US and Europe, it was concluded that evidence supported the consumption of vegetables including legumes, but not fruit, as conferring protective effects for cognitive decline with age [57]. Associations have also been found in other populations; for example, vegetable and legume consumption was associated with slower cognitive decline among the 5000 participants (who were aged 65 years and over) in the Chinese Longitudinal Health Longevity study [58]. Evidence for the impact of other food groups on cognitive performance among older adults is both limited and inconsistent. For instance, in contrast with findings regarding the intake of unsaturated fat [49], another US study of community-dwelling older people identified a dose–response association between dietary intake of cheese and lower prevalence of cognitive impairment [59]. A recent systematic review of evidence from 37 prospective cohort studies (aged 65 years and older) concluded that the consumption of vegetables and fish has a beneficial effect on cognitive performance, whereas a diet high in saturated fat resulted in an increased risk of dementia [60].

In terms of dietary patterns, and aligned with the suggested role of n-3 LCPs and the effect of fish and vegetable consumption identified in populations studies, research has mainly focused on the impact of the Mediterranean diet. For instance, a large US prospective study that identified associations between vegetable and fish consumption and lower cognitive decline over a 6-year follow-up period [61,62], subsequently examined adherence to the Mediterranean dietary pattern and a healthy eating index, based on US dietary guidelines. After adjusting for a wide range of confounders, their findings showed a dose response, with a traditional Mediterranean diet associated with slower rates of cognitive decline, and this has been shown in similar studies [63].

Not all population studies have identified cognitive benefits of a Mediterranean diet. Adherence to a Mediterranean diet by participants in Bordeaux, who were part of the prospective Three City Cohort study in France, was associated with higher scores for only one of the cognitive tests applied and not for an overall cognitive measure [64]. An Australian longitudinal study found no evidence for a protective effect of a Mediterranean diet against cognitive decline over a 4-year period, although there was an association between excessive caloric intake and increased cognitive decline [65]. These inconsistent results suggest a number of potential issues, including the measurement of the Mediterranean diet, which in a number of studies does not distinguish between saturated and unsaturated fat, fish and oily fish. However, adherence to the Mediterranean dietary pattern in these studies does not necessarily mean that intakes of, for instance olive oil or fish, are equivalent to those in Greece, the reference culture for the Mediterranean diet [66].

Few longitudinal studies can examine the impact of dietary patterns on change in cognitive capability through midlife, while controlling for a wide range of other socioeconomic factors.

A recent study has shown that 'healthy dietary choice' at 36 and 43 years, based on a simple index for basic food choices and intakes of white or wholemeal bread and the number of portions of fresh fruit and vegetables, were associated with slower memory decline over 20 years, after adjusting for smoking and exercise, as well as socioeconomic position, sex, prior cognitive ability, and symptoms of anxiety and depression [67].

An alternative approach to an *a priori* determination of dietary patterns via a specified index is to use a data driven or *a posteriori* analysis to determine the clustering of foods into dietary patterns [68]. In a recent French study, where diet was first assessed in midlife (aged 45 years or more), two main dietary patterns were identified and labelled as 'healthy' and 'traditional' [69]. The 'healthy' diet was characterized by consumption of fruit (fresh and dried), whole grains, fresh dairy products, vegetables, breakfast cereal, tea, vegetable fat, nuts, and fish and was negatively correlated with meat and poultry, refined grains, animal fat, and processed meat intake. The findings showed that adherence to the 'healthy' pattern in middle-age, while sustaining controlled energy intake, was related to higher cognitive performance 13 years later, particularly verbal memory, than the 'traditional' dietary pattern.

Other research using the Whitehall II study has provided similar findings also using *a posteriori* analysis to investigate the effect of dietary patterns on cognitive deficit, defined as being in the lowest sex-specific quintile of cognitive performance. The findings suggested that a 'whole food' pattern (rich in fruit, vegetables, dried legume, and fish) was associated with lower odds of cognitive deficit, and a 'processed food' pattern (rich in processed meat, chocolates, sweet desserts, fried food, refined cereals, and high-fat dairy products) with higher odds. However, adjustment for education considerably attenuated these associations, indicating that education may be an important confounder in the association between nutrition and cognition [70].

16.5 Role of early diet on physical and cognitive capability and ageing

There have been no studies that have been able to define the role of early diet and nutrition on the ageing process consistently. Breastfeeding is found to be important for a range of physical and cognitive outcomes in childhood [71–74]. A recent review has highlighted that investigation of nutrition and diet in early life may clarify those factors that lead to a higher peak of physical capability attained in midlife, which acts as a baseline for subsequent decline in physical capability during later life (Chapter 2). Dietary patterns have been found to 'track' through childhood, and overall evidence suggests that early childhood diet affects physical capability, especially muscular strength, in later life [20]. There is limited evidence for the effect of dietary patterns during infancy, beyond breastfeeding, on subsequent cognitive performance; however, the influence of excessive weight gain in adolescence has been shown to be negatively associated with cognitive outcomes into adulthood [75].

16.6 Challenges and future directions

Overall there has been more longitudinal research investigating the effects of nutrients than of food groups and dietary patterns on physical and cognitive capability, but the evidence is often inconsistent. There is evidence to suggest that a role of some components of diet, such as fresh vegetables and oily fish as part of a 'healthy' or Mediterranean dietary pattern, is likely to have some beneficial effects on healthy ageing. At this time, however, it is not possible to move beyond that position to make other recommendations. For instance, there is insufficient evidence to support universal supplementation of older people to promote healthy ageing, though supplements may be prescribed as part the treatment of specific conditions. The first priority is to ensure that older people maintain a healthy diet with sufficient intakes to avoid inadequacy in dietary components.

The study of the effects of diet on healthy ageing highlights some of the issues fundamental to observational studies. Given that conditions such as dementia can take decades to develop, the effects of dietary intake may also need to accumulate over a similar or longer time frame, and this is a major limitation of randomized trials. Even where associations may have been detected, findings from observational studies on diet are greatly limited in terms of the implications for inferring causality. Cross-sectional studies provide a snapshot view and typically rely on retrospective data recalled by participants, although analysis of repeat data from cohort studies nevertheless provides evidence of association rather than causality. However evidence of a dose response association between exposure and outcome obtained from cohort studies will help strengthen the case that the association is indicative of a causal pathway.

Since diet and nutrition are a deeply embedded part of daily life and influenced by a broad array of social, cultural, and economic factors, this may mean that confounding and potential bias are particularly serious issues for observational studies. For instance, it may be difficult to unravel the influence of specific nutrients from more global measures of diet since intakes of food groups tend to correlate or cluster with each other, whereby individuals with high fruit and vegetable consumption are also more likely to have low saturated fat intake, which also leads to clustering of nutrient intakes such as the antioxidants beta-carotenes and vitamin C. Davey Smith illustrated the point with respect to the evidence from observational studies of a positive association between vitamin E and vitamin C intake and the reduced risk of coronary heart disease, associations that were not replicated in randomized controlled trials [76]. As he points out, the associations identified in the British Women's Heart and Health study were largely attenuated, once the confounding factors across life were controlled for.

Reverse causation is another well recognized issue with cross-sectional studies; for instance participants may have adopted an unhealthy diet as a result of early cognitive decline (prior to its clinical diagnosis). The problem remains with prospective cohort studies. For instance, as Richards [77,78] has pointed out children with higher cognitive capability may, as adults, choose to have better diets; even if the study controls for the family social background or other socioeconomic factors the possibility of reverse causation will not be eliminated. Evidence of an association may also reflect a common cause for both the explanatory and outcome variable, in this case some characteristic of diet, and an indicator of healthy ageing. A plausible example may be the influence of socioeconomic deprivation leading to not only a poor diet but also depression, lack of social engagement, and hence risk of increased cognitive decline [79].

Over the last decade, a number of innovative approaches have emerged that, although restricted in the scope of their application, attempt to address some of these limitations of conventional observational studies. These include Mendelian randomization studies, epigenetic studies and cross cohort studies (Chapters 5 and 15). In addition, there have been substantial advances in the use of biomarkers to provide more objective markers for certain nutritional exposures.

Epidemiological research on diet and healthy ageing would still benefit substantially from improvements in existing cohort studies and new observational studies. The current state of evidence suggests these changes should include:

♦ repeated measures of dietary intake and physical and cognitive capability across the life course, since effects may be modest and cumulative

♦ use of established measurement methods and variables, such as for food intakes and classification of dietary patterns, so that they are comparable across studies

♦ dietary intakes from food diaries that are complemented by the collection of biological markers for nutritional components

♦ inclusion of wide-ranging potential confounders, so that the effects of diet can be identified in context of other lifestyle factors and the broader socioeconomic environment

♦ a focus on data collection in early midlife and with respect to parenting, to capture information about intergenerational dietary influences.

16.7 **Conclusions**

Research on healthy ageing is framed around the notion of a trajectory for physical and cognitive capability that rises in early life and reaches its peak in adulthood, that acts as a reserve of capability, and that needs to be maintained in midlife with the aim of slowing the progressive rate of decline with age. However many findings with respect to the influence of diet still rely on research that focuses on risk factors to reduce chronic disease in later life, rather than to optimize healthy ageing. Considerable further research is also needed to investigate the effect of diet on the shape of this trajectory, for instance the different rates of decline of the various domains of physical and cognitive capability in midlife and later life.

Another theme that has emerged from this overview is that if dietary effects are both modest and cumulative, then the research needed to provide a more robust evidence base with causal pathways identified for the role of diet on healthy ageing may lie beyond the resolution of many current cohort and clinical studies.

It is not surprising therefore that, in terms of healthy ageing outcomes, there is little evidence for intakes *beyond* current guidelines for healthy diets and avoidance of inadequacy in dietary components; and also beyond what might be already prescribed for treatment of specific chronic disease, such as supplementation of vitamin D among the elderly to improve bone health. The balance of evidence does appear to suggest that aspects of healthy diets, as specified in guidelines for dietary patterns, could be highlighted for additional benefits for healthy ageing:

♦ long-term benefits of breastfeeding and healthy childhood nutrition

♦ an emphasis on consumption of vegetables, particularly cruciferous vegetables

♦ an emphasis on the consumption of fish, especially oily fish.

To the extent that the Mediterranean dietary pattern is distinguished from the above, it may have further protective effects in slowing some aspects of physical and cognitive decline, although the evidence is far from unequivocal.

Even though diet may only result in modest effects for an individual over the long term, it has the potential to aggregate to substantial benefits for the population, and for worthwhile public health policy, with little indication of negative consequences. The effects may also increase with greater understanding of the interaction and optimal combinations of dietary and other lifestyle interventions, such as physical activity. Above all, epidemiological research should recognize that dietary patterns are deeply embedded in social and cultural context, rather than view these aspects just as potential confounders for effects of diet on healthy ageing. The Mediterranean diet, in a traditional sense, signifies far more than the consumption of certain foods, but a lifestyle that celebrates visiting markets to select fresh seasonal vegetables, fish, and other ingredients for home cooked meals; in other words, an opportunity for regular social engagement, cognitive stimulation, and physical activity.

References

1 **Stanner SA, et al.** A review of the epidemiological evidence for the 'antioxidant hypothesis'. *Public Health Nutr* 2004;7:407–22.

2 **Kant AK.** Dietary patterns and health outcomes. *J Am Diet Assoc* 2004;**104**:615–35.

3 **United States Department of Agriculture.** Food Guide Pyramid 2012. Available from <http://www.choosemyplate.gov/food-groups/downloads/MyPyramid_Food_Intake_Patterns.pdf>

4 United States Department of Agriculture. Choosemyplate 2012. Available from: <http://www.choosemyplate.gov>

5 **National Health Service U.** The eatwell plate 2012. <http://www.nhs.uk/livewell/goodfood/pages/eatwell-plateaspx>.

6 **Australian Government National Health and Medical Research 2012.** <http://www.nhmrc.gov.au/_files_nhmrc/publications/attachments/n31.pdf>

7 **Canada's food guide to healthy eating 2007.** <http://www.hc-sc.gc.ca/fn-an/food-guide-aliment/index-eng.php>

8 **Trichopoulou A, et al.** Adherence to a Mediterranean diet and survival in a Greek population. *New Engl J Med* 2003;**348**:2599–608.

9 **Sofi F, et al.** Adherence to Mediterranean diet and health status: meta-analysis. *BMJ* 2008;**337**:a1344

10 **Lennox AMBJ, Buttriss JL, Gibson-Moore H.** Maternal nutrition and infant feeding: current practice and recommendations. In: British Nutrition Foundation and Buttris JL, editors. Nutrition and Development: Long and Short Term Consequences for Health. A Report of the British Nutrition Foundation Task Force. West Sussex: Wiley Blackwell; 2013.

11 **Barker DJP.** Fetal and Infant Origins of Adult Disease. London: BMJ Books; 1992.

12 **Nieuwenhuizen WF, et al.** Older adults and patients in need of nutritional support: review of current treatment options and factors influencing nutritional intake. *Clin Nutr* 2010;**29**:160–9.

13 **Furst T, et al.** Food choice: a conceptual model of the process. *Appetite* 1996;**26**:247–65.

14 **Falk LW, et al.** Food choice processes of older adults: a qualitative investigation. *J Nutr Educ* 1996;**28**: 257–65.

15 **Edstrom KM, Devine CM.** Consistency in women's orientations to food and nutrition in midlife and older age: a 10-year qualitative follow-up. *J Nutr Educ* 2001;**33**:215–23.

16 **Devine CM, et al.** Food choices in three ethnic groups: interactions of ideals, identities, and roles. *J Nutr Educ* 1999;**31**:86–93.

17 **Locher JL, et al.** A multidimensional approach to understanding under-eating in homebound older adults: the importance of social factors. *Gerontologist* 2008;**48**:223–34.

18 **Hughes G, et al.** Old and alone: barriers to healthy eating in older men living on their own. *Appetite* 2004;**43**:269–76.

19 **Locher JL, et al.** The effect of the presence of others on caloric intake in homebound older adults. *J Gerontol A Biol Sci Med Sci* 2005;**60**:1475–8.

20 **Robinson S, et al.** Nutrition and sarcopenia: a review of the evidence and implications for preventive strategies. *J Aging Res* 2012;**2012**:510801.

21 **Paddon-Jones D, et al.** Role of dietary protein in the sarcopenia of aging. *Am J Clin Nutr* 2008;**87**: 1562S–6S.

22 **Wolfe RR, et al.** Optimal protein intake in the elderly. *Clin Nutr* 2008;**27**:675–84.

23 **Kim JS, et al.** Dietary implications on mechanisms of sarcopenia: roles of protein, amino acids and antioxidants. *J Nutr Biochem* 2010;**21**:1–13.

24 **Lord C, et al.** Dietary animal protein intake: association with muscle mass index in older women. *J Nutr Health Aging* 2007;**11**:383–7.

25 **Pennings B, et al.** Amino acid absorption and subsequent muscle protein accretion following graded intakes of whey protein in elderly men. *Am J Physiol Endocrinol Metab* 2012;**302**:E992–9.

26 **Katsanos CS, et al.** A high proportion of leucine is required for optimal stimulation of the rate of muscle protein synthesis by essential amino acids in the elderly. *Am J Physiol Endocrinol Metab* 2006;**291**:E381–7.

27 **Wall BT, et al.** Leucine co-ingestion improves post-prandial muscle protein accretion in elderly men. *Clin Nutr* 2013;**32**:412–9.

28 **Houston DK, et al.** Dietary protein intake is associated with lean mass change in older, community-dwelling adults: the Health, Aging, and body Composition (Health ABC) study. *Am J Clin Nutr* 2008;**87**: 150–5.

29 **Beasley JM, et al.** Protein intake and incident frailty in the Women's Health Initiative Observational study. *J Am Geriatr Soc* 2010;**58**:1063–71.

30 **Tieland M, et al.** Protein supplementation improves physical performance in frail elderly people: a randomized, double-blind, placebo-controlled trial. *J Am Med Dir Assoc* 2012;**13**:720–6.

31 **Mulla UZ, et al.** Adult macronutrient intake and physical capability in the MRC National Survey of Health and Development. *Age Ageing* 2013;**42**:81–7.

32 **Arnal MA, et al.** Protein pulse feeding improves protein retention in elderly women. *Am J Clin Nutr* 1999;**69**:1202–8.

33 **Arnal MA, et al.** Protein feeding pattern does not affect protein retention in young women. *J Nutr* 2000;**130**:1700–4.

34 **Arnal MA, et al.** Pulse protein feeding pattern restores stimulation of muscle protein synthesis during the feeding period in old rats. *J Nutr* 2002;**132**:1002–8.

35 **Calder PC.** n-3 polyunsaturated fatty acids, inflammation, and inflammatory diseases. *Am J Clin Nutr* 2006;**83**:1505S–19S.

36 **Berbert AA, et al.** Supplementation of fish oil and olive oil in patients with rheumatoid arthritis. *Nutrition* 2005;**21**:131–6.

37 **Fulle S, et al.** The contribution of reactive oxygen species to sarcopenia and muscle ageing. *Exp Gerontol* 2004;**39**:17–24.

38 **Robinson SM, et al.** Diet and its relationship with grip strength in community-dwelling older men and women: the Hertfordshire cohort study. *J Am Geriatr Soc* 2008;**56**:84–90.

39 **Cesari M, et al.** Antioxidants and physical performance in elderly persons: the Invecchiare in Chianti (InCHIANTI) study. *Am J Clin Nutr* 2004;**79**:289–94.

40 **Lauretani F, et al.** Low plasma carotenoids and skeletal muscle strength decline over 6 years. *J Gerontol A Biol Sci Med Sci* 2008;**63**:376–83.

41 **Alipanah N, et al.** Low serum carotenoids are associated with a decline in walking speed in older women. *J Nutr Health Aging* 2009;**13**:170–5.

42 **Bischoff-Ferrari HA, et al.** Fracture prevention with vitamin D supplementation: a meta-analysis of randomized controlled trials. *JAMA* 2005;**293**:2257–64.

43 **Grimaldi AS, et al.** 25(OH) Vitamin D is associated with greater muscle strength in healthy men and women. *Med Sci Sports Exerc* 2013;**45**:157–62.

44 **Stockton KA, et al.** Effect of vitamin D supplementation on muscle strength: a systematic review and meta-analysis. *Osteoporos Int* 2011;**22**:859–71.

45 **Milaneschi Y, et al.** Mediterranean diet and mobility decline in older persons. *Exp Gerontol* 2011;**46**:303–8.

46 **Tomey KM, et al.** Dietary intake related to prevalent functional limitations in midlife women. *Am J Epidemiol* 2008;**167**:935–43.

47 **Stafford M, et al.** Behavioural and biological correlates of physical functioning in middle aged office workers: the UK Whitehall II study. *J Epidemiol Community Health.* 1998;**52**:353–8.

48 Plassman BL, et al. Systematic review: factors associated with risk for and possible prevention of cognitive decline in later life. *Ann Intern Med* 2010;**153**:182–93.

49 Morris MC, et al. Dietary fat intake and 6-year cognitive change in an older biracial community population. *Neurology* 2004;**62**:1573–9.

50 Dangour AD, et al. Fish consumption and cognitive function among older people in the UK: baseline data from the OPAL study. *J Nutr Health Aging* 2009;**13**:198–202.

51 Dangour AD, et al. Omega 3 fatty acids and cognitive health in older people. *Br J Nutr* 2012;**107**:S152–8.

52 Kesse-Guyot E, et al. Adherence to nutritional recommendations and subsequent cognitive performance: findings from the prospective Supplementation with Antioxidant Vitamins and Minerals 2 (SU.VI.MAX 2) study. *Am J Clin Nutr* 2011;**93**:200–10.

53 van de Rest O, et al. Intakes of (n-3) fatty acids and fatty fish are not associated with cognitive performance and 6-year cognitive change in men participating in the Veterans Affairs Normative Aging study. *J Nutr* 2009;**139**:2329–36.

54 Harrison FE. A critical review of vitamin C for the prevention of age-related cognitive decline and Alzheimer's disease. *J Alzheimers Dis* 2012;**29**:711–26.

55 Bowman GL, et al. Nutrient biomarker patterns, cognitive function, and MRI measures of brain aging. *Neurology* 2012;**78**:241–9.

56 Daviglus ML, et al. National Institutes of Health state-of-the-science conference statement: preventing Alzheimer disease and cognitive decline. *Ann Intern Med* 2010;**153**:176–81.

57 Loef M, Walach H. Fruit, vegetables and prevention of cognitive decline or dementia: a systematic review of cohort studies. *J Nutr Health Aging* 2012;**16**:626–30.

58 Chen X, et al. Lower intake of vegetables and legumes associated with cognitive decline among illiterate elderly Chinese: a 3-year cohort study. *J Nutr Health Aging* 2012;**16**:549–52.

59 Rahman A, et al. Dietary factors and cognitive impairment in community-dwelling elderly. *J Nutr Health Aging* 2007;**11**:49–54.

60 Lee Y, et al. Systematic review of health behavioral risks and cognitive health in older adults. *Int Psychogeriatr* 2010;**22**:174–87.

61 Morris MC, et al. Associations of vegetable and fruit consumption with age-related cognitive change. *Neurology* 2006;**67**:1370–6.

62 Morris MC, et al. Fish consumption and cognitive decline with age in a large community study. *Arch Neurol* 2005;**62**:1849–53.

63 Scarmeas N, et al. Mediterranean diet and mild cognitive impairment. *Arch Neurol* 2009;**66**:216–25.

64 Feart C, et al. Adherence to a Mediterranean diet, cognitive decline, and risk of dementia. *JAMA* 2009;**302**:638–48.

65 Cherbuin N, Anstey KJ. The Mediterranean diet is not related to cognitive change in a large prospective investigation: the PATH Through Life study. *Am J Geriatr Psychiatry* 2012;**20**:635–9.

66 Tangney CC, et al. Adherence to a Mediterranean-type dietary pattern and cognitive decline in a community population. *Am J Clin Nutr* 2011;**93**:601–7.

67 Cadar D, et al. The role of lifestyle behaviors on 20-year cognitive decline. *J Aging Res* 2012;**2012**:304014.

68 Mishra G, et al. Dietary patterns of Australian adults and their association with socioeconomic status: results from the 1995 National Nutrition Survey. *Eur J Clin Nutr* 2002;**56**:687–93.

69 Kesse-Guyot E, et al. A healthy dietary pattern at midlife is associated with subsequent cognitive performance. *J Nutr* 2012;**142**:909–15.

70 Akbaraly TN, et al. Education attenuates the association between dietary patterns and cognition. *Dement Geriatr Cogn Disord* 2009;**27**:147–54.

71 Artero EG, et al. Longer breastfeeding is associated with increased lower body explosive strength during adolescence. *J Nutr* 2010;**140**:1989–95.

72 **Robinson SM, et al.** Variations in infant feeding practice are associated with body composition in childhood: a prospective cohort study. *J Clin Endocrinol Metab* 2009;**94**:2799–805.

73 **Anderson JW, et al.** Breast-feeding and cognitive development: a meta-analysis. *Am J Clin Nutr* 1999;**70**:525–35.

74 **Richards M, et al.** Long-term effects of breast-feeding in a national birth cohort: educational attainment and midlife cognitive function. *Public Health Nutr* 2002;**5**:631–5.

75 **Richards M, et al.** Birthweight, postnatal growth and cognitive function in a national UK birth cohort. *Int J Epidemiol* 2002;**31**:342–8

76 **Davey Smith G.** Use of genetic markers and gene-diet interactions for interrogating population-level causal influences of diet on health. *Genes Nutr* 2011;**6**:27–43.

77 **Richards M.** Childhood intelligence and being a vegetarian. *BMJ* 2007;**334**:216–7.

78 **Richards M, et al.** Health returns to cognitive capital in the British 1946 birth cohort. *Longit Life Course Stud* 2010;**1**:281–96.

79 **Shatenstein B, et al.** Diet quality and cognition among older adults from the NuAge study. *Exp Gerontol* 2012;**47**:353–60.

Chapter 17

Lifetime lifestyles II: physical activity, the life course, and ageing

Ulf Ekelund

17.1 Introduction

17.1.1 Physical activity—a key factor for lifelong health

Physical activity is one of the most powerful modifiable lifestyle factors affecting health across life. Substantial evidence has emerged over the last 50 years clearly demonstrating that low levels of physical activity are one of the major contributors to morbidity and mortality from non-communicable diseases. Importantly, this is not limited to developed countries but also extends to developing countries. Based on this evidence, the World Health Organization has recognized physical inactivity as the fourth leading risk factor for premature mortality after high blood pressure, tobacco use and high blood glucose levels [1]. Considering the beneficial effects of physical activity on blood pressure, blood glucose levels, and other metabolic risk factors this estimate is likely conservative.

The benefits from physical activity also extend beyond physical health. Regular physical activity is associated with better self-rated quality of life, improved sleep, reduced stress, as well as stronger relationships with friends and social interactions [2]. While much of our understanding of the health benefits associated with physical activity are derived from observational and exercise training studies in middle-aged adults, evidence clearly suggests that physical activity is positively associated with health outcomes across life.

17.1.2 Key definitions

Key definitions of physical activity, exercise, sedentary behaviour, energy expenditure and related concepts are summarized in the text box (Box 17.1). *Physical activity* is distinct from *exercise* as the latter is only a sub-component of physical activity done with a specific purpose (e.g. to improve health or fitness). Physical activity *intensity* is the physiological effort associated with physical activity and can be defined as multiples of resting energy expenditure, so called metabolic equivalent tasks (MET). One MET is equal to resting energy expenditure (REE) and moderate intensity physical activity (MPA) is defined as 3–4 METs (i.e. 3–4 times REE), whereas vigorous intensity physical activity (VPA) is performed at an intensity >6 METs. *Physical inactivity* should not be used interchangeably with *sedentary behaviour*. Physical inactivity refers to individuals or groups of people who do not meet current recommendations for public health whereas sedentary behaviour is any behaviour characterized by low energy expenditure while sitting or reclining. *Exercise capacity* refers to the ability to be physically active and is mainly determined by the individual's *maximal cardiorespiratory fitness*. The possibility to improve or maintain a high level of

Box 17.1: Useful definitions

Physical activity* (PA): body movement by skeletal muscles which increase energy expenditure above resting levels.

Exercise*: a subcomponent of PA, which is structured, repetitive, and performed with the purpose to improve physical function, health or wellbeing.

Physical inactivity: usually defined as not meeting physical activity recommendations for public health.

Sedentary behaviour: any waking behaviour characterized by low energy expenditure (<1.5 times REE) while sitting or reclining (Sedentary Behaviour Research Network. Standardized use of the terms 'sedentary' and 'sedentary behaviours'. *Appl Physiol Nutr Metab* 2012;**37**: 540–42).

Intensity: the physiological demand (work load) associated with activity usually defined as multiples of REE, so called *metabolic equivalents* (METs).

Resting energy expenditure (REE): amount of energy required for maintaining body functions during rest. REE is similar to basal metabolic rate (BMR) which is defined as the minimal amount of energy required for maintaining body functions following an overnight fasting rest.

Total energy expenditure (TEE): total amount of energy expended per unit of time, usually per day and measured as MJ/day.

Physical activity energy expenditure (PAEE): amount of energy expended in physical activity calculated as TEE minus REE.

Physical fitness*: a set of attributes an individual has or achieves that relate to the ability to be physically active. Physical fitness is usually categorized into performance related fitness and health related fitness.

Health related fitness*: includes components such as cardiorespiratory fitness (CRF), muscular strength, flexibility and endurance.

Cardiorespiratory fitness (CRF)*: the body's function to utilize oxygen to generate energy for work. Limiting factors for CRF include the heart's ability to deliver blood (cardiac output) and the enzyme systems in the mitochondrion involved in ATP generating processes.

Endurance: the ability to perform physical activity continuously for extended periods of time without interruption.

cardiorespiratory fitness (i.e. trainability) across life is associated with longevity, wellbeing and independence in later life.

17.2 **Measurement of physical activity**

While cardiorespiratory fitness can be precisely measured in the laboratory, free-living measurements of physical activity in large population-based samples are more complicated. Assessment of physical activity can be undertaken using self-report or objective monitoring, the latter either by direct measurement of body movement (e.g. by accelerometry), by a physiological response to body movement (e.g. change in heart rate), or a combination of both.

17.2.1 **Self-report methods**

Self-report methods of physical activity assessment, for example questionnaires, are the cheapest and arguably simplest method of assessing physical activity and may be the only feasible method in the majority of large observational studies.

However, all self-report methods have some unavoidable limitations, as they are subject to recall bias. This can be intentional or accidental false recall, missed recall or differential reporting accuracy of different intensities (usually sub-categorized into sedentary, light, moderate and vigorous intensity), and domains (e.g. work, transport, recreational and domestic related activity) of activity. The subjective classification of intensity is also a problem with all self-report methods, and contributes to the large variation in error in between-individual estimates of physical activity.

Another limitation of many questionnaires is that they tend to measure only one aspect of physical activity such as sport participation or time spent in moderate to vigorous physical activity (MVPA). Participation in discrete activities (e.g. structured exercise) is generally more accurately recalled by self-report methods, as the individual has made a conscious decision to carry out that activity in a defined period of time. However, habitual or total everyday physical activity is much more difficult to capture accurately with self-report methods; it is generally considered that self-report methods are inaccurate for individual and group estimation of physical activity energy expenditure (PAEE) as they either over- or underestimate PAEE [3]. Despite these limitations, many recently developed questionnaires have been shown to be valid for categorizing individuals into discrete groups of activity (i.e. inactive, moderately inactive, moderately active, and active) and for ranking individuals [4]. The reader is referred to recent systematic reviews for a more detailed description of the reliability and validity of various self-reported methods to assess physical activity [3,4].

17.2.2 **Objective measurement of physical activity**

17.2.2.1 Accelerometry

Acceleration is a change in velocity over time ($m \cdot s^{-2}$) and therefore quantifies the frequency, duration, and intensity of body movement. Acceleration is measured in one (vertical), two (vertical and medio-lateral), or three directions. Most commonly used accelerometers are placed around the waist (close to the body's centre of gravity), but can be attached to other body segments (e.g. wrist, ankle, or thigh). Accelerometry can accurately determine time spent in ambulatory activities, time spent in different activity intensities, and time spent sedentary. However, accelerometry cannot accurately capture the limited vertical movement of some activities, such as cycling, and is also unable to assess an increase in energy expenditure while carrying an external load. Attempts have been made to use accelerometer data as the basis for developing PAEE prediction equations. The key issue here is whether laboratory-derived prediction equations can be generalized to the everyday, free-living situation. This, in turn, is dependent on the range of activities included in the laboratory study that produced the prediction equations. The majority of studies have used sedentary activities and activities with mainly vertical movements to derive the prediction equations, which appear to be valid in laboratory settings but not necessarily in free living [5].

One of the biggest challenges facing researchers is to choose the most accurate and appropriate method for interpreting accelerometry data due to the wide range of published methods. There is no consensus on how to define thresholds for different intensity levels based on accelerometry output. Accelerometry intensity thresholds are levels of movement (counts per minute; cpm) that are equivalent to different activity intensities (e.g. moderate and vigorous intensity activity). Unfortunately, the wide range of different thresholds used affects comparability between studies.

For example, the lower cut-point for moderate intensity activity varies by a factor of 17 in different studies of adults [6]. When these different cut-points were applied in the same population they provided substantially different estimates of both time spent in different intensity levels and the proportion of the population categorized as physically active, despite the same underlying data [5].

17.2.2.2 Heart rate monitoring and combined heart rate and movement sensing

Increased heart rate is a physiological response to an increase in physical activity and thereby indicates energy expenditure. The principle underlying the heart rate method of assessing physical activity is the linear relationship between heart rate and energy expenditure during aerobic exercise when using large muscle groups (e.g. legs while walking). The primary outcome measure is heart rate, which can be used to estimate time spent in different intensity levels of activity (e.g. moderate and vigorous intensity) using absolute heart rate data (i.e. above a predetermined heart rate threshold) or relative to the individual's maximal heart rate. A secondary outcome measure is PAEE estimated using regression equations derived from individual or group calibrations. Assessment of physical activity using heart rate is problematic at low levels of activity, as the assumption of a linear relationship between heart rate and physical activity is more often met at higher intensities of activity. A number of techniques have been devised to overcome the limitations of heart rate monitoring including individual calibration, and the use of heart rate indices [7].

Both heart rate monitoring and accelerometry have known errors when used to assess free-living physical activity. As these errors are not positively correlated, it has been suggested that combining heart rate monitoring with measurement of body movement by accelerometry may overcome some of these limitations [8]. For example, at lower intensity levels, heart rate is less accurate at estimating energy expenditure whereas at low intensity levels accelerometery has low error. Conversely, activities performed at high intensity are assessed with greater uncertainty by accelerometry. Further, activities not measured well by accelerometry such as cycling, walking on an incline, carrying weights, and those involving predominantly upper-body work are captured well by heart rate monitoring [9,10]. Additionally, the heart rate signal can be used to detect non-wearing time segments, since differentiating between inactivity and a monitor not worn is impossible using the acceleration signal alone.

Both accelerometry and combined heart rate and movement sensing have recently been used to assess free-living physical activity in relatively large epidemiological studies of children and adults. These have begun to contribute to our understanding of population levels of activity and their associations with health outcomes. For further details on additional methods, their feasibility, reliability and validity the reader is referred to the Medical Research Council toolkit for dietary and physical activity assessment <http://dapa-toolkit.mrc.ac.uk/index.html>.

17.3 Age-related changes in physical activity, sedentary time, and cardiorespiratory fitness

17.3.1 Variation in physical activity and sedentary time by age

Descriptive surveillance data comparing differences in physical activity by age and sex from different sources are consistent in two ways. First, physical activity levels decline by age in adulthood; and second, men are more active than women across age groups. These observations appear generalizable across cultures and ethnic groups regardless of whether physical activity has been assessed by self-report or objectively.

Data on objectively measured physical activity levels from large observational studies of young people in Europe and North America suggest a consistent decline in physical activity from childhood through to puberty [11,12]. One of the most comprehensive datasets available on self-reported physical activity in adulthood is the World Health Organization (WHO) global health observatory data repository which combines data from 122 countries representing approximately 89% of the world population [13]. Using this dataset, a consistent linear decline by age in the proportion of adults who were physically active was observed, although the differences between geographical regions were substantial. For example, older adults (>60 years) from South East Asia were considerably more active than individuals of the same age from other regions and were also more active than younger adults (15–29 years) from most other regions [13]. The overall declines by age were also observed for vigorous intensity physical activity and for walking.

Similar age-related differences in physical activity are also observed when using objectively measured data from population-based samples from Norway, Portugal, UK and the US [14–17]. Figure 17.1 displays the mean time spent in MVPA in these populations by age-group. Data from Norway were averaged into two groups (20–64 year and >64 years) whereas data from other countries were stratified into age bands. While significant heterogeneity across countries is evident, declining MVPA levels by age are substantial and remarkably pronounced in British and American populations. For example, middle-aged British and American men and women accumulated about three to four times as much time in MVPA compared to older men and women. Another striking difference when comparing the data from different countries is that older adults in Norway and Portugal accumulated about twice as much time in MVPA compared with those in the UK and US. While selection bias and measurement differences may explain some of the differences between studies, cultural and environmental differences are likely to be the main contributors to the observed population differences.

Age-related patterns of time spent sedentary are not equally consistent. Data on objectively measured time spent sedentary in a representative US sample suggest that on average about 55% of time during the day is spent sedentary with the greatest proportions of time spent sedentary observed in older adolescents and older adults (> 60 years). Sedentary time increased linearly in both men and women from about age 30 reaching close to 75% of daytime in those older than 75 [18]. Similar data obtained by accelerometry from Portugal confirmed the increase in sedentary time between ages 10 and 17 years, with a levelling off between 18 and 29 and small increases thereafter with those aged > 65 spending more than 70% of the daytime sedentary [15]. In contrast smaller age-related increases in sedentary time have been reported in Norway [14]. In summary, data on objectively measured sedentary time by accelerometry indicate high levels of sedentariness during adolescence and in older adults post retirement.

17.3.2 Time trends in physical activity

Mechanization, urbanization and technological developments have led to remarkable changes in the way we live our lives and our behaviours, including physical activity. Many of the current generation of older adults grew up in an environment characterized by manual labour and active transportation completely different from today's modern society which is characterized by automobile dependence, traffic congestion, and sedentary occupations. Unfortunately, robust data on population trends in physical activity over long time periods are scarce.

In a comprehensive review of the available time trend data from the US [19] it was concluded that leisure time physical activity has increased slightly over the last 50 years whereas physical activity in all other domains including work, home and transportation have declined, suggesting an overall decline in total physical activity. Major contributors to this trend included changes to

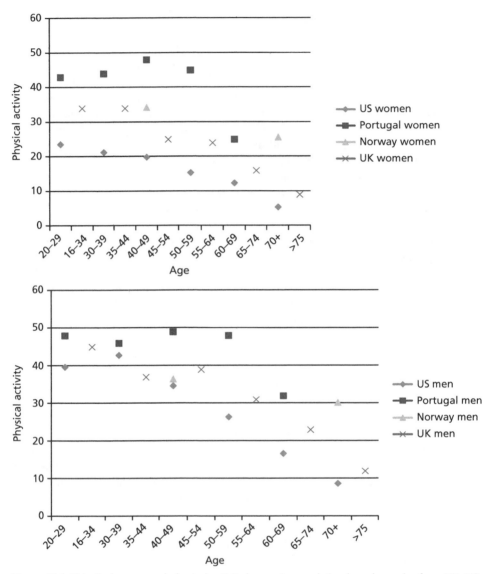

Figure 17.1 Objectively measured physical activity by age in population-based samples from UK, US, Norway, Portugal, in women and men.

Source: data from Hansen BH, et al. Accelerometer-determined physical activity in adults and older people, *Medicine and Science in Sports and Exercise*, Volume **44**, Issue 2, pp. 266–72, Copyright © 2012; Baptista F, et al. Prevalence of the Portuguese population attaining sufficient physical activity. *Medicine and Science in Sports and Exercise*, Volume **44**, Issue 4, pp. 466–73, Copyright © 2012; Troiano RP, et al. Physical activity in the United States measured by accelerometer, *Medicine and Science in Sports and Exercise*, Volume **40**, Issue 1, pp. 181–8, Copyright © 2008 and Townsend N, et al, Physical Activity Statistics, British Heart Foundation, London, Copyright © 2012.

the built environment and an increasing proportion of the population being sedentary [19]. These observations are supported by more recent US data suggesting that work-related physical activity energy expenditure has fallen by more than 100 kcal per day over the last 50 years [20]. Although consistent increases over time in leisure time physical activity including sport participation at all ages, including older age groups, have been reported in several countries [21–26] it is unclear whether this compensates for the decline in activity in other domains. Further, these results should be interpreted in light of the overall low levels of physical activity in older adults.

While temporal trend data on sedentary behaviours are scarce, available evidence from Australia suggests that small increases in transport related sedentary time have occurred between 1997 and 2006 whereas leisure sedentary time has remained stable [27]. In this study about 10–12% of women and 16–18% of men were reported to spend more than 2 hours of sitting time in cars each day [27]. Repeated cross-sectional surveys in representative samples of the population using precise assessment methods are required to properly understand future time trends in physical activity and sedentary behaviour.

17.3.3 **Variation in cardiorespiratory fitness by age**

Maximal cardiorespiratory fitness is measured by indirect calorimetry during an exercise test to exhaustion or estimated from a sub-maximal test (e.g. step test) and is one of the most important factors influencing an individual's ability to exercise, participate in recreational activities and engage in active living.

Cardiorespiratory fitness is largely determined by age, sex, body composition, lifestyle and heritability. It is one of the strongest predictors of all-cause mortality with risk estimates comparable to those for hypertension, smoking, elevated cholesterol levels and chronic illness [28]. In normal healthy individuals, data suggest that maximal cardiorespiratory fitness increases by age up to about 20 to 30 years and thereafter declines by about 8–10% per decade [29]. Longitudinal studies have suggested a steeper rate of decline which accelerates to about 20% to 25% per decade in healthy older men and women aged 70 and above [30]. Reduced physical activity contributes to this decline but similar rates of decline are observed among highly active individuals even though the cardiorespiratory fitness of those who exercise regularly is substantially higher than that of inactive peers in all age groups [30]. A cardiorespiratory fitness of about 18–20 mlO_2/kg/min distinguishes between high and low physical functioning in adults older than 65 years and when the intensity of an activity exceeds an individual's maximal cardiorespiratory fitness, the activity has to be terminated. Indeed, if the activity is performed for longer duration the intensity has to be substantially lower not to exceed 50% of maximal cardiorespiratory fitness. Thus, the ability to maintain a high aerobic capacity at old age is a major determinant of functional independence in daily living.

Given the importance of maintaining a high level of cardiorespiratory fitness across life, what is the evidence that this is affected by physical activity and exercise? While exercise training improves aerobic capacity in children by up to 10% there are no observed associations with habitual physical activity [31]. In contrast, numerous observational studies have demonstrated that habitual physical activity and exercise are associated with higher levels of cardiorespiratory fitness in adults. For example, cardiorespiratory fitness was about 30–40% higher in 60 to 80 year-old distance runners compared with their age-matched active peers and similar to those 20 to 30 years younger [32]. This observation is at least partly explained by genetic factors due to the inter-individual differences in response to exercise training. Data from the Heritage study showed that sedentary individuals of all ages increased their cardiorespiratory fitness by an average of 15–20%

following a 20-week structured endurance exercise programme [33]. However, the between-individual response to exercise training was substantial, with some individuals demonstrating no response and others showing an increase of up to 1000 mL O_2/min. Importantly, cardiorespiratory fitness is also modifiable by exercise training in older adults with improvements comparable to those observed in younger adults. A meta-analysis of training studies in persons aged 60 and older found a mean increase in cardiorespiratory fitness of 16% [34]; exercise of higher intensity and longer duration elicited greater improvement.

17.4 Factors influencing lifetime physical activity

Understanding why people are physically active or inactive is important when planning public health interventions. Factors associated with physical activity include demographic, biological, psychosocial, behavioural, social, cultural, and environmental factors. Further, regional and national policies, and global trends affect activity levels across life. In this section some of the most consistent findings on factors influencing physical activity across life are briefly summarized and gaps in the current knowledge are highlighted.

17.4.1 Early life

Animal models suggest that *in utero* growth restriction reduces locomotor activity [35,36]. Very low birthweight infants appear to have lower self-reported levels of physical activity in early adulthood [37,38]. A recent meta-analysis examining the associations between birthweight and self-reported physical activity observed lower levels of activity at both extremes of the birthweight spectrum [39]. However, this observation was not confirmed when physical activity was measured objectively [40,41]. While physical activity may not be reduced during childhood in those born with low or very low birthweight, data in adults suggest that activity levels are reduced in those with low birthweight compared with those born normal weight [37,38]. No studies have definitively explained why activity levels decline after childhood in those with low and very low birthweight. However, smaller body size and late maturation may delay development of motor skills and may have long-lasting influences on exercise capacity.

Earlier infant motor development, as indicated by younger age at standing unaided and walking, has been linked with higher activity levels in adolescence [42]. Understanding whether early motor development is associated with physical activity and sedentary behaviour in adulthood and whether the influence of infant motor development extends to long-term influences on body composition, obesity and metabolic risk need further examination.

17.4.2 Childhood and adolescence

Except for the non-modifiable determinants of sex and age, few factors have been consistently linked with physical activity during childhood and adolescence. One of the psychosocial factors most consistently shown to be associated with physical activity in childhood and adolescence is self-efficacy (i.e. confidence in the ability to be physically active). Further, the perception of the ability to be physically active, perceived behavioural control, and previous physical activity appear to influence activity levels in youth [43]. Support from family and peers also appears to influence activity levels in children (parental support) and in adolescents (peer support) [43]. Environmental factors influencing young peoples' activity levels include how friendly an area is for walking (walkability), traffic volume (negatively), availability to destinations such as shops (land-use mix) and residential density (Chapter 18) [44].

17.4.3 **Adults**

Similar to findings in young people, the most consistent psychosocial factor associated with higher levels of physical activity in adulthood is self-efficacy [43]. Previous history of physical activity and the intention to be physically active also appears to be important [43,45]. Not surprisingly, individual factors such as perceived stress and poor health status are consistently associated with lower levels of physical activity in adulthood [43,45], whereas higher levels of education and occupational class are associated with higher levels of leisure time physical activity. Social factors associated with physical activity include social support but not marital status [43] whereas occupational factors such as job strain, working hours, and overtime are negatively associated with physical activity [46]. Among major life events retirement appears to be associated with higher levels of MVPA whereas widowhood is unrelated to physical activity [47]. However, according to a recent systematic review, there is insufficient evidence to make conclusions about the determinants of physical activity and exercise in older adults [48]. The authors highlighted the need for additional research on individual determinants of activity in older adults and recommended the use of objective methods for assessing physical activity [48].

Few environmental factors have been associated with physical activity in adults; however the ability to walk from home to nearby destinations appears to be associated with transport related physical activity whereas no consistent environmental correlates of physical activity have been identified in older adults (Chapter 18) [43].

17.4.4 **Is physical activity stable across life?**

Previous history of physical activity has been identified as a determinant of current physical activity which raises the question of whether physical activity habits are formed at a young age and remain stable across life. Physical activity appears to be fairly stable or track (maintaining a position within a group) during childhood, adolescence, and adulthood in men, whereas in women the level of tracking is lower [49]. In both men and women, tracking is lower during life transitional phases (e.g. from childhood to adolescence). Generally, studies with repeated measures of physical activity at different time points report lower tracking with increasing length of follow-up [50]. One study with a very long follow-up time (11 to 67 years) observed significant but low tracking in men ($r = 0.14$) and women ($r = 0.12$) [51]. Additional research on tracking of physical activity including long-term follow-up and objective measures of physical activity is warranted. In addition, more research is needed to investigate the influence of significant life transitions such as marriage and retirement on tracking.

17.5 **Physical activity and healthy ageing**

17.5.1 **Survival**

A seminal study conducted in the early 1950s by Morris and colleagues [52] showed that London bus drivers were at higher risk of cardiac events than their more active conductor peers. Since then, numerous studies including work by Paffenbarger and colleagues [53,54] have demonstrated an inverse relationship between physical activity and all-cause and coronary heart disease (CHD) mortality [55]. A recent conservative estimate suggests that physical inactivity causes 9% of premature mortality and more than five million deaths per year worldwide. The risk of premature death associated with being physically inactive is similar to the risk associated with established risk factors such as smoking and obesity [56].

The protective effect of higher levels of physical activity on all-cause and cardiovascular mortality is consistent in men and women, across age groups and ethnicity. Data suggest that being more physically active or fit is associated with up to a 50% reduction in risk of mortality in men [57]. Similar results were observed in women, with up to a 52% increase in all-cause mortality and a doubling in cardiovascular mortality in physically inactive women compared with their active peers. In combined analysis including more than 116,000 women from the Nurses' Health Study in the US, higher levels of physical activity were associated with reduced risk of all-cause mortality regardless of adiposity level, but did not eliminate the increased risk associated with obesity [58]. These results suggest that physical activity is protective against premature death independently of adiposity but being both normal weight and active confer the greatest benefits.

Moreover, it seems that people who are active and fit yet have other risk factors for cardiovascular disease may be at lower risk compared with those who are unfit and without these other risk factors [57]. The survival advantages from exercise also extend to total physical activity in daily living in older adults [59,60]. A study in healthy community-dwelling older men and women aged 70–82 showed that an increase in free-living PAEE of 287 kcal/day (equivalent to about one hour of walking) was associated with a 32% lower risk of mortality [59]. This study is unique, as daily PAEE was precisely measured using the doubly-labelled water method. Additional evidence for the benefits of being physically active in old age are provided by a study of 893 men and women with a mean age of 82 in which physical activity was measured by accelerometry. After 4 years of follow-up, the risk of death was 29% lower in the high active group (90th percentile of PAEE) compared to the low active group (10th percentile) [60]. The effect of physical activity on mortality appears graded and suggests additional benefits in a dose–response manner. However, the protective effect of physical activity is already observed at relatively low levels of physical activity. Wen and colleagues [61] recently demonstrated that walking for about 15 minutes per day was associated with a 14% reduced risk of all-cause mortality and an increase in life expectancy of 3 years. Finally, a number of randomized controlled trials have demonstrated the effectiveness of exercise as secondary prevention, in that regular exercise can attenuate or reverse the disease process in patients with cardiovascular disease [55].

There is incontrovertible evidence accumulated over more than 60 years of research to suggest that regular physical activity is associated with reduced risk of premature death. The association appears to be linear and graded; the most active people are at the lowest risk. The greatest improvements are observed when people who are sedentary and least fit become physically active. Importantly, the beneficial effects of physical activity on survival also extend to older adults who become physically active in later life, and small increases in daily physical activity, of as little as 15 to 20 minutes of walking each day, appear to be associated with substantial gains in life expectancy.

While there is substantial evidence to suggest that physical activity is one of the most important lifestyle factors associated with longevity, the question arises whether higher levels of physical activity also delay onset of chronic diseases and disability.

17.5.2 Avoidance of chronic diseases

The risk of chronic diseases, including obesity and metabolic diseases, is influenced by factors from conception onwards with low birthweight consistently linked with increased risk for metabolic diseases such as type 2 diabetes in adulthood [62]. Further, high birthweight and rapid weight gain in infancy appear to be associated with increased risk of later obesity [63]. Higher levels of physical activity are associated with lower levels of adiposity and favourable metabolic risk factors already in childhood [64]. However, longitudinal studies in which physical activity has been measured objectively in childhood and related to metabolic risk in adulthood are lacking which leaves us with uncertainty about whether higher levels of physical activity in earlier life have effects on metabolic health later in life.

Higher levels of physical activity improve optimal functioning and wellbeing throughout life (Chapters 2, 3, and 4). Here, the available evidence on whether physical activity prevents the development of obesity and type 2 diabetes in adults is briefly summarized and the potential modifying or mediating role of adiposity on the associations between physical activity and diabetes discussed. The rationale for focusing on obesity and diabetes is: (1) the high prevalence of these two conditions; (2) the predicted increase in incident diabetes and associated dramatic increase in healthcare costs; (3) their association with cardiovascular morbidity and mortality; (4) the important role of lifestyle factors such as diet and physical activity in preventing these conditions; and (5) the potential mediating role of obesity and type 2 diabetes in associations of physical activity with physical capability, cognitive capability, and wellbeing.

17.5.2.1 Physical activity and obesity

Physical activity increases energy expenditure and maintains or increases muscle mass, which may result in an increased basal metabolism and an increased capacity for utilizing fat during rest and exercise. There is compelling evidence of a strong inverse cross-sectional association between physical activity and body weight, fat mass, and obesity [65]. However, cross-sectional observational studies cannot be used to infer causality or determine the direction of association. Prospective cohort studies, in which physical activity and body weight/obesity are measured at baseline and body weight/obesity is assessed again at follow-up, are better placed to suggest the direction of association between activity and gain in body weight. Recent systematic reviews on this topic [66–68] have suggested that either there is inconsistent evidence of a predictive effect of baseline physical activity on gain in body weight [66]; that physical activity, in general, is not associated with subsequent excess weight gain and obesity [67]; or that low levels of activity are only weakly associated with future weight gain [68].

Physical activity may be differentially associated with general and central obesity. Data from the European Prospective Investigation into Nutrition and Cancer Study (EPIC) in more than 288,000 men and women from 10 European countries suggested an independent inverse association between baseline activity levels and abdominal adiposity in both normal weight, overweight and obese men and women. However, no association between physical activity and weight gain was observed [69].

Only a few studies are available that have used objective measures of PAEE when examining the association between baseline PAEE and gain in body weight [70–72]. Results from these studies, although relatively small in sample size, do not support the notion that low levels of physical activity contribute to gain in body weight and development of obesity, and so it is tempting to speculate that energy intake may play a greater role than PAEE in influencing weight gain. Some have also suggested that the association between baseline physical activity and body weight may be reversed or bi-directional [73,74]; that is, high body weight and obesity limit the ability to be physically active and therefore predict lower levels of activity at follow-up.

In summary, the nature of the prospective associations between physical activity and subsequent gain in body weight is complex and may be bi-directional. Furthermore, the association is complicated by the influence of energy intake on energy balance, an exposure even more difficult to measure accurately than physical activity in observational studies (Chapter 16). Future studies combining the most accurate methods to assess physical activity and dietary intake in combination with body composition are needed to understand the combined effects of activity and dietary intake on energy balance across life.

17.5.2.2 Physical activity and type 2 diabetes

Numerous observational studies have shown that physical activity is associated with a decreased risk of type 2 diabetes in men and women [75,76]. Increasing physical activity by about 500 kcal per week was associated with a 6% reduction in the risk of incident diabetes [75]. However, obesity appears to be a stronger risk factor for incident type 2 diabetes than physical inactivity. Therefore, it is important to understand whether physical activity is also protective in those who are obese. A recent study examining the combined effects of physical activity and general and central adiposity on incident diabetes showed that physical activity was associated with a reduction in the risk of developing type 2 diabetes across body mass index categories in men and women, as well as in abdominally lean and obese men and women [77]. An increase of about 100 to 150 kcal per day in PAEE, equivalent to about 20 to 30 minutes of brisk walking, was associated with a 13% and 7% relative reduction in risk of type 2 diabetes independent of adiposity and other confounders, in men and women respectively [77]. The protective effect of physical activity on diabetes risk also extends to older men [78]. Even light intensity activity reduced the risk of diabetes especially among those who were overweight or obese, and increasing physical activity or maintaining at least moderate levels of physical activity was strongly protective against diabetes [78].

Physical activity is also beneficial for secondary and tertiary prevention of diabetes. For example, results from the Diabetes Prevention Programme [79] and the Finish Diabetes Prevention Study [80] have demonstrated that lifestyle interventions reduced the risk of type 2 diabetes by 58% compared with 38% for medication [79]. Further, an intensive supervised exercise intervention in middle-aged adults with type 2 diabetes and the metabolic syndrome demonstrated clinically meaningful improvements in all cardiovascular risk factors measured. In contrast, counselling alone increased self-reported physical activity but did not affect any of the risk factors suggesting that a greater volume of exercise than recommended may be needed for secondary prevention of type 2 diabetes [81].

Higher levels of physical activity have numerous effects on metabolism that contribute to the observed inverse associations with metabolic morbidity. These include improved blood lipid profile, reduction in blood pressure, improved insulin sensitivity, fibrinolysis, and endothelial function. Importantly, physical activity has direct effects on metabolic parameters independent of adiposity and while the optimal combination of high levels of physical activity and normal weight is preferable, the health gains of being physically active extend to overweight and obese individuals and those with central obesity.

17.5.3 Physical activity guidelines for adults

Supported by compelling evidence from observational research and well conducted exercise interventions demonstrating a positive effect of higher levels of physical activity on numerous health outcomes in men and women, in all age groups and ethnicities, physical activity recommendations for public health have been developed.

The WHO physical activity guidelines for health [82] state that adults aged 18–64 years should: (1) participate in at least 150 minutes of MVPA, such as walking, dancing, gardening, hiking, swimming, cycling, per week or at least 75 min of vigorous intensity activity (e.g. sports, planned aerobic exercise) or an equivalent combination of both; (2) these aerobic activities should be performed in bouts of at least 10 minutes; (3) additional benefits are achieved by increasing MVPA time to 300 minutes or vigorous intensity activity to 150 minutes per week, or an equivalent combination; (4) muscle strengthening activities should be done at least twice per week.

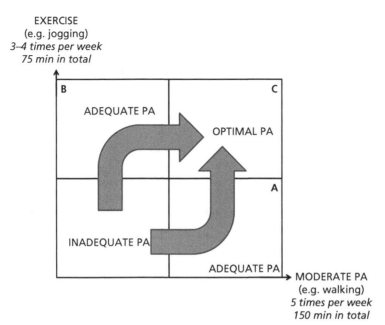

Figure 17.2 Two modalities of physical activity (PA) adequate to give health benefits. **A**: physical activity of moderate intensity, for example walking, cycling and playing, with a frequency of five times per week and a total of 150 minutes per week. **B**: exercise of moderate to vigorous intensity, for example jogging, swimming, tennis, resistance training, and circuit training, three to four times per week and a total of 75 minutes per week. **C**: the *optimal* activity dose may be the combination of **A** and **B**, i.e. both moderate physical activity and moderate to vigorous exercise.

The same recommendations apply for older adults (i.e. >65 years) with two important additions: (1) older adults with poor mobility should perform physical activity to enhance balance and prevent falls on 3 or more days per week; and (2) when older adults cannot do the recommended amounts of physical activity due to health conditions, they should be as physically active as their abilities and conditions allow.

A dose–response association is implicated and higher levels of physical activity likely confer additional health benefits. Figure 17.2 suggests two equivalent but different modalities of obtaining health benefits from physical activity according to the present recommendations.

While the current recommendations state that activity should be performed in bouts of at least 10 minutes, evidence is emerging that accumulating MVPA throughout the day regardless of whether the activity is performed in 10 minute bouts may have positive effects on metabolic risk factors [83]. This observation is further supported by the inverse association between PAEE, a measure of total physical activity, and mortality in the elderly [59]. Before reformulating the current recommendations, additional research on the health benefits of total physical activity, PAEE, and total accumulated time in MVPA compared with continuous 10 minutes bouts is needed.

17.6 **Future research directions**

In this chapter I have summarized the most common methods for assessing physical activity in large population-based samples, discussed how physical activity varies by age, summarized the current knowledge on factors associated with physical activity across life, and discussed physical activity in terms of healthy ageing with a specific focus on survival to old age, and the role of physical activity in relation to obesity and diabetes.

While much knowledge has been generated in the area of physical activity and how it relates to health across life there are some important gaps in our current knowledge that need to be addressed in the future. First, population level trend data in physical activity assessed objectively are needed to understand how activity levels change over time and across age groups. Second, there is a paucity of data on individual and collective determinants of physical activity, especially factors influencing physical activity in older adults. Further, it is unknown whether specific factors in early life such as motor development have long-lasting influences on later physical activity. Finally, the detailed dose–response associations between physical activity and health outcomes can only be addressed by increasing the precision of the measurements of physical activity.

This knowledge is needed when designing population-based interventions, targeted interventions for specific groups and when redefining physical activity guidelines for public health.

References

1 **World Health Organization.** WHO Physical Inactivity: a Global Public Health Problem. Geneva: World Health Organization; 2011.

2 **Landers DM, Shawn SM.** Physical activity and mental health. In Tenenbaum G, Eklund RC, editors. Handbook of Sport Psychology. 3rd ed. New Jersey: John Wiley; 2007:469–91.

3 **Prince SA, et al.** A comparison of direct versus self-report measures for assessing physical activity in adults: a systematic review. *Int J Behav Nutr Phys Act* 2008;**5**:56.

4 **Helmerhorst HJF, et al.** A systematic review of reliability and objective criterion-related validity of physical activity questionnaires. *Int J Behav Nutr Phys Act* 2012;**9**:103.

5 **Corder K, et al.** Assessment of physical activity in youth. *J Appl Physiol* 2008;**105**:977–87.

6 **Matthews C.** Calibration of accelerometer outputs for adults. *Med Sci Sports Exerc* 2005;**37**:S512–22.

7 **Logan N, et al.** Resting heart rate definition and its effect on apparent levels of physical activity. *Med Sci Sports Exerc* 2000;**32**:162–6.

8 **Brage S, et al.** Branched equation modeling of simultaneous accelerometry and heart rate monitoring improves estimate of directly measured physical activity energy expenditure. *J Appl Physiol* 2004;**96**: 343–51.

9 **Brage S, et al.** Reliability and validity of the combined heart rate and movement sensor Actiheart. *Eur J Clin Nutr* 2005;**59**:561–70.

10 **Strath SJ, et al.** Integration of physiological and accelerometer data to improve physical activity assessment. *Med Sci Sports Exerc* 2005;**37**:S563–71.

11 **Riddoch CJ, et al.** Physical activity levels and patterns of 9 and 15 year old European children. *Med Sci Sports Exerc* 2004;**36**:86–92.

12 **Nader PR, et al.** Moderate-to-vigorus physical activity from ages 9 to 15 years. *JAMA* 2008;**300**:295–305.

13 **Hallal PC, et al.** Global physical activity levels: surveillance progress, pitfalls, and prospects. *Lancet* 2012;**380**:258–71.

14 **Hansen BH, et al.** Accelerometer-determined physical activity in adults and older people. *Med Sci Sports Exerc* 2012;**44**:266–72.

15 **Baptista F, et al.** Prevalence of the Portuguese population attaining sufficient physical activity. *Med Sci Sports Exerc* 2012;**44**:466–73.

16 **Troiano RP, et al.** Physical activity in the United States measured by accelerometer. *Med Sci Sports Exerc* 2008;**40**:181–8.

17 **Townsend N, et al.** Physical Activity Statistics. London: British Heart Foundation; 2012

18 Matthews CE, et al. Amount of time spent in sedentary behaviors in the United States, 2003–2004. *Am J Epidemiol* 2008;**167**:875–81.

19 Brownson RC, et al. Declining rates of physical activity in the United States: What are the contributors? *Annu Rev Public Health* 2005;**26**:421–43.

20 Church TS, et al. Trends over 5 decades in US occupation-related physical activity and their associations with obesity. *PLoS One* 2011;**6**:e19657.

21 Knuth AG, Hallal PC. Temporal trends in physical activity: a systematic review. *J Phys Act Health* 2009;**6**:548–59.

22 Juneau CE, Potvin L. Trends in leisure-, transport-, and work-related physical activity in Canada 1994–2005. *Prev Med* 2010;**51**:384–6.

23 Palacios-Cena D, et al. Time trends in leisure time physical activity and physical fitness in elderly people: 20 year follow-up of the Spanish population national health survey (1987–2006). *BMC Public Health* 2011;**11**:799.

24 Sjol A, et al. Secular trends in acute myocardial infarction in relation to physical activity in the general Danish population. *Scand J Med Sci Sports* 2003;**13**:224–30.

25 Stamatakis E, Chaudhury M. Temporal trends in adults' sports participation patterns in England between 1997 and 2006: the Health Survey for England. *Br J Sports Med* 2008;**42**:901–8.

26 Chau JY, et al. Cross-sectional associations between occupational and leisure-time sitting, physical activity and obesity in working adults. *Prev Med* 2012;**54**:195–200.

27 Sugiyama T, et al. Prolonged sitting in cars: prevalence, socio-demographic variations, and trends. *Prev Med* 2012;**55**:315–8.

28 Blair SN, et al. Influences of cardiorespiratory fitness and other precursors on cardiovascular disease and all-cause mortality in men and women. *JAMA* 1996;**276**:205–10.

29 Fleg JL, Lakatta EG. Role of muscle loss in the age–associated reduction in VO2max. *J Appl Physiol* 1988;**65**:1147–51.

30 Fleg JL, et al. Accelerated longitudinal decline of aerobic capacity in healthy older adults. *Circulation* 2005;**112**:674–82.

31 Armstrong N, et al. Aerobic fitness and its relationship to sport, exercise training and habitual physical activity during youth. *Br J Sports Med* 2011;**45**:849–58.

32 Fleg JL, et al. Cardiovascular responses to exhaustive upright cycle exercise in highly trained older men. *J Appl Physiol* 1994;**77**:1500–6.

33 Bouchard C, et al. Familial aggregation of VO(2max) response to exercise training: results from the HERITAGE Family Study. *J Appl Physiol* 1999;**87**:1003–8.

34 Huang G, et al. Controlled endurance exercise training and VO_{2max} changes in older adults: a meta-analysis. *Prev Cardiol* 2005;**8**:217–25.

35 Vickers MH, et al. Sedentary behavior during postnatal life is determined by the prenatal environment and exacerbated by postnatal hypercaloric nutrition. *Am J Physiol Regul Integr Comp Physiol* 2003;**285**:R271–3.

36 Bellinger L, et al. Exposure to undernutrition in fetal life determines fat distribution, locomotor activity and food intake in ageing rats. *Int J Obes* 2006;**30**:729–3.

37 Rogers M, et al. Aerobic capacity, strength, flexibility, and activity level in unimpaired extremely low birth weight (<or = 800 g) survivors at 17 years of age compared with term-born control subjects. *Pediatrics* 2005;**116**:e58–65.

38 Hovi P, et al. Glucose regulation in young adults with very low birth weight. *N Engl J Med* 2007;**356**:2053–63.

39 Andersen LG, et al. Birth weight in relation to leisure time physical activity in adolescence and adulthood: meta-analysis of results from 13 Nordic cohorts. *PLoS One* 2009;**4**:e8192.

40 Mattocks C, et al. Early life determinants of physical activity in 11 to 12 year olds: cohort study. *BMJ* 2008;**336**:26–9.

41 **Ridgway CL, et al.** Does birth weight influence physical activity in youth? A combined analysis of four studies using objectively measured physical activity. *PLoS One* 2011;**6**:e16125.

42 **Ridgway C, et al.** Infant motor development predicts sport participation at age 14 years: northern Finnish birth cohort of 1966. *PLoS One* 2009;**4**:e6837.

43 **Bauman AE, et al.** Correlates of physical activity: why are some people physically active and others not? *Lancet* 2012;**380**:258–71.

44 **Ding D, et al.** Neighborhood environment and physical activity among youth: a review. *Am J Prev Med* 2011;**41**:442–55.

45 **Van Stralen MM, et al.** Determinants of initiation and maintenance of physical activity among older adults: a literature review. *Health Psychol Rev* 2009;**3**:147–207.

46 **Kirk MA, Rhodes RE.** Occupation correlates of adults' participation in leisure-time physical activity: a systematic review. *Am J Prev Med* 2011;**40**:476–85.

47 **Koeneman MA, et al.** Do major life events influence physical activity among older adults: the Longitudinal Aging Study Amsterdam. *Int J Behav Nutr Phys Act* 2012;**9**:147.

48 **Koeneman MA, et al.** Determinants of physical activity and exercise in healthy older adults: a systematic review. *Int J Behav Nutr Phys Act* 2011;**8**:142.

49 **Telama R.** Tracking of physical activity from childhood to adulthood: a review. *Obesity Facts* 2009;**3**: 187–95.

50 **Telama R, et al.** Physical activity from childhood to adulthood: a 21-year tracking study. *Am J Prev Med* 2005;**28**:267–73.

51 **Friedman HS, et al.** Stability of physical activity across the lifespan. *J Health Psychol* 2008;**13**:1092–104.

52 **Morris J, et al.** Coronary heart disease and physical activity of work. *Lancet* 1953;**262**:1111–20.

53 **Paffenbarger RS Jr, et al.** Energy expenditure, cigarette smoking, and blood pressure level as related to death from specific diseases. *Am J Epidemiol* 1978;**108**:12–8.

54 **Paffenbarger RS, Hale WE.** Work activity and coronary heart mortality. *N Engl J Med* 1975;**292**:545–50.

55 **Warburton DE, et al.** Health benefits of physical activity: the evidence. *CMAJ* 2006;**174**:801–9.

56 **Lee IM, et al.** Effect of physical inactivity on major non-communicable diseases worldwide: an analysis of burden of disease and life expectancy. *Lancet* 2012;**380**:219–29.

57 **Myers J, et al.** Fitness versus physical activity patterns in predicting mortality in men. *Am J Med* 2004;**117**:912–8.

58 **Hu FB, et al.** Adiposity as compared with physical activity in predicting mortality among women. *N Engl J Med* 2004;**351**:2694–703.

59 **Manini TM, et al.** Daily activity energy expenditure and mortality among older adults. *JAMA* 2006;**296**:171–9.

60 **Buchman AS, et al.** Total daily physical activity and longevity in old age. *Arch Intern Med* 2012;**172**: 444–6.

61 **Wen CP, et al.** Minimum amount of physical activity for reduced mortality and extended life expectancy: a prospective cohort study. *Lancet* 2011;**378**:1244–53.

62 **Whincup PH, et al.** Birth weight and risk of type 2 diabetes. A systematic review. *JAMA* 2008;**300**: 2886–97.

63 **Druet C, et al.** Prediction of childhood obesity by infancy weight gain: an individual-level meta-analysis. *Paediatr Perinat Epidemiol* 2012;**26**:19–26.

64 **Ekelund U, et al.** Moderate to vigorous physical activity and sedentary time and cardiometabolic risk factors in children and adolescents. *JAMA* 2012;**307**:704–12.

65 **Besson H, et al.** A cross-sectional analysis of physical activity and obesity indicators in participants of the EPIC-PANACEA study. *Int J Obes* 2009;**33**:497–506.

66 **Fogelholm M, Kukkonen-Harjula K.** Does physical activity prevent weight gain—a systematic review. *Obes Rev* 2000;**1**:95–111.

67 **Summerbell CD.** Results by exposures–5.6 Physical activity. *Int J Obes* 2009;**33**:S57–73

68 **Wareham NJ, et al.** Physical activity and obesity prevention: a review of the current evidence. *Proc Nutr Soc* 2005;**64**:229–47.

69 **Ekelund U, et al.** Physical activity and gain in abdominal adiposity and body weight: prospective cohort study in 288,498 men and women. *Am J Clin Nutr* 2011;**93**:826–35.

70 **Tataranni PA, et al.** Body weight gain in free-living Pima Indians: effect of energy intake vs expenditure. *Int J Obes Relat Metab Disord* 2003;**27**:1578–83.

71 **Ekelund U, et al.** Physical activity energy expenditure predicts changes in body composition in middle-aged healthy whites: effect modification by age. *Am J Clin Nutr* 2005;**81**:964–9.

72 **Luke A, et al.** Energy expenditure does not predict weight change in Nigerian or African-American women. *Am J Clin Nutr* 2009;**89**:169–76.

73 **Ekelund U, et al.** Sedentary time and weight gain in healthy adults; reverse or bidirectional causality? *Am J Clin Nutr* 2008;**88**:612–7.

74 **Golubic R, et al.** Rate of weight gain predicts change in physical activity levels: a longitudinal analysis of the EPIC-Norfolk cohort. *Int J Obes (Lond)* 2013;**37**:404–9.

75 **Helmrich SP, et al.** Physical activity and reduced occurrence of non-insulin-dependent diabetes mellitus. *N Engl J Med* 1991;**325**:147–52.

76 **Manson JE, et al.** Physical activity and incidence of non-insulin-dependent diabetes mellitus in women. *Lancet* 1991;**338**:774–8.

77 **The InterAct Consortium.** Physical activity reduces the risk of incident type 2 diabetes in general and abdominally lean and obese men and women: the EPIC-InterAct study. *Diabetologia* 2012;**55**:1944–52.

78 **Jefferis BJ, et al.** Longitudinal associations between changes in physical activity and onset of type 2 diabetes in older British men: the influence of adiposity. *Diabetes Care* 2012;**35**:1876–83.

79 **Knowler WC, et al.** Reduction in the incidence of type 2 diabetes with lifestyle modification or metformin. *N Engl J Med* 2002;**346**:393–403.

80 **Tuomilehto J, et al.** Prevention of type 2 diabetes mellitus by changes in lifestyle among subjects with impaired glucose tolerance. *N Engl J Med* 2001;**344**:1343–50.

81 **Balducci S, et al.** Effect of an intensive exercise intervention strategy on modifiable cardiovascular risk factors in subjects with type 2 diabetes mellitus. *Arch Intern Med* 2010;**170**:1794–1803.

82 **World Health Organization.** Global recommendations on physical activity for health. <http://www.who.int/dietphysicalactivity/factsheet_recommendations/en/index.html>

83 **Glazer NL, et al.** Sustained and shorter bouts of physical activity are related to cardiovascular health. *Med Sci Sports Exerc* 2013;**45**:109–15.

Chapter 18

Lifetime lifestyles III: where we live, the life course, and ageing

Emily T Murray and Mai Stafford

18.1 What is known about ageing and residential area

Sizeable socioeconomic inequalities in healthy ageing have been noted in Chapters 1, 2, and 3, with those in the least advantaged socioeconomic positions having the greatest risk of early death, disability, and poorer physical and cognitive capability. Over the last decade, there has been a renewed emphasis in epidemiology on links between where individuals reside and their health. With advances in statistical methods and data linkage, multilevel approaches to demonstrate the health effects of living in different kinds of areas have been made possible. Over and above a resident's own socioeconomic characteristics, reviews show that residence in a more deprived area is associated with a moderately increased risk of mortality and morbidity [1–4].

Just as individual social and economic circumstances in childhood and adulthood are related to capability many decades later (Chapters 2 and 3), so characteristics of the places people live in childhood and throughout their adult life might influence their prospects for ageing well in later life. A life course approach would suggest that the particular features of residential areas that influence ageing might vary across life and that the importance of residential areas, versus other contexts, for ageing might also depend on the life stage. There are reasons to hypothesize that the link between residential area characteristics and health outcomes will be stronger among older compared with younger people, although this has not yet been empirically demonstrated in any systematic way. These reasons have been clearly laid out elsewhere [5] and are briefly summarized here. One is that older people may simply have been exposed to their residential environment for a longer period of time. A second is that the biological, psychological and cognitive processes associated with ageing might render older people more vulnerable to their residential environment. Thirdly, the residential environment might assume greater importance as other settings (notably the workplace) no longer feature heavily in older people's daily lives. On the other hand, intimate ties that are not necessarily geographically close, may assume greater importance for the health and wellbeing of older people [6].

The ageing of the population and concerns about how and where to provide formal and informal health and social care have generated a literature concerned with older people and place, ageing in place and the role of the home and residential area in ageing well as research topics [7–9]. According to life course models of ageing, factors that potentially determine outcomes in older age may operate at any point including the prenatal, childhood, adolescent, early, and later adulthood periods (Chapter 1). Outcomes in later life reflect trajectories and processes that may have been operating for decades and those processes may have been influenced by features in the residential area. However, quantitative studies of area effects are predominantly cross-sectional, or consider area characteristics at only a single time point. Residential mobility of individuals and physical, social, and economic changes in areas over time mean that such studies could mis-estimate area effects. Examples of studies which have investigated life course area effects using data on area in childhood/early adulthood and later in life – including effects on self-rated health [10], blood pressure [11], long-term illness [12], sub-clinical atherosclerosis [13], ischaemic heart disease [14], mortality [12,15,16], and, through the Healthy Ageing across the Life Course research collaboration (HALCyon), physical and cognitive capability [17,18] – are relatively small in number.

This chapter aims to bring a life course perspective to research into residential environments and healthy ageing. Of course a single chapter cannot hope to cover such a broad topic and so we focus on physical and cognitive capability as key components of ageing. We develop a conceptual model that we hope can be used to guide empirical work. In doing so, we illustrate some of the ways in which areas across life can contribute to healthy ageing and the considerable practical and methodological challenges that need to be addressed as this branch of work moves forward. We begin with a brief section on the challenges of defining and measuring residential areas before going on to review what is already known about residential area and physical and cognitive capability in later life.

18.2 **Assessment of residential areas**

There are primarily two sources of data to describe the characteristics of an area, namely internal (or same-source), where survey residents themselves are asked how they perceive a specified area around their residence, or external, where an outside data source is used to characterize the area. External data about the area may be based on perceptions (for example, aggregates of percep-tions from people living in the same area as the survey resident) [19,20] or on objective data (for example, counts of the number of people classified as unemployed) [21–23]. Studies using objec-tive measures of the area have typically used aggregated census data indicating the proportion of socioeconomically disadvantaged or advantaged residents. Other administrative sources, such as recorded crime statistics and land use records, have also been used. An alternative approach is to systematically observe the residential area, using trained observers and protocols which permit replication, to capture features such as land use, the physical condition of buildings, physical dis-order [24] or the urban built environment [25].

A key challenge for studies of area effects on health is to appropriately define the residential area to avoid biases arising from the use of arbitrary or inappropriate boundaries. Several approaches have been taken including allowing the survey resident to conceptualize their own boundary without guidance or restriction, giving the survey resident a guide (such as referring to the area within about a 10 minute walk of their home), using the knowledge of local stakeholders (such as service providers) to define boundaries, using a specified buffer zone around the survey resident's home, and using administrative boundaries (such as those derived for collection of census data or mail distribution). Individually-specified boundaries differ between residents and from census-based boundaries [26], as the quotes below from a qualitative study of 60 study members from the MRC National Survey of Health and Development (NSHD) and Hertfordshire Cohort Study collected as part of HALCyon illustrate [27]:

'And it was nice because we had double summer time then and it was sunny until about 10 o'clock at night; it was lovely, it really was. And my mother used to have to come over the fields looking for us to go to bed, you know. No child does that these days, which is very sad I think.'

'Yes there was but it was a fair walk away. Battersea Park, it was a lovely park and it still is, and I used to live probably a 10 minute walk from there; 5, 10 minute walk, and that was probably—, there was that *at the end of the borough and at the other end was Clapham Common and there wasn't—, but in the immediate vicinity, no.'*

Many have used census tracts, census wards or equivalent census boundaries assumed to approximate the settings in which residents interact with each other and with local infrastructure. There is no simple solution and the selection depends on the research question to be addressed, among other factors. The choice is further complicated in longitudinal studies, because over time individuals may move around between different areas, and areas may change over time.

'It is, it's quite, quite different so yeah the decision to change to a town was a good one . . . I'd like to live in the country again but living in a town is entirely different and very satisfactory . . . '

'There's no shops at all now; we used to have a post office come shop which is now closed but we've now got a post office that opens two mornings a week in, hmmm, in part of the village hall. We've got a village hall which is very well used.'

In addition, even when data to characterize features of areas, such as the level of material deprivation, are available over a long time series, they are likely to have changed in meaning and/or measurement and the administrative boundaries used to measure the exposure change over time as well. For example, the UK census has included items on household amenities since 1951 [28], enabling calculation of the proportion of households in an area lacking amenities, though the list of amenities considered has changed in subsequent censuses. Also, the smallest geographic level at which amenity data are available for the 1951 census is the Local Government District, which is approximately a third the population of Local Government Districts in the 2001 census [29].

A few databases do exist where historical census data have been configured to be comparable to modern census boundaries, namely the Office for National Statistics Longitudinal Study in the UK [30] and the Neighborhood Change Database in the US [31]. However, taken together with factors such as individuals self-selecting themselves into areas and close links between individual socioeconomic position and residence, more work is needed to disentangle the relationships between individuals, their residence and their health over life to test whether associations are true effects of areas or artefacts of residential selection.

18.3 Residential area and physical capability in later life

18.3.1 Areas assessed at a single occasion

Physical capability, or the ability to perform physical tasks of daily living [32], can also be measured objectively or subjectively (Chapter 2). Only two studies of which we are aware have investigated links between a person's residential environment and objectively assessed physical performance. Of those, Lang and colleagues concentrated solely on the socioeconomic environment, using the English Longitudinal Study of Ageing (ELSA) to show that residence in a more deprived area, as measured by the index of multiple deprivation, was cross-sectionally associated with slower walking speed, independent of individual socioeconomic position, health behaviours and health status [33].

A study conducted by Brown and colleagues (2008) assessed the built environment of the East Little Havana area of Miami, Florida in the US, with trained student raters who coded architectural features theorized to facilitate visual and social contacts. In their population-based sample of Hispanic elders aged 70 to 100 who resided in the rated area, those living on blocks with front entrance features such as porches, stoops and being elevated above the pavement had better physical capability 2 years later than older people who lived in blocks with fewer of these features. Findings were robust to adjustment for age, gender, and income [34].

Several cross-sectional studies have also assessed self-reported measures of physical capability and area characteristics. Using area characteristics assessed internally to the study, results are quite consistent with residents with higher self-reported disability also reporting more perceived problems in their local area [35–38], less perceived amenities [36–38], feeling less safe [36,39–41], and lower perceptions of social cohesion [36–38,41,42]. With one exception [42], all studies adjusted for at least one indicator of individual socioeconomic position, usually income or education.

However, findings where both exposure and outcome are based on self-reported data and internal to the study are potentially biased, because of the tendency for individuals to report in a consistently positive or negative manner, and for perceptions of the residential area to differ according to demographic characteristics of individuals that are known to be related to physical capability, such as socioeconomic position [43]. Studies using external assessments do not have this limitation. For one measure of the social environment—crime—objective measures of assessment using the census and other administrative data confirmed those found with the subjective assessment (internal to the study) of feeling less safe [42,44]. In further analysis, the authors of those papers attributed associations entirely to misdemeanour arrests, suggesting that results reflected feelings of safety by residents rather than overall crime.

Census-derived measures of area deprivation are also consistently related with cross-sectional self-rated measures of physical health. In the UK, this was true for outcomes of physical functioning in those aged 35 to 65 from the Whitehall II study [45] and functional limitations in those 65 and older participating in the Medical Research Council Cognitive Function and Ageing Study (MRC CFAS) [46]. Two US studies, one a nationally representative sample of 55 to 64 year-olds [42] and the other aged 65 and older from New York City alone [44], found associations with general disability. Additionally, in a 2000–2001 British cross-sectional population survey of people aged 65-plus living at home, area deprivation was associated with disability independently of perceived area problems, safety, neighbourliness, and amenities [36].

Results for socioeconomic area effects on longitudinal changes in physical health are less consistent. One study using data from ELSA found that after adjusting for health, lifestyle, and sociodemographic confounders, area deprivation was related to 2-year incidence of mobility disability [33]. However, two studies with longer follow-up did not find a relationship. One of these was a 10-year follow-up of SF-36 physical component summary from the Whitehall II study [45]. The other, a nationally representative sample of those aged 45-plus from the Americans' Changing Lives Study, followed people over 15 years from 1986 to 2001 to assess the incidence of difficulty walking several blocks [40]. For the latter, results are difficult to interpret as they were only shown after adjustment for a host of individual level socioeconomic, demographic, and health characteristics, and area-level measures of population density, age structure, and objective built environment census measures.

The Americans' Changing Lives Study did however find that the percentage of car-based commuters, compared to walking or public transport commuters, was significant in the full model, although only for those greater than 75 [40]. These results are consistent with earlier studies showing that a higher presence of 'walk ability'-related urban design factors were associated with instrumental activities of daily living (IADL) [42,44,47]. Whether associations between area deprivation and mobility are explained by land use differences in poorer compared to better areas is unclear. Freedman and colleagues (2008) found that area economic advantage, disadvantage, and street connectivity were all independently related to lower body limitations and disability [44], suggesting that there are multiple explanatory pathways linking area of residence to disability. Further studies are needed with comparable area-level economic and built environment measures to be able to draw conclusions.

18.3.2 **Longitudinal and lifetime areas**

One of the challenges in investigating the impact of area conditions over the life course on health in later life is identifying suitable data. Studies need to have area identifiers collected for each individual at multiple dates over a long period, corresponding area-level exposure data (such as area deprivation) for each date, and individual health outcomes in later adulthood. Although retrospective data on addresses throughout life can be collected [13], the accuracy of the address data may not be optimal and may result in a lower rate of successful geocoding to area-level exposure data compared with prospective collection. For ageing outcomes such as dementia, or where individuals have moved considerably over their lifetime, this method of data collection may be particularly difficult.

Prospectively collected residential addresses of participants in the NSHD were linked to census data in 1951, 1971, and 1999 on various area socioeconomic measures [29]. This provided area socioeconomic data for study members at ages 4, 26, and 53 years, respectively. Using a multilevel regression model to partition the variance in objectively assessed physical capability at age 53, chair rise time, standing balance time, and grip strength were each found to vary significantly between areas in childhood, early adulthood, and midlife [17]. For example, at age 53, 9% of differences in standing balance time occurred between areas and the remaining 91% between individuals in the same area. However, using a more sophisticated cross-classified model to account for area of residence across all three ages, the variation in standing balance time was higher, at 13% of the total. The authors concluded that the simpler model resulted in underestimation of the total contribution of area across life. This study also found that areas with a higher percentage of working age residents employed in manual occupations at age 4, 26, or 53 had on average a lower standing balance time (Figure 18.1). The associations at ages 4 and 53 persisted on adjustment for childhood and adult individual socioeconomic position for standing balance time, though not for chair rise time or grip strength [17]. One limitation of this study is that the lowest level of aggregation consistently available at all time points was local government district level and, in addition to the changes in district level population size as noted earlier, this underestimates the contribution of area of residence to physical capability compared with lower level units. Despite the limitations, these findings suggest that for the promotion of higher physical capability in later life we need to consider not only individual characteristics but also the socioeconomic environments in which people reside.

18.4 **Residential area and cognitive capability in later life**

Studies assessing associations of adult area characteristics with cognitive capability (Chapter 3) have mainly examined socioeconomic characteristics of the environment. Eight studies have found cross-sectional links between census-derived summary deprivation indices and two different tests of cognitive functioning: the Mini-Mental State Examination (MMSE) [46,48–51] and the Telephone Interview for Cognitive Status (TICS) [52–54]. These findings seem robust given that studies were conducted across many different geographic regions in the US [49–54] and England [46,48], and used a range of composite measures of area socioeconomic conditions including percentage employed, housing characteristics, and tenure.

Most studies also adjusted for individual socioeconomic factors, such as occupational class and education, with associations reduced but not eliminated [46,48,49,51,53,54]. In one of the American studies [52], researchers went a step further, stratifying analyses by the individual wealth of their nationally representative sample of 55 to 64 years-olds, to discover that a summary measure of area disadvantage (comprising percentage low education, receiving public assistance,

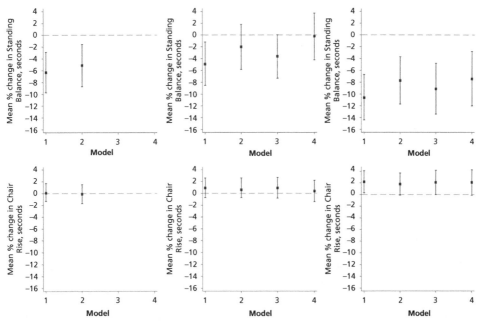

Figure 18.1 Associations of area deprivation at ages 4, 26, and 53 years with physical capability measures of standing balance and chair rise times at age 53 years (MRC National Survey of Health and Development, 1946–1999) [17]. Mean percentage change, and 95% confidence intervals, of physical capability measures at age 53 years for a 1-standard deviation increase in area deprivation in 1950, 1972 and 1999, from cross-classified models. Left column is aged 4 years (1950), middle column aged 26 years (1972) and right column aged 53 years (1999). Models: **1**, unadjusted (n = 2300); **2**, adjusted for cross-sectional individual socioeconomic position (SEP) (i.e. area deprivation 1950 adjusted for childhood SEP only); **3**, adjusted for prior area deprivation (i.e. area deprivation in 1972 adjusted for 1950); **4**, full model fitted for all prior area deprivation and current and prior individual SEP (i.e. area deprivation in 1999 adjusted for area deprivation in 1950 and 1972, and individual SEP in 1950, 1972, and 1999 (ages 4, 26, and 53 years). Area deprivation was measured as the percentage of occupied persons in an area with partly skilled or unskilled occupations. Due to missing data, models adjusting for individual SEP (models **2** and **4**) contain n < 2300.

poverty, and unemployment) had an especially large association with the cognitive function of individuals who had little personal wealth themselves. Similarly, differences in cognition between individuals of high and low educational attainment were greater in areas with a greater percentage of low educational attainment. These findings suggest that poor cognitive outcomes may be the product of interactions between individual and environmental conditions.

In addition, two of the previous eight studies, both samples of elderly Hispanic populations from western US communities [49–51], assessed area socioeconomic effects on decline in cognitive functioning in elderly populations. Whereas the Sacramento Area Latino Study on Aging (SALSA) [49] found area effects on both baseline and 10-year cognitive decline, area disadvantage was only related to baseline cognitive functioning in the Hispanic Established

Populations for Epidemiologic Studies of the Elderly (HEPESE) study and not decline over 5 years of follow-up [51].

Clarke and colleagues went a step further by not only examining effects of census socioeconomic affluence on cognitive functioning, but also investigating what other individual and area-level factors these relationships may have been acting through [53]. In their representative survey of community-dwelling adults (50 years and older) in Chicago, higher area affluence, as measured by census tract median home value, percentage college achievement, percentage in professional or managerial occupations, and percentage aged 30 to 39 years, was related to better cognitive functioning. For white residents this association could be partly explained by a greater density of institutional resources, such as schools, churches, libraries, and community centres. For African Americans and Hispanics the reverse was true, with residence in areas with greater institutional resources associated with lower cognitive functioning. Physical activity explained a small part of the association between institutional resources and cognition in white residents, suggesting access to those resources may provide white older adults with physical activity opportunities, which may lead to better cognitive functioning.

Two studies have examined social aspects of residential areas in relation to cognitive capability, both cross-sectional. The first study, a representative sample of US adults aged 70 and older in 1993, showed that the higher the proportion of residents in a census tract without a high school diploma, the lower their average TICS scores, even after adjustment for individual education, wealth, income, marital status, ethnicity, self-reported disability, depression, and co-morbidities [55]. The second study, a population-based sample of adults aged 65 and over in Baltimore, Maryland in the US [54], showed lower processing speed and executive function for persons residing in areas with higher hazard score (12 items from the US 2000 census representing social disorganization, public safety, physical disorder, and economic deprivation). However, further analysis revealed the association only existed for those with a particular genetic variant (Apo lipoprotein E epsilon-4 allele), a strong predictor of Alzheimer's disease. These findings, as well as the above study demonstrating a significant cross-level interaction [52], suggest that poor conditions in the area of residence are interacting with individual risk factors to produce differential cognitive ability at older ages.

Paralleling the analysis of physical capability described in Section 18.3.2, associations of area-level characteristics across life with cognitive capability at 53 years have also been investigated in the NSHD [18]. Statistically significant variation between different local government districts at ages 26 and 53, but not at age 4, was found for verbal ability and verbal memory. Consistent with this, failure to consider areas across life resulted in only a small degree of underestimation of the contribution of area to cognition in later life. Area low social class at ages 4 and 53, defined as the percentage of residents in manual occupations, explained a significant amount of the area variation in verbal memory independently of each other, and of concurrent individual socioeconomic position. Thus it seems that characteristics of areas at earlier ages are associated with both cognitive and physical capability in later life, though the specific life stage at which areas may exert their influence, if causal, could vary by outcome.

18.5 **Summary of existing literature on area effects on capability**

Existing studies have made a start on documenting whether area characteristics are associated with physical and cognitive capability in childhood and (mostly) in older age. Only a handful of quantitative, multilevel studies have examined simultaneous effects on later life morbidity and/or mortality of area in childhood/early adulthood and in later life. None have data to adequately characterize areas of residence in early and later life to help us understand the features of area that we need to intervene on. This is a challenge even for studies of concurrent area effects on health and much more so when seeking to isolate features of childhood areas using retrospective or historical administrative data. Furthermore, no studies have developed and tested a model which articulates multiple social, economic and behavioural pathways linking residential environment across a lifetime to healthy ageing; though this is increasingly being attempted in cross-sectional and short run longitudinal studies of area effects. However, given what we know so far about the key determinants of physical and cognitive capability in later life (Chapters 2 and 3), it is clear that the residential environment has a potentially important role throughout life, as we seek to illustrate in Section 18.6.

18.6 **Conceptual framework**

An important influence in the discipline of environmental gerontology has been the ecological model of ageing developed by Lawton [56]. According to this model, the balance between the demands of the environment and a person's ability to cope with those demands determine behaviour, disability and wellbeing. Although Lawton proposed that physical and social features of the environment are important in this model, the pathways were not elaborated. This model has subsequently been developed and extended as an aid to understanding more about the specific pathways on which area features might influence health and capability in older people [6,57–59].

Several conceptual papers and reviews have summarized the numerous pathways by which the area environment may influence morbidity and mortality [60–62]. Here we focus on pathways that may potentially influence physical capability. Figure 18.2 builds on the environmental mechanism schematic laid out by Diez Roux and Mair [22], and Chapters 2 and 3, to aid discussion of how area contexts across life may promote or constrain capability. Capability in older age depends on the rate of development, peak attainment, and the rate of decline in later life (Chapter 2) [63]. Area characteristics may impact on each of these elements of the physical capability trajectory to result in inequalities in capability in later life.

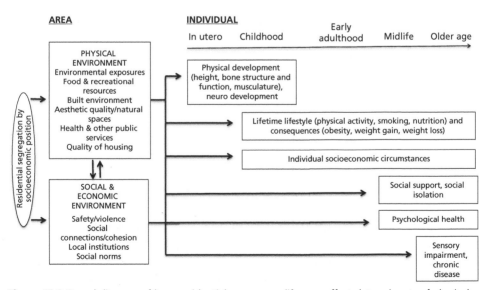

Figure 18.2 Causal diagram of how residential area across life may affect determinants of physical capability level and decline in older age.

18.6.1 **Applying the conceptual framework to physical capability**

Major risk factors for low level or declining physical capability in older age include physical and cognitive development in childhood [64], lower levels of physical activity, smoking, increased and decreased body mass index, chronic disease, low frequency of social contacts, vision impairment, and depression [65,66]. Taking each of these in turn, there is evidence for a possible influence of area factors across life. Higher rates of child maltreatment, a risk factor for poor growth, have been seen in areas characterized by high levels of socioeconomic deprivation and low levels of pre-school childcare [67]. Social cohesion, sense of belonging and local friendship networks are among the area social characteristics that are associated with childhood cognitive development, possibly operating partly through better maternal mental health and more nurturing and stimulating parenting practices in more advantaged areas [68,69]. Poor quality housing and overcrowding may also lead to increased levels of stress, and as a result people may turn to unhealthy behaviours as a coping mechanism [70–72].

The way areas are designed—particularly in terms of proximity and connectivity to local destinations such as schools and parks—has been implicated in physical activity of children [73,74]. Multiple studies across a range of ages have identified characteristics of the built environment that could have an influence on the ability and desirability of walking or taking public transit to work among adults [40,42,44,48]. Negative street characteristics [42,44], perceptions of fewer amenities [36,37,41], and high crime [36,37,41,42,44] in an area could keep individuals from utilizing their area for physical activity [75].

The social environment may also play a part in the development of physical capability inequalities through social norms for health-related behaviours. Living in certain areas may promote adoption and maintenance of behaviours from others in the area practicing the same behaviours. These collective norms may be health promoting or downward levelling [76,77] and may operate in childhood or adulthood. Thus the preponderance of people from manual occupations or with lower levels of education in more deprived areas may be linked to norms of unhealthy behaviours, such as being less physically active and smoking more, thus increasing the risk of poor physical capability [78,79].

Effects of nutrition on physical capability in older age have been somewhat neglected in the literature [66] but numerous studies exist documenting how food environments in both children and adults are related to obesity [80,81], a prime risk factor for poor physical capability later in life. More socioeconomically deprived areas have been consistently associated with 'obesogenic' dietary behaviours in adults [80] though the pathways by which this occurs are unclear. For example, some studies have found correlations between the area socioeconomic environment and less 'availability' of health-promoting area amenities [82,83] and concentration of health-damaging environmental factors, such as fast food chains [84]. However, findings are not consistent across all types of area amenities or across countries [82–86].

Public spaces provide opportunities for local social interactions and social support [87] and some evidence that levels of psychological distress are lower in more socially cohesive areas [88].

18.6.2 **Applying the conceptual framework to cognitive capability**

The life course model of cognition is similar to that of physical capability and both depend on neurodevelopmental and neurodegenerative processes. Cognitive ability tends to correlate well with skeletal growth in childhood [89] and physical capability tests that rely to some degree on the central nervous system [90], and it may be hypothesized that the same built and social environment processes described for physical capability may also affect cognitive capability.

Experimental evidence indicates that boys in families who were randomly assigned to assistance to move into a low poverty area had higher achievement test scores than controls who remained in public housing in a high poverty area [91]. Homework time and school safety partially accounted for programme effects.

The educational and occupational environment may play a part in cognitive development and maintenance. Associations between area deprivation and cognition [55] and between area educational level and cognition[53,55] may reflect increased exposure to cognitively stimulating resources [92,93] in more socioeconomically advantaged areas. Clarke and colleagues' finding that area affluence, partly comprised of educational variables, was explained by a greater density of institutional resources such as schools, libraries, and community centres supports this explanation [53]. Area deprivation and lack of resources in the area are also associated with children's behaviour, school attendance and educational attainment [94–96], which have implications for adult cognition independently of childhood cognition.

18.7 **Conclusions**

The literature on area effects on ageing has begun to document associations between features of the areas people live in childhood as well as throughout adulthood on health outcomes in later life. Replication is needed, along with exploration of whether areas across life are important for when and how quickly capability declines and if so, what particular features of areas are relevant at each life stage. Despite these challenges, we hope that we have illustrated that evidence points towards an association between residential area in childhood or early adulthood and healthy ageing in later life.

As with all life course models, conceptual models will need to carefully distinguish individual-level confounders from mediators and multilevel studies will need to use statistical modelling strategies that do not underestimate area effects by controlling for individual characteristics that may have been impacted by area of residence earlier in life [97].

Identifying ageing studies where survey members have well characterized areas of residence throughout life is a challenge. For most older age groups alive today, surveys of neighbouring residents or interviewer-rated assessments would not have been done historically. Although census and other administrative data sources are not optimal, we are at present largely reliant on these to characterize historical areas. Longitudinal studies started now could employ teams of area raters at regular intervals or link to new technologies, such as Google Earth, to make repeated area assessments; but pertinent health data on ageing could not be collected for decades and would involve great expense.

Recognition of the importance of supporting the health and social needs of the ageing population within policy circles is clear. Recent strategic documents have set out approaches to ensuring that local areas as well as homes will provide for lifetime changes and needs [98]. Designing communities for active ageing continues to be a stated public health priority in the UK and internationally [99,100]. In many cities, planning for communities that are inclusive of all ages rather than age segregated is seen as the way forward. What is needed further is a better understanding of the pathways by which man-made environmental characteristics affect our bodies over the life course and how these structural factors can help promote healthy active ageing long into later life.

Acknowledgements

We thank the other members of the HALCyon area-based work package for all of their hard work and expert knowledge: Rebecca Hardy, Yoav Ben-Shlomo, Kate Tilling, Humphrey Southall, and Paula Aucott.

We also thank Sam Parsons and Jane Elliott for their work in collecting in-depth information on samples of birth cohort study members and for providing the quotes included within this chapter as part of the HALCyon programme.

References

1 **Diez Roux AV.** Neighborhoods and health: where are we and where do we go from here? *Rev Epidemiol Sante Publique* 2007;**55**:13–21.

2 **Meijer M, et al.** Do areas affect individual mortality? A systematic review and meta-analysis of multi-level studies. *Soc Sci Med* 2012;**74**:1204–12.

3 **Riva M, et al.** Toward the next generation of research into small area effects on health: a synthesis of multilevel investigations published since. *J Epidemiol Community Health*, 1998;**61**:853–61.

4 **Pickett KE, Pearl M.** Multilevel analyses of area socioeconomic context and health outcomes: a critical review. *J Epidemiol Community Health* 2001;**55**:111–22.

5 **Glass TA, Balfour JL.** Neighborhoods, aging, and functional limitations. In: Kawachi I, Berkman LF, editors. Neighborhoods and Health Oxford: Oxford University Press: 2003:303–34.

6 **Carstensen LL, et al.** Taking time seriously: a theory of socioemotional selectivity. *Amer Psychol* 1999;**54**:165–81.

7 **Andrews GJ, Phillips DR.** Ageing and Place: Perspectives, Policy, Practice. London and New York: Routledge; 2005.

8 **Bowling A.** Ageing Well: Quality of Life in Old Age. England and New York: Open University Press; 2005.

9 **Wahl HW, Weisman GD.** Environmental gerontology at the beginning of the new millennium: reflections on its historical, empirical, and theoretical development. *Gerontologist* 2003;**43**:616–27.

10 **Johnson RC, et al.** Health disparities in mid-to-late life: the role of earlier life family and neighborhood socioeconomic conditions. *Soc Sci Med* 2012;**74**:625–36.

11 **Elford J, et al.** Migration and geographic variations in blood pressure in Britain. *BMJ* 1990;**300**:291–5.

12 **Curtis S, et al.** Area effects on health variation over the life-course: analysis of the longitudinal study sample in England using new data on area of residence in childhood. *Soc Sci Med* 2004;**58**:57–74.

13 **Carson AP, et al.** Cumulative socioeconomic status across the life course and subclinical atherosclerosis. *Ann Epidemiol* 2007;**17**:296–303.

14 **Elford J, et al.** Migration and geographic variation in ischemic heart disease in Great Britain. *Lancet* 1989;**8634**:343–6.

15 **Leyland AH, Naess O.** The effect of area of residence over the life course on subsequent mortality. *J R Statistic Soc A* 2009;**172**:555–78.

16 **Strachan DP, et al.** Mortality from cardiovascular disease among interregional migrants in England and Wales. *BMJ* 1995;**310**:423–7.

17 **Murray ET, et al.** Area deprivation across the life course and physical capability in mid-life: findings from the 1946 British birth cohort. *Am J Epidemiol* 2013;**178**:441–50.

18 **Murray ET, Stafford M.** The way we live: what's new from a life course approach? Changing social context and ageing. London, England: paper presented at a pre-meeting symposium for the Society for Social Medicine annual scientific meeting; 2012.

19 **Mujahid MS, et al.** Assessing the measurement properties of neighborhood scales: from psychometrics to ecometrics. *Am J Epidemiol* 2007;**165**:858–67.

20 **Auchincloss AH, et al.** Neighborhood resources for physical activity and healthy foods and incidence of type 2 diabetes mellitus: the Multi-Ethnic study of Atherosclerosis. *Arch Intern Med* 2009;**169**:1698–704.

21 **Riva M, et al.** Toward the next generation of research into small area effects on health: a synthesis of multilevel investigations published since July 1998. *J Epidemiol Community Health* 2007;**61**:853–61.

22 **Diez Roux AV, Mair C.** Neighborhoods and health. *Ann N Y Acad Sci* 2010;**1186**:125–45.

23 **Naess O, Leyland AH.** Analysing the effect of area of residence over the life course in multilevel epidemiology. *Scand J Public Health* 2010;**38**(Suppl 5):119–26.

24 **Sampson RJ, Raudenbush SW.** Systematic social observation of public spaces: a new look at disorder in urban neighborhoods. *Amer J Sociol* 1999;**105**:603–51.

25 **Weich S, et al.** Measuring the built environment: validity of a site survey instrument for use in urban settings. *Health Place* 2001;**7**:283–92.

26 **Coulton CJ, et al.** Mapping residents' perceptions of neighborhood boundaries: a methodological note. *Am J Community Psychol* 2001;**29**:371–81.

27 **Elliott J, et al.** The design and content of the halcyon qualitative study: a qualitative substudy of the National Study of Health and Development and the Hertfordshire Cohort Study. CLS Working Paper Series. London: Centre for Longitudinal Studies; 2011/5.

28 Housing: percentage of households with all amenities. In: A Vision of Britain through Time. <http://www.visionofbritain.org.uk/atlas/nat_data_theme_page.jsp?data_theme=T_HOUS> (accessed 2 Feb 2013).

29 **Murray ET, et al.** Challenges in examining area effects across the life course on physical capability in mid-life: findings from the 1946 British birth cohort. *Health Place* 2012;**18**:366–74.

30 **Norman P, et al.** Selective migration, health and deprivation: a longitudinal analysis. *Soc Sci Med* 2005; **60**:2755–71.

31 Geolytics Inc. (2006). Normalized data—neighborhood change database (NCDB) tract data from 1970–2000. <http://www.geolytics.com/USCensus,Neighborhood-Change-Database-1970-2000,Products.asp> (accessed 02 Feb 2013).

32 **Jette M.** Toward a common language for function, disability, and health. *Phys Ther* 2006;**86**:726–34.

33 **Lang IA, et al.** Area deprivation and incident mobility disability in older adults. *Age Ageing* 2008;**37**:403–10.

34 **Brown SC, et al.** Built environment and physical functioning in Hispanic elders: the role of "eye on the street". *Environ Health Perspect* 2008;**116**:1300–7.

35 **Balfour JL, Kaplan GA.** Neighborhood environment and loss of physical function in older adults: evidence from the Alameda county study. *Am J Epidemiol* 2002;**155**:507–15.

36 **Bowling A, Stafford M.** How do objective and subjective assessments of area influence social and physical functioning in older age? Findings from a British survey of ageing. *Soc Sci Med* 2007;**64**: 2533–49.

37 **Bowling A, et al.** Do perceptions of area environment influence health? Baseline findings from a British survey of aging. *J Epidemiol Community Health* 2006;**60**:476–83.

38 **Pampalon R, et al.** Perception of place and health: differences between areas in the Quebec City region. *Soc Sci Med* 2007;**65**:95–111.

39 **Clark CR, et al.** Perceived neighborhood safety and incident mobility disability among elders: the hazards of poverty. *BMC Public Health* 2009;**9**:162.

40 **Clarke P, et al.** Urban built environments and trajectories of mobility disability: findings from a national sample of community-dwelling American adults (1986–2001). *Soc Sci Med* 2009;**69**:964–70.

41 **Martin KR, et al.** Associations of perceived neighborhood environment on health status outcomes in persons with arthritis. *Arthritis Care Res (Hoboken)* 2010;**62**:1602–11.

42 **Beard JR, et al.** Neighborhood characteristics and disability in older adults. *J Gerontol B Psychol Sci Soc Sci* 2009;**64**:252–7.

43 **Kamphius CB, et al.** Why do poor people perceive poor areas? The role of objective area features and psychosocial factors. *Health Place* 2010;**16**:744–54.

44 **Freedman VA, et al.** Neighborhoods and disability in later life. *Soc Sci Med* 2008;**66**:2253–67.

45 **Stafford M, et al.** Area characteristics and trajectories of health functioning: a multilevel prospective analysis. *Eur J Public Health* 2008;**18**:604–10.

46 Basta NE, et al. Community-level socio-economic status and cognitive and functional impairment in the older population. *Eur J Public Health* 2008;**18**:48–54.

47 Clarke P, George LK. The role of the built environment in the disablement process. *Am J Public Health* 2005;**95**:1933–9.

48 Lang IA, et al. Neighborhood deprivation, individual socioeconomic status, and cognitive function in older people: analyses from the English Longitudinal Study of Ageing. *J Am Geriatr Soc* 2008;**56**:191–8.

49 Al Hazzouri AZ, et al. Neighborhood socioeconomic context and cognitive decline among older Mexican Americans: results from the Sacramento area latino study on aging. *Am J Epidemiol* 2011;**174**: 423–31.

50 Sheffield KM, Peek MK. Neighborhood context and cognitive decline in older Mexican Americans: results from the Hispanic Established Populations for Epidemiologic Studies of the Elderly. *Am J Epidemiol* 2009;**169**:1092–101.

51 Shih RA, et al. Neighborhood socioeconomic status and cognitive function in women. *Am J Public Health* 2011;**101**:1721–8.

52 Aneshensel CS, et al. The urban neighborhood and cognitive functioning in late middle age. *J Health Soc Behav* 2011;**52**:163–79.

53 Clarke PJ, et al. Cognitive function in the community setting: the area as a source of 'cognitive reserve'? *J Epidemiol Community Health* 2012;**66**:730–6.

54 Lee BK, et al. Neighborhood psychosocial environment, apolipoprotein E genotype, and cognitive function in older adults. *Arch Gen Psychiatry* 2011;**68**:314–21.

55 Wight RG, et al. Urban neighborhood context, educational attainment, and cognitive function among older adults. *Am J Epidemiol* 2006;**163**:1071–8.

56 Lawton MP. Competence, environmental press, and the adaptation of older people. In: Lawton MP, et al, editors. Ageing and the Environment: Theoretical Approaches. New York: Springer; 1982:33–59.

57 Wahl HW, et al. Aging well and the environment: toward an integrative model and research agenda for the future. *Gerontologist* 2012;**52**:306–16.

58 Lynch JW, et al. Why do poor people behave poorly? Variation in adult health behaviours and psycho-social characteristics by stages of the socioeconomic lifecourse. *Soc Sci Med* 1997;**44**:809–19.

59 Cummins S, et al. Understanding and representing 'place' in health research: a relational approach. *Soc Sci Med* 2007;**65**:1825–38.

60 Diez-Roux AV. Bringing context back into epidemiology: variables and fallacies in multilevel context. *Am J Public Health* 1998;**88**:216–22.

61 Kawachi I, Berkman LF. Neighborhoods and Health: an Overview. Oxford: Oxford University Press; 2003.

62 Macintyre S, et al. Place effects in health: how can we conceptualise, operationalize and measure them? *Soc Sci Med* 2002;**55**:125–39.

63 Ben-Shlomo Y, Kuh D. A life course approach to chronic disease epidemiology: conceptual models, empirical challenges and interdisciplinary perspectives. *Int J Epidemiol* 2002;**31**:285–93.

64 Kuh D, et al. Developmental origins of midlife physical performance: evidence from a British birth cohort. *Am J Epidemiol* 2006;**164**:110–21.

65 Stuck AE, et al. Risk factors for functional status decline in community-living elderly people: a systematic literature review. *Soc Sci Med* 1999;**48**:445–69.

66 Craigie AM, et al. Tracking of obesity-related behaviors from childhood to adulthood: a systematic review. *Maturitas* 2011;**70**:266–84.

67 Klein S. The availability of area early care and education resources and the maltreatment of young children. *Child Maltreat* 2011;**16**:300–11.

68 Cutrona CE, et al. Direct and moderating effects of community context on the psychological well-being of African American women. *J Pers Soc Psychol* 2000;**76**:1088–101.

69 **Barnes J, Cheng H.** Do parental area perceptions contribute to child behaviour problems? A study of disadvantaged children. *Vulnerable Children and Youth Studies: An International Interdisciplinary Journal for Research, Policy and Care* 2006;**1**:2–14.

70 **Stead M, et al.** "It's as if you're locked in": qualitative explanations for area effects on smoking in disadvantaged communities. *Health Place* 2001;**7**:333–43.

71 **Shohaimi S, et al.** Residential area deprivation predicts smoking habit independently of individual educational level and occupational social class. A cross sectional study in the Norfolk cohort of the European Investigation into Cancer (EPIC-Norfolk). *J Epidemiol Community Health* 2003;**57**:270–6.

72 **De Vriendt T, et al.** European adolescents' level of perceived stress is inversely related to their diet quality: the healthy lifestyle in Europe by nutrition in adolescence study. *Br J Nutr* 2012;**108**:371–80.

73 **Giles-Corti B, et al.** Encouraging walking for transport and physical activity in children and adolescents: how important is the built environment? *Sports Med* 2009;**39**:995–1009.

74 **Millstein RA, et al.** Home, school, and neighborhood environment factors and youth physical activity. *Pediatr Exerc Sci* 2011;**23**:487–503.

75 **Yang W, et al.** Evaluation of personal and built environment attributes to physical activity: a multilevel analysis on multiple population-based data sources. *J Obes* 2012;**2012**:548910.

76 **Portes A.** Social capital: its origins and applications in contemporary sociology. *Ann Rev Sociol* 1998;**24**:1–24.

77 **Portes A, Landolt P.** Unsolved mysteries; the Tocqueville files II: the downside of social capital. *The American Prospect* 1996;**7**:26.

78 **Chuang YC, et al.** Effects of area socioeconomic status and convenience store concentration on individual level smoking. *J Epidemiol Community Health* 2005;**59**:568–73.

79 **Matheson FI, et al.** Influence of neighborhood deprivation, gender and ethno-racial origin on smoking behavior of Canadian youth. *Prev Med* 2011;**52**:376–80.

80 **Giskes K, et al.** A systematic review of environmental factors and obesogenic dietary intakes among adults: are we getting closer to understanding obesogenic environments? *Obes Rev* 2011;**12**:e95–e106.

81 **Rahman T, et al.** Contributions of built environment to childhood obesity. *Mt Sinai J Med* 2011;**78**: 49–57.

82 **Macintyre S, et al.** Do poorer people have poorer access to local resources and facilities? The distribution of local resources by area deprivation in Glasgow, Scotland. *Soc Sci Med* 2008;**67**:900–14.

83 **Smith DM, et al.** Area food environment and area deprivation: spatial accessibility to grocery stores selling fresh fruit and vegetables in urban and rural settings. *Int J Epidemiol* 2010;**39**:277–84.

84 **Macdonald L, et al.** Area fast food environment and area deprivation—substitution or concentration? *Appetite* 2007;**49**:251–4.

85 **Pearce J, et al.** Are socially disadvantaged areas deprived of health-related community resources? *Int J Epidemiol* 2007;**36**:348–55.

86 **Macdonald L, et al.** The food retail environment and area deprivation in Glasgow city, UK. *Int J Behav Nutr Phys Act* 2009;**6**:52.

87 **Cattell V, et al.** Mingling, observing, and lingering: everyday public spaces and their implications for well-being and social relations. *Health Place* 2008;**14**:544–61.

88 **De Silva MJ, et al.** Social capital and mental illness: a systematic review. *J Epidemiol Community Health* 2005;**59**:619–27.

89 **Richards M, et al.** Birthweight, postnatal growth and cognitive function in a national UK birth cohort. *Int J Epidemiol* 2002;**31**:342–8.

90 **Kuh D, et al.** Lifetime cognitive performance is associated with midlife physical performance in a prospective national birth cohort study. *Psychosom Med* 2009;**71**:38–48.

91 **Leventhal T, Brooks-Gunn J.** A randomized study of neighborhood effects on low-income children's educational outcomes. *Dev Psychol* 2004;**40**:488–507.

92 **Compton DM, et al.** Age-associated changes in cognitive function in highly educated adults: emerging myths and realities. *Int J Geriatr Psychiatry* 2000;**15**:78–85.

93 **Wilson RS, et al.** Assessment of lifetime participation in cognitively stimulating activities. *J Clin Exp Neuropsychol* 2003;**25**:634–42.

94 **Molnar BE, et al.** Effects of neighborhood resources on aggressive and delinquent behaviors among urban youths. *Am J Public Health* 2008;**98**:1086–93.

95 **Leventhal T, Dupere V.** Moving to opportunity: does long-term exposure to 'low-poverty' neighborhoods make a difference for adolescents? *Soc Sci Med* 2011;**73**:737–43.

96 **Sampson RJ, et al.** Durable effects of concentrated disadvantage on verbal ability among African-American children. *Proc Natl Acad Sci USA* 2008;**105**:845–52.

97 **Morenoff JD, Lynch JW.** What makes a place healthy? Neighborhood influences on racial/ethnic disparities in health over the life course. In: Anderson NB, Bulatao RA, Cohen B, editors. National Research Council (US) Panel on Race, Ethnicity, and Health in Later Life. Critical Perspectives on Racial and Ethnic Differences in Health in Late Life. Washington, DC: US National Academies Press; 1994: Section 11.

98 **Communities and Local Government** (2008). Delivering lifetime homes, lifetime areas: a national strategy for housing in an ageing society. <http://www.housinglin.org.uk/Topics/browse/HousingOlderPeople/OlderPeopleStrategy/NationalHousingStrategy/?parent=3669&child=4938>

99 **Department of Health** (2010). Healthy lives, healthy people: our strategy for public health in England. <http://www.dh.gov.uk/en/Publicationsandstatistics/Publications/PublicationsPolicyAndGuidance/DH_121941>

100 **World Health Organization (WHO)**(2002). Active ageing: a policy framework. <http://www.who.int/ageing/publications/active_ageing/en/index.html>

Chapter 19

What have we learnt for future research and knowledge exchange?

Diana Kuh, Rachel Cooper, Rebecca Hardy,
James Goodwin, Marcus Richards,
and Yoav Ben-Shlomo

19.1 Introduction

This concluding chapter draws on the preceding chapters to highlight key findings and themes in life course research on healthy ageing. It places these within a knowledge transfer framework, given that the overriding reason for seeking to identify factors that influence health at older ages is to guide the design and implementation of preventive and therapeutic interventions. The rapidly increasing numbers of older people across the world lends urgency to communicating that research evidence quickly and effectively to stakeholders. At its simplest, life course research should offer pointers about where and when to intervene to optimize function and wellbeing in older people.

19.2 Knowledge translation and research on ageing

Knowledge translation (KT) refers to bridging the gap between 'what is known' and 'what is done', and is defined by the World Health Organization (WHO) as 'the synthesis, exchange and application of knowledge by relevant stakeholders to accelerate the benefits of global and local innovation in strengthening health systems and improving people's health' [1]. Government bodies and research funders have expressed growing concerns that the findings of investments in health research are not reaching policymakers, practitioners, or the general public and so are not leading to evidence-based policies and practices, thereby limiting any potential impact on human health. There has been much discussion of the translational model for clinical research (e.g. Cooksey's model, from bench to bedside), but less for public health [2,3]. The research findings brought together in this book are most relevant to the non-linear and inter-sectoral interfaces of the translational framework for public health.

The climate or context, at the international, national and local level, determines whether there will be a receptive audience for our research findings and any related policy or practice change. Certainly the economic and social implications of an ageing society are high on the agenda of most governments. The Madrid International Plan of Action on Ageing, adopted at the United Nations Second World Assembly in April 2002, sets the global context with the 'key challenge of building a society for all ages' [4]. Although not legally binding, this plan has been agreed upon by 159 governments. Its principal goals are: recognizing the social, cultural, economic, and political contribution of older persons; enabling older persons to continue with income-generating work for as long as they want and can do so productively; advancing health and wellbeing in ageing, including utilizing life course approaches; enabling 'ageing in place' through a supportive environment, including housing and transportation; promoting positive images of ageing; and reducing neglect, abuse, and violence.

Within this context, the WHO published its Knowledge Translation on Ageing and Health: a Framework for Policy Development 2012 [5]. This initiative evaluated nine KT frameworks for knowledge transfer and highlighted seven key elements: (1) the climate or context for research use; (2) linkage and exchange efforts that build relationships between researchers and users; (3) creation of new knowledge that is timely and relevant; (4) 'push' efforts from the knowledge creators; (5) 'pull' efforts that enable policymakers to identify relevant research; (6) 'pull' efforts to draw the relevant evidence into policy making; and (7) evaluation of KT impact.

This book is primarily concerned with knowledge creation and dissemination, i.e. the 'push' effort, with a particular focus on the findings from observational cohort studies. We briefly reflect on the role of such studies in KT, summarize the key research findings and themes that have emerged from the previous chapters, and then consider the most relevant messages for research users.

19.2.1 The role of cohort studies in knowledge translation

There are substantial challenges of translating research findings from observational studies into practice or policy-relevant messages for healthy ageing or for other health outcomes. Researchers face a tension between being cautious in extrapolating findings from such studies, and being faced with growing demands from research funders to demonstrate impact. It is therefore not surprising that researchers may make practice or policy recommendations on insufficient evidence [6].

However, cohort studies can play a valuable role in illuminating likely causal relationships under certain conditions, helping research users judge when to take action (Chapter 5) [7]. These conditions include a carefully considered study design and appropriate methods of analysis to maximize the chances of reaching reliable conclusions; and guidelines have been developed to strengthen the reporting from observational studies in epidemiology [8], and extended to molecular epidemiology [9]. Findings from observational studies need to be replicated and systematically reviewed to assess their robustness and generalizability, and evidence across different types of study should be synthesized before investing in policy and practice change. However, design and methodological challenges remain (Chapter 5), including how often to repeat assessments, when to invest in emerging technologies that provide more refined and dynamic measures but are still comparable with earlier measures, and how best to investigate the relationship between multiple trajectories (Chapters 6 and 7). Cross-national designs may be particularly relevant for generating hypotheses about the differential impact of past policies, and can enhance confidence in causal relationships when exposure–outcome patterns are seen in populations which have different confounding structures [10]. Comparing findings within and between family members can also strengthen causal inference. The use of genetic instruments (Mendelian Randomization), where available, also avoids reverse causation and confounding but requires large sample sizes and therefore large collaborative consortia. Data on secular trends and natural experiments [11] can provide insights into the effects of varying social exposures (e.g. unemployment) that may have major public health impact. This is particularly useful if embedded within a cohort study with individual level data on participants before and after the exposure, facilitating tests for interactive effects, rather than simply using repeat cross-sectional data (e.g. whether pre-morbid psychological distress interacts with economic recession in having a far greater negative effect on health).

Contrary to earlier comments [12], we have not suggested that it should eventually be possible to understand individual determinants of health fully even with a large life course 'fantasy' cohort capturing all exposures from birth until death. We agree that at an individual level there would still be predictive uncertainty, given the important role of stochastic events across life and especially in ageing [13]. However such a cohort would allow us to have a far better understanding of the natural history of risk factors and their trajectories as well as identifying at risk subgroups that may benefit from earlier intervention. For example, the often contradictory findings seen with cortisol levels and outcomes may reflect differences in the natural history of cortisol dysregulation which may transition through different stages with both phases of over and underactivity (Chapter 10).

Finally, cohort studies can justify the need for an intervention, such as a trial, suggest effect sizes on which to base its size, provide evidence on possible subgroup effects, and provide a set of intermediate outcomes [14]. However, long-term trials that reflect life course exposures present a particularly challenging scenario, and may not be practical or ethical, which is another reason to strengthen causal inference from observational studies.

19.3 Common and emerging themes in a life course approach to healthy ageing

19.3.1 Healthy ageing is a complex phenotype

The broad principles of life course research on ageing were described in Chapter 1: interdisciplinary research to understand the lifetime determinants of, and inter-relationships between wellbeing and biological ageing at the individual, body system and molecular and cellular levels, and the consequences for daily activities, participation, and quality of life. The subsequent chapters showed conceptual and measurement challenges in most aspects of these domains.

Chapter 1 also drew attention to the lack of an agreed definition of healthy ageing, although it seems clear that this should encompass health preservation, not just the development of disease risk [15]. Our definition included survival to older age, minimal risk of clinical disorders and disease risk, optimal functioning at the individual and at the body system level for as long as possible, and wellbeing. Standardized measures would clearly facilitate cross cohort studies, and more refined measures [16] would facilitate aetiological insights. However, we are not advocating at this stage a composite measure of healthy ageing (Section 19.3.3). Rather we felt a broad conceptual framework was required to indicate how these different ageing outcomes relate to each other and to potential risk and protective factors operating across life. It remains to be seen how useful the framework described in Chapter 1 will be: the extent to which it helps to generate and operationalize new hypotheses and leads to greater clarity on the most important connections and likely causal models.

Contributors to subsequent chapters reported on many of the relationships embedded in our framework and commented on the strengths and limitations of the available studies (see also Section 19.3.4 on risk factors). There is strong evidence that objective measures of physical and cognitive capability and wellbeing were related to subsequent mortality; and the evidence relating them to subsequent morbidity is growing. There is bidirectionality in that chronic conditions and functional markers of preclinical disease are also risk factors for decline in capability and/or wellbeing. For example, lower physical capability levels have been linked to future risk of fracture, and osteoporosis and fractures have been related to subsequent declines in physical capability. This example also highlights the important interrelationships between bone and muscle which require further research (Chapter 12).

In respect of interrelationships between our three chosen healthy ageing indicators at the individual level, Gale and colleagues found evidence relating wellbeing to capability which was more extensive than evidence relating capability to future wellbeing. Space precluded a discussion about the dynamic relationship between physical and cognitive capability, despite our conceptual framework assuming an intimate relationship between mind and body. We refer readers to our HALCyon/IALSA systematic review which explored existing literature on these dynamic relationships [17]. Clouston and colleagues identified only seven studies that had investigated associations of *change* in fluid cognition with *change* in physical capability; such an analysis is methodologically challenging (Chapters 6 and 7). Overall, findings were not sufficiently strong or consistent to support a common cause mechanism, and lack of standardized measurement protocols limited comparability. Whilst many regard ageing as a loss of responsiveness and maintenance of function across a broad array of body systems, this disjunction between cognitive and physical domains is of great interest, and understanding why some subgroups decline in both whilst others maintain good function in one but not the other may provide important aetiological insights.

In respect of underlying biology, few candidate genes that influence physical or cognitive capability have been identified (Chapter 14) although conventional heritability studies and novel analytic approaches indicate a significant genetic component for both (Chapters 2 and 3). Studies relating telomere length, and change in telomere length, to capability are weak and inconsistent. According to Martin-Ruiz and von Zglinicki (Chapter 13), telomere length is unlikely to be a robust marker of biological ageing. They argue a biomarker index may be more fruitful but the strongest current contenders when comparing relationships of different potential biomarkers with subsequent risk of disability, institutionalization and death are physiological measures such as lung function, muscle strength, and verbal memory rather than markers at the molecular or cellular levels. This is consistent with our use of these functional measures as indicators of healthy ageing. Somewhat more positive were the results of the relationships between markers of the HPA axis and physical and cognitive capability (Chapter 10) where prospective studies and a meta-analysis suggested that the ability to mount a good stress-induced response may be a marker of a more reactive and healthier HPA axis, with implications for functional ageing.

19.3.2 Natural history of biological systems: extending functional trajectories

A life course approach to healthy ageing focuses on maximizing functional reserve at maturity and delaying onset and slowing the rate of functional decline. Several contributors mentioned the limited information on lifetime trajectories, secular trends and cohort effects in the components of healthy ageing, and the underlying biological functions on which they depend. Gale and colleagues confirmed that the lifetime trajectory of wellbeing was unlike the trajectories of many biological functions. Wellbeing appears to plateau in older people and may show a decline much closer to the end of life than the decline in capability, perhaps when functional decline and activity limitations accelerate and impact more clearly on quality of life. The apparently different life course trajectories of some cardio-metabolic functions, such as the midlife increase in blood pressure (Chapter 11), can be reconceptualized as reflecting age related loss in arterial wall elasticity due to wear and tear from repeated pulsatile expansion and contraction [18]. Trajectories are often inferred from cross-sectional studies, with little empirical evidence on the extent of tracking over long time periods and whether timing or rate of change in earlier periods influence timing or rate of change in later periods. Aspects of cardiovascular function are an exception as a number of long-established cohort studies have many repeat measures, although surprisingly little use has been made of these data to characterize trajectories and investigate the factors that affect change (Chapter 11). Mean changes in trajectories may well hide considerable individual variation. We raised in Chapters 6 and 7 some of the analytical challenges and study design requirements of adequately measuring within-person change and identifying points when acceleration or deceleration occur. Such turning points are of great interest for potential intervention. From the design aspect, few studies in young participants have some of the key measures (such as physical capability) and the specific tests may need to be modified to avoid ceiling and floor effects and to detect meaningful variation.

19.3.3 Use of composite indices versus individual components

In a number of chapters, the use of composite indices, such as overall measures of healthy ageing, frailty and summary physical performance scores in studies of ageing was highlighted. Such indices may, from a clinical or prognostic perspective, have utility and promote person-centred care. However, as the individual components of these indices often represent slightly differing underlying constructs because they test different body system functions, aetiological insights may be better served by studying the life course determinants of each component separately, especially as important effects specific to individual components may otherwise be disguised. For example, early life growth patterns predict some but not all physical performance tests (Chapter 2), and similarly dysregulation in cortisol production was associated with slower walking speed but not with grip strength (Chapter 10).

19.3.4 Lifetime risk factors for healthy ageing

The evidence to date points to a broad set of conventional risk factors for chronic diseases that also reduce the chance of optimizing capability and/or wellbeing. These include socioeconomic circumstances, body size, health status and health behaviours; however, the pattern of associations, including the effect of exposure timing may be different, and reflect different underlying pathways. The life course perspective encourages researchers to focus on the impact on healthy ageing of: childhood socioeconomic position (SEP) as well as adult SEP at the individual and area-based level; growth and developmental trajectories as well as adult changes in body size, and composition; health histories as well as current health status; and on the early acquisition of lifestyle and its cumulative effects.

Contributors provided robust evidence that childhood as well as adult socioeconomic circumstances matter for functional ageing (Chapters 2, 3, and 11), and emerging evidence for adult wellbeing (Chapter 4), suggesting that causal factors may operate from early life. In Chapter 18, Murray and Stafford highlighted how socioeconomic characteristics of the neighbourhood in which participants grew up, as well as where they lived in adulthood, also affected the chance of healthy ageing. These area-level characteristics may mould individual risk factors, act over and above such factors, or be part of the explanation for links between individual socioeconomic factors and ageing.

In terms of body size, there is robust evidence that those of higher birthweight have better muscle strength and higher bone mineral content and bone area in later life; those with higher levels of adult adiposity have worse physical performance; and that these adult effects are stronger in women and non-linear, primarily affecting those at the highest levels of adiposity (Chapters 2 and 12). While the evidence is more limited on the postnatal growth trajectory, single cohort studies suggest that pre-pubertal height and weight gain are generally associated with better adult physical capability, but from puberty onwards the associations are generally negative, at least for physical performance (Chapter 2). There is clear evidence that adiposity and change in adiposity across life is a risk factor for adult vascular and metabolic function (Chapter 11). Evidence linking adiposity to adult cognitive capability and wellbeing is much less clear-cut (Chapters 3 and 4).

We have already noted the probable bidirectional relationships between capability, wellbeing and chronic health conditions; more prospective studies of these factors, ideally reaching back into childhood would be informative for understanding how these dynamic interrelationships unfold.

Most epidemiological studies of ageing focus on the characteristics of the participating study member and pay less attention to the lives of those who either care for, or who are cared for by, the participant. The importance of linked and interdependent lives [19] in relation to healthy ageing was brought home forcibly by the narrative biographies in Chapter 9. Carpentieri and Elliott showed that caring for others may provide a sense of purpose and meaning but an excessive care burden impacts on the chance of healthy ageing. In particular this chapter showed the importance of the partner's health and functional decline on the wellbeing of participants. Cohort investigators should consider collecting more quantitative information on this topic.

Modifiable lifestyle factors, such as diet and physical activity are thought to be important for physical and cognitive capability. We found limited and inconsistent evidence from cross cohort studies in respect of diet and capability, and little support from the findings of randomized trials (Chapter 16). Limited evidence of the role of nutrition for bone health was also presented (Chapter 12). Differing measures of diet and nutrition across cohorts is one factor that limits comparisons and may contribute to inconsistent findings. For example, creating harmonized dietary measures from food frequency questionnaires and dietary diaries in the HALCyon cohorts was very challenging and limited the ability to carry out meta-analyses. Diet is also heavily confounded by socioeconomic circumstances; the use of genetic instrumental variables or biomarkers where possible provides one way forward. There is more robust evidence from observational studies and randomized controlled trials of the importance of physical activity for physical and cognitive capability (Chapters 2 and 3) and other ageing outcomes (Chapters 12 and 17).

The strength and even the direction of associations between some risk factors and ageing outcomes may change with age and by birth cohort. For example weight loss in later life, particularly if it is non-intentional, is often associated with poorer health outcomes, including physical and cognitive capability and physical frailty, and osteoporosis (Chapters 1 and 2). Health status may be a more important risk factor for wellbeing at younger ages, whereas the impact of social relationships becomes stronger at older ages (Chapter 4).

Studies with repeat data on risk factors across life are rarely the same studies with repeat data on ageing outcomes. Most existing work has thus either related risk factors across life to ageing outcomes, measured at one point in time, or related risk factors during one period in life (usually midlife or later) to changes in function and health status in later life. However, as repeat measures of lifetime risk factors and ageing outcomes become more widely available in the same studies it will be possible to investigate how changing risk factors drive changes in ageing outcomes, although this will bring new methodological challenges.

The life course perspective also encourages researchers to investigate the earlier life factors that shape these risk factors. There is strong evidence that adult socioeconomic circumstances, body size, lifestyle, and many health conditions are established or shaped by factors acting during childhood and adolescence. This research needs to be applied to risk factor trajectories and longitudinal profiles.

19.4 **When to intervene to promote healthy ageing?**

The life course perspective, drawing on evidence from research in birth cohorts and other cohort studies, has already influenced policy documents of relevance for healthy ageing. In the UK for example, the life course perspective has infiltrated policy widely, such as in relation to obesity [20,21], health inequalities [22], mental capital and wellbeing [23], and women's health [24]. Importantly, and consistent with the overall emphasis of the present book, this perspective emphasizes the importance of human capital investment during biological, psychological and social development, but also the value of interventions right across life.

A growing number of policy documents emphasize the importance of early life for laying down the foundations for lifelong health [22,25]. There are moral, ethical and economic arguments for early childhood interventions to improve child health, development and social circumstances [26], and such interventions may also improve the chance of healthy ageing. We found strong evidence for early life influences on adult physical and cognitive capability, but there was more limited and weaker evidence for wellbeing. A review of prenatal and preschool health promotion interventions found strong evidence for effectiveness of reducing exposure to tobacco and unintentional injuries, but evidence was limited in the cases of mental health and obesity [27]. There are good practice models for early intervention that show improved social, educational and health outcomes in childhood and adolescence [28,29]; and a few with long-term follow-up show that there may be continuing benefits into adult life. Indicators of healthy ageing such as mental wellbeing and physical and cognitive capability should be included as outcomes in long-term follow-ups and future evaluations where possible.

Life course epidemiology from the start also emphasized the importance of adolescence as another vulnerable social and biological transition—a time of rapid brain development, changing body composition, sexual and reproductive maturation, and the establishment of many health behaviours, educational investments, and social influences beyond the family. For these reasons adolescence is also increasingly being described as a foundation for future health [30,31], and a growing body of knowledge about effective preventive strategies during this period is being built up [32]. As with early childhood interventions, long-term evaluation should include indicators of healthy ageing.

In adulthood there are also times of heightened physiological or behavioural plasticity during later biological and social transitions, for example during pregnancy, becoming a parent, or during the menopause and retirement transitions, when interventions to promote health may also have long-term benefits for healthy ageing; but there is still a paucity of research in this area (Chapter 11). There is increasing evidence, however, that earlier adult onset or faster changes in risk factors such as high blood pressure and obesity result in poorer cardiovascular health (Chapter 11) and may also affect other ageing outcomes.

More specific to healthy ageing research is whether we can identify early markers of an accelerated trajectory of functional decline or a worsening longitudinal risk profile, and target interventions at these susceptible subgroups. This requires health care systems capable of monitoring individuals over time using comparable instruments. We need to evaluate whether simple and regular performance assessments, as used for objective measures of physical and cognitive capability, could be used by practitioners to identify those most vulnerable to accelerated ageing. Can suitable thresholds be identified? Do the different tests provide added value?

Our suggestions are consistent with the call for earlier and more rigorously maintained risk factor management [15], that takes into account risk factor trajectories, though we accept that whether this represents the most cost-effective strategy needs further evaluation. Which risk factors and intermediate markers should we pay most attention to? We suggest those that provide the greatest population attributable risk, where effective interventions exist, and/or where secular trends, based on cohort or period effects, suggest that risk factors are changing in an adverse direction. An obvious current contender, based on these criteria, is obesity. But risk factors often cluster together and interventions designed to modify several of them, using a variety of different strategies may be an attractive option.

While focusing on the most effective times to intervene earlier in life to improve healthy ageing, this is not to downplay the importance of intervening in later life to promote health and wellbeing and of providing good quality, integrated health and social care that meets the complex needs of older people. We found consistent evidence of associations between physical activity and healthy ageing outcomes, and effective interventions have been identified. Meta-analyses of results from intervention studies have shown benefits of fitness training for cognition [33], and wellbeing, the latter with positive consequences for cardiovascular status, strength, and functional capacity [34]. The Lifestyle Interventions and Independence for Elders (LIFE)-pilot study provided evidence that a physical activity intervention programme can improve physical performance in the short term in an older high risk group [35], with the full study currently testing whether this intervention can also delay onset of mobility disability [36]. In addition, evidence has also shown that multifactorial interventions targeting older populations provide an effective preventive strategy for falls, with such findings being translated into clinical practice [37,38]. However, not all interventions in this age group are equally successful; we refer readers to a review [39] of interventions in primary care and community settings to promote health and wellbeing in later life, including complex interventions, interventions to prevent falls and promote physical activity and improved nutrition, and interventions using information and communication technology. With some notable exceptions, this review generally found weak and conflicting evidence for the beneficial effects of intervention, along with areas of unknown effectiveness, and identified few studies with long-term follow-up. There is clearly further work to be done on designing, implementing, and evaluating evidence-based interventions at all stages of life to increase the chance of healthy ageing.

Structural approaches that modify or regulate the environment to improve healthy ageing are also important to consider, and are emphasized in the Madrid International Plan noted at the beginning of this chapter, in particular those that enable 'ageing in place'. As well as accessible housing and transportation, this involves neighbourhood features such as crime prevention surveillance, pedestrian/traffic segregation, and street topography [40] and is potentially amenable to change at local or national level. The National Institute for Health and Clinical Excellence, having considered the evidence, has produced public health guidance on the promotion and creation of physical environments that support increased levels of physical activity [41]. Repeat time trend data highlight the large short-term health impacts of changes in the policy or political context [42,43].

The WHO KT framework requires researchers to take responsibility for pushing the knowledge out to research users, including the provision of actionable messages. The researchers contributing to this book have drawn on cohort studies to investigate risk and protective factors for healthy ageing. The messages for policymakers are about the key factors that need to change and the timing of interventions; how best to intervene is beyond the scope of this book. Intervention studies need to be well-designed and evaluated, and this is methodologically challenging, particularly for complex interventions [44]. There is increasing recognition that going beyond dissemination to changing policy and practice requires the involvement of health professionals, older people themselves, and those with expertise in implementation science [45]; this will be necessary to reduce the gap between research findings on healthy ageing and applications of innovations to improve population health. Of relevance here are the 'What Works Centres' that were announced by the UK government in March 2013 to provide robust, comprehensive evidence to guide decision making on public spending; these include a 'What Works Centre for Early Intervention' and a 'What Works Centre for Ageing Better'. We are working with AgeUK as an intermediary to produce a summary of the key findings of this book, and to repackage the knowledge on healthy ageing so that it is adapted to particular contexts and situations and fine-tuned for different user groups, in line with the WHO KT framework. The brochure can be downloaded from the HALCyon website, along with supplementary material from this book.

19.5 **Future research directions**

Rapid technological developments are facilitating more detailed and longitudinal phenotypes and environmental exposures. The blossoming field of epigenetics applied to life course designs [46] has potential to reveal the biological mechanisms underlying associations between early life exposures and healthy ageing indicators (Chapter 15). Metabolomics is also being undertaken increasingly in cohort studies, allowing the assessment of a wide array of lipid proteins rather than simple cholesterol levels, and combining this with more dynamic assessments. Similarly, proteomic patterns may enable a better characterization of how toxic exposures influence health [47]. The need to capture multiple and richer measures over time requires dynamic techniques that are not too burdensome for participants. 'Omics' technologies represent one example; others include the use of mobile phone applications and the internet; all present new analytical challenges in handling complex data.

This feeds into the perennial debate about the benefits of cohorts that are large but thin (fewer measures on large samples) compared with the benefits of cohorts that are small but fat (where the whole sample or at least selected subgroups are phenotyped far more intensively). Clearly both approaches have merit and should be undertaken if funding permits. Initial large scale studies or consortia enable selective sampling of extreme genotypes or phenotypes in sufficient numbers (e.g. recall by extremes of functional genotypes) or phenotypic discordance (e.g. participants who are obese but with good metabolic profiles).

The life course model we present in this book has evolved from our earlier version by highlighting the importance of compensatory reserve and adaptations, and how they may or may not help restore function after an adverse exposure. This will help further explain the variability in exposure–outcome relationships, since the ability to compensate may fully or partially mitigate exposure effects. We are aware of few studies that have measured these phenomena. For example, one elegant study testing the potentially adverse psychological effects of being a carer used a vaccination paradigm to demonstrate that carers were less able to mount a satisfactory immune response [48].

The adaptations older people make to their behaviour or the environment to maintain wellbeing, activities, and autonomy in the face of functional decline and health challenges is also a growing area of research where life course studies could make a particular contribution, by examining to what extent adaptability is shaped by earlier exposures and experiences. Of particular interest for developing possible novel interventions are the characteristics of subgroups functioning well or having high wellbeing despite an increased lifetime risk burden.

There are a growing number of networks bringing together cohort investigators and experts from a range of biomedical, psychological, and social science disciplines to act as a catalyst for these research developments and apply them to the study of human development and ageing.

HALCyon, FALCon, IALSA, introduced in Chapter 1, and a new network CLOSER (Cohorts and Longitudinal Studies Enhancement Resources) are four such networks that are developing joint research infrastructure for further scientific collaborations, capacity building, cohort enhancements and knowledge translation. These include retrospective and prospective data harmonization, shared hypotheses, study designs, and data analysis, and the development of more effective 'push' and 'pull' efforts with intermediary organisations to get the key messages out to research users.

References

1 **Pablos-Mendez A, Shademani R.** Knowledge translation in global health. *J Contin Educ Health Prof* 2006;**26**:81–6.

2 **Green LW, et al.** Diffusion theory and knowledge dissemination, utilization, and integration in public health. *Annu Rev Public Health* 2009;**30**:151–74.

3 **Ogilvie D, et al.** A translational framework for public health research. *BMC Public Health* 2009;**9**:116.

4 **United Nations.** Political declaration and Madrid International Plan of Action on Ageing. New York: United Nations; 2002.

5 **World Health Organization.** Knowledge translation on ageing and health: a framework for policy development. Geneva: World Health Organization; 2012. <http://www.who.int/ageing/publications/knowledge_translation_en.pdf>

6 **Prasad V, et al.** Observational studies often make clinical practice recommendations: an empirical evaluation of authors' attitudes. *J Clin Epidemiol* 2013;**66**:361–6.

7 **Academy of Medical Sciences Working Group (Chair Rutter M).** Identifying the environmental causes of disease: how should we decide what to believe and when to take action? London: Academy of Medical Sciences; 2007.

8 **Von Elm E, et al.** The strengthening the reporting of observational studies in epidemiology (STROBE) statement: guidelines for reporting observational studies. *PLoS Med* 2007;**4**:e296.

9 **Gallo V, et al.** STrengthening the Reporting of OBservational studies in Epidemiology–Molecular Epidemiology STROBE-ME: an extension of the STROBE statement. *J Clin Epidemiol* 2011;**64**:1350–63.

10 **Brion MJ, et al.** What are the causal effects of breastfeeding on IQ, obesity and blood pressure? Evidence from comparing high-income with middle-income cohorts. *Int J Epidemiol* 2011;**40**:670–80.

11 **Medical Research Council.** Using natural experiments to evaluate population health interventions: guidance for producers and users of evidence. London: MRC; 2011.

12 **Davey Smith G.** Lifecourse epidemiology of disease: a tractable problem? *Int J Epidemiol* 2007;**36**:479–80.

13 **Kirkwood TB.** Commentary: ageing—what's all the noise about? Developments after Gartner. *Int J Epidemiol* 2012;**41**:351–2.

14 **Guralnik JM, Kritchevsky SB.** Translating research to promote healthy aging: the complementary role of longitudinal studies and clinical trials. *J Am Geriatr Soc* 2010;**58**:S337–42.

15 **Barondess JA.** Toward reducing the prevalence of chronic disease: a life course perspective on health preservation. *Perspect Biol Med* 2008;**51**:616–28.

16 **Kivimaki M, Ferrie JE.** Epidemiology of healthy ageing and the idea of more refined outcome measures. *Int J Epidemiol* 2011;**40**:845–7.

17 **Clouston SAP, et al.** The dynamic relationship between physical function and cognition in longitudinal aging cohorts. *Epidemiol Rev* 2013;**35**:33–50.

18 **McEniery CM, et al.** An analysis of prospective risk factors for aortic stiffness in men: 20-year follow-up from the Caerphilly prospective study. *Hypertension* 2010;**56**:36–43.

19 **Elder GH, Jr, Shanahan MJ.** The life course and human development. In: Damon W, Lerner RM. The Handbook of Child Psychology. Volume 1. 6th ed. Hoboken, New Jersey: Wiley; 2006:1–98.

20 **Butland B, et al.** Foresight: tackling obesities: future choices—project report. UK Government's Foresight Programme, London: Government Office for Science; 2007.

21 **Department of Health.** Healthy lives, healthy people: a call to action on obesity in England. London: DOH; 2011. <https://www.gov.uk/government/uploads/system/uploads/attachment_data/file/213720/dh_130487.pdf>

22 **Marmot M.** Fair Society, Healthy Lives: The Marmot Review. London: UCL Institute of Health Equity; 2010.

23 **Foresight Mental Capital and Wellbeing Project.** Final project report. London: The Government Office for Science; 2008.

24 **Scientific Advisory Committee.** Opinion paper 27: Why should we consider a life course approach to women's health care? London: Royal College of Obstetricians and Gynaecologists; 1-8-2011.

25 **Center on the Developing Child at Harvard University.** The foundations of lifelong health are built in early childhood. 2010. <http://developingchild.harvard.edu>

26 **Boyce WT, Keating D.** Should we intervene to improve childhood circumstances? In: Kuh D, Ben-Shlomo Y, editors. A Life Course Approach to Chronic Disease Epidemiology. 2nd ed. Oxford: Oxford University Press; 2004:415–46.

27 **Guyer B, et al.** Early childhood health promotion and its life course health consequences. *Acad Pediatr* 2009;**9**:142–9.

28 **Karoly LA, et al.** Early Childhood Interventions: Proven Results, Future Promise. Santa Monica, California: RAND Corporation; 2005. <http://www.rand.org/content/dam/rand/pubs/monographs/2005/RAND_MG341.pdf>

29 **Burr J, Grunewald R.** Lessons learned: a review of early childhood development studies. 2006. <http://www.minneapolisfed.org/publications_papers/studies/earlychild/lessonslearned.pdf>

30 **Sawyer SM, et al.** Adolescence: a foundation for future health. *Lancet* 2012;**379**:1630–40.

31 **Santelli JS, et al.** Adolescent risk-taking, cancer risk, and life course approaches to prevention. *J Adolesc Health* 2013;**52**:S41–4.

32 **Catalano RF, et al.** Worldwide application of prevention science in adolescent health. *Lancet* 2012;**379**: 1653–64.

33 **Colcombe S, Kramer AF.** Fitness effects on the cognitive function of older adults: a meta-analytic study. *Psychol Sci* 2003;**14**:125–30.

34 **Netz Y, et al.** Physical activity and psychological well-being in advanced age: a meta-analysis of intervention studies. *Psychol Aging* 2005;**20**:272–84.

35 **Pahor M, et al.** Effects of a physical activity intervention on measures of physical performance: results of the Lifestyle Interventions and Independence for Elders pilot (LIFE-P) study. *J Gerontol A Biol Sci Med Sci* 2006;**61**:1157–65.

36 **Fielding RA, et al.** The Lifestyle Interventions and Independence for Elders study: design and methods. *J Gerontol A Biol Sci Med Sci* 2011;**66**:1226–37.

37 **Tinetti ME, et al.** A multifactorial intervention to reduce the risk of falling among elderly people living in the community. *N Engl J Med* 1994;**331**:821–7.

38 **Tinetti ME, Kumar C.** The patient who falls: "It's always a trade-off". *JAMA* 2010;**303**:258–66.

39 **Frost H, et al.** Promoting health and wellbeing in later life. Interventions in primary care and community settings. Edinburgh: Scottish Collaboration for Public Health Research and Policy; 2010. <www.SCPHRP.ac.uk> ISBN: 978=0-9565655-5-6.

40 **Burton EJ, et al.** Good places for ageing in place: development of objective built environment measures for investigating links with older people's wellbeing. *BMC Public Health* 2011;**11**:839.

41 **National Institute for Health and Clinical Excellence.** Physical activity and the environment: NICE Public Health Guidance 8; 2008.

42 Franco M, et al. Population-wide weight loss and regain in relation to diabetes burden and cardiovascular mortality in Cuba 1980–2010: repeated cross sectional surveys and ecological comparison of secular trends. *BMJ* 2013;**346**:f1515.

43 Shkolnikov V, et al. Changes in life expectancy in Russia in the mid-1990s. *Lancet* 2001;**357**:917–21.

44 Craig P, et al. Developing and evaluating complex interventions: the new Medical Research Council guidance. *BMJ* 2008;**337**:a1655.

45 Lobb R, Colditz GA. Implementation science and its application to population health. *Annu Rev Publ Health* 2013;**34**:235–51.

46 Ng JW, et al. The role of longitudinal cohort studies in epigenetic epidemiology: challenges and opportunities. *Genome Biol* 2012;**13**:246.

47 Patel CJ, et al. Systematic evaluation of environmental factors: persistent pollutants and nutrients correlated with serum lipid levels. *Int J Epidemiol* 2012;**41**:828–43.

48 Vedhara K, et al. Chronic stress in elderly carers of dementia patients and antibody response to influenza vaccination. *Lancet* 1999;**353**:627–31.

Index

Note: page locators in italics denote illustrations